The Therapeutic Potential of

MARIHUANA

The Therapeutic Potential of
MARIHUANA

Edited by

Sidney Cohen

University of California
Los Angeles, California

and

Richard C. Stillman

National Institute on Drug Abuse
Rockville, Maryland

Plenum Medical Book Company · New York and London

Library of Congress Cataloging in Publication Data

Main entry under title:

The Therapeutic potential of marihuana.

Includes index.
1. Marihuana—Therapeutic use—Congresses. 2. Marihuana—Physiological effect—Congresses. 3. Tetrahydrocannabinol—Therapeutic use—Congresses. 4. Tetrahydrocannabinol—Physiological effect—Congresses. I. Cohen, Sidney, 1910   II. Stillman, Richard C.
RM666.C266T47   615'323'962   76-17106
ISBN 0-306-30955-6

Proceedings of a conference on The Therapeutic Potential of
Marihuana held at the Asilomar Conference Center in Pacific
Grove, California, November, 1975

Conference and Proceedings Organized and Produced
by Plog Research, Inc. for the National Institute
on Drug Abuse, under Contract No. 271-75-3015

This book was coedited by Richard Stillman in his private capacity. No official
support or endorsement by the NIDA is intended or should be inferred.

© 1976 Plenum Publishing Corporation
227 West 17th Street, New York, N. Y. 10011

Plenum Medical Book Company is an imprint of Plenum Publishing Corporation

Printed in the United States of America

Foreword

Scientific information about cannabis and its components has grown exponentially during the past decade. Certain of the findings have led to exploratory studies into the therapeutic utility of the drug. At the present time, a number of areas of usefulness have been investigated, with some showing greater promise than others.

At what point should these data be collected and presented? Should it be early, after some initial impressions have been obtained? Or should it come later, following confirmatory studies by others? Both stages of development are represented in this volume. In a number of instances, the papers consist of hitherto unpublished material.

It seemed worthwhile to bring together the investigators working in a wide variety of disciplines who had in common their research activities in the therapeutic aspects of the cannabinoids and related synthetic compounds. This was done at the Asilomar Conference Center in Pacific Grove, California during November, 1975. The papers presented and the ensuing discussion constitute the contents of this volume. It is the Editors' hope that the book will stimulate further involvement in the therapeutic studies.

It should not be expected, nor is it anticipated that some cannabinoid will be available commercially in the near future. The nature of the approval process is such that years elapse between initial testing, however promising, and final approval for marketing. This is particularly true for a completely new chemical entity, and even more so for one with a checkered reputation. Cannabis, itself, will never be adopted for medical indications. It contains dozens of constituents, some of which have undesirable effects. Delta-9-tetrahydrocannabinol is a possible candidate, but it is more likely that a synthetic analogue, tailored to intensify the desired action and to avoid the undesired ones, will be preferred.

We are grateful to the National Institute on Drug Abuse for granting support and assistance for the meeting. Dr. Stephen Szara provided continuing help and invaluable advice. A special note of appreciation is due Dr. Michael Rolnick, whose great enthusiasm for the goals of this conference were critical in its formation.

Dr. Stanley Plog of Plog Research, Inc. planned and executed the logistical support which resulted in a stimulating experience. We are grateful to Jean Eggen of Plog Research who organized the editing and final production of this document. Assisting her in this effort were Rebecca Bohlinger and Elizabeth Korbonski. To the speakers, the chairpersons, and the discussants we offer thanks for their stimulating contributions.

Sidney Cohen, M. D.
Westwood, California

Richard Stillman, M. D.
Rockville, Maryland

Contents

TUMOR PROBLEMS

ANTICONVULSANT ACTIVITY

SYNTHETIC CANNABINOID-LIKE COMPOUNDS

Introduction

Sidney Cohen

University of California

Los Angeles, California

The fact that a plant had been extensively used as a folk medicine in a wide array of ailments is far from a guarantee of its efficacy. Nevertheless, pharmaceutical firms have been known to consult with curanderas and shamans in the hope that promising leads might be uncovered which could be exploited in a technologically advanced society. And well they might. Many of the major therapeutic advances were evolved from such botanicals as arrow poisons, toxic berries used to catch fish, and deadly nightshade, the Borgia's "Saturday Night Special." The ordeal bean opened up anticholinesterase therapy, a penicillinase mold has prime responsibility for our antibiotic era, and a purple fungus that spoils rye grain provided the first oxytocic and anti-migraine compounds. The contributions of digitalis, red squill, the seaweed, ephedra, and the Oriental poppy are long past, and we do not think about them anymore. Then there was the coca leaf which led to an array of synthetic local anesthetics, and the Indian snakeroot which was the immediate forerunner of certain tranquilizers and antihypertensives. The list is much longer, but it need not be recited here.

The constituents of Indian hemp have unusual chemical configurations, and these are coming under scientific scrutiny after millennia of trial-and-error traditional usage. The possible utility of cannabis seems to derive from two general pharmacologic activities: its mind-altering properties and its physiologic action. In the first instance the euphoriant, relaxed state is exploited in attempts to treat tension, depression, and other noxious affects. In the second instance, the subjective psychic symptoms are unnecessary; in fact, they often become undesired side effects. Rather, it is bronchopulmonary, cardiovascular, or ophthalmic physiology that merits attention.

Cannabis is a controversial plant these days. It evokes the widest spectrum of emotional reaction from adoration to revulsion that I have ever witnessed in response to a weed. We must be aware of the debate, if only because it makes our findings more newsworthy than they are. Of course, we are deeply interested in any report of adverse effects about cannabis because it relates to our current and future work with the agent. But beyond that, we cannot allow the extreme value judgments from either polar group to affect our studies. There is an appropriate Latin epigram whose author I do not remember. Translated it goes:

> "Nothing is of itself good or evil; only the manner of usage makes it so."

CHAPTER 1

CROSS-CULTURAL PERSPECTIVES ON THERAPEUTIC USES OF CANNABIS

Vera Rubin

Research Institute for the Study of Man

New York, New York

An Associated Press dispatch, headlined "Pot the Health Food," reported that a young man charged with possession of ten pounds of marihuana claimed that he was a vegetarian and protested the seizure of his food supply. This was described in the news item as "a novel defense" (New York Post, August 13, 1975).

Use of cannabis in the dietary may be a "novel legal defense" in our courts, but it is an old practice; hemp porridge was a customary part of the diet in monasteries in Eastern Europe during the Middle Ages, and folk use in the dietary is undoubtedly much earlier. The ingestion of cannabis in various forms is linked to therapeutic uses of the plant since ancient times.

According to Schultes (1973), cannabis is one of the oldest plants known to man and was cultivated for fiber, food, and medicine thousands of years before it became the "superstar" of the drug culture. Schultes has also pointed out that only about twenty of the approximately sixty known plant species that have been used as "intoxicants" may be considered of major importance; and "only a very few of these species -- coca, the opium poppy, cannabis, and tobacco -- are numbered among the world's commercially important plants" (Schultes, 1969: 5). Cannabis is undoubtedly the most extraordinary of these plants in the diversity of its traditional uses over the millennia.

One of the few psychoactive plants not indigenous to the Americas, cannabis probably originated in Asia, and the oldest recorded references to its use are in the ancient literature of China, India, and the Near East. While traditional folk use of cannabis undoubtedly has the greatest antiquity in these areas, the multipurpose use of the plant spread with its diffusion over the centuries to other world areas.

Cannabis researchers are now familiar with the recorded therapeutic attributes of the plant cited in recent literature, and it would be redundant to review them at this conference, except to cite a few of the general references.

A good deal of information is to be found, en passant, in the Report of the Indian Hemp Drugs Commission, 1893-1894 (Great Britain, 1969). Grinspoon (1971), Snyder (1971), and Mikuriya (1973), among others, have provided historical reviews of therapeutic uses of cannabis.

It is salutary to be reminded that Rabelais, amateur botanist [1] and physician as well as author, anticipated by over 400 years the Yugoslav report (Radosevic, Kupinic and Grlic, 1962) on the antibiotic qualities of cannabis:

> The juice of this herb [Pantagruelion [2]] ...kill every kind of vermin...[it is] a prompt remedy for horses with colic and broken wind. Its root, boiled in water, softens hardened sinews, contracted joints, sclerotic gout, and gouty swellings. If you want quickly to heal a scald or burn, apply some Pantagruelion raw. [Grinspoon, 1971: 397-398]

This paper will briefly indicate some unpublished materials on traditional and experimental therapeutic uses of cannabis. One source of information about early extensive folk-medicinal uses of the plant stems from a series of papers presented at an international multidisciplinary conference on Cross-Cultural Perspectives on Cannabis, held in August, 1973 (Rubin, in press).

There are several types of evidence to indicate the importance of cannabis in prehistoric times. Archeological evidence of the use of cannabis by the Scythians, corroborating the account by Herodotus, has recently been established by S. I. Rudenko, a Soviet archeologist (Emboden, 1972). There is also archeological evidence of the use of cannabis in northeast Asia, during the neolithic period, about 6,000 years ago. Hui-Lin Li (in press) writes that

> cannabis had multitudinal uses in ancient times in China.... attesting to its antiquity as a cultivated species...The medicinal properties were first recorded in the classical herbal Pen Ts'oo Ching, compiled in the first or second century A.D., but undoubtedly based on traditions passed down from prehistoric times.

The Pen Ts'oo Ching, the earliest pharmacopoeia in existence, records medicinal uses of cannabis; among other uses, ma-fei-san (boiled hemp compound) was given to surgical patients as an anesthetic. A tenth-century work records that ma fen (an infusion of the "fruit" of hemp) is used "for waste disease and injuries; it clears blood and cools temperature; it relieves fluxes; it undoes rheumatism; it discharges pus." The temperate Chinese also warned against excessive, intoxicating uses of the plant, although they accepted the use of opium, introduced in the eighth century A. D. (Li, in press).

Cannabis was probably introduced to southeast Asia around the sixteenth century, as Dr. Marie Martin, a French ethnobotanist, notes in a paper which reports on current therapeutic usage in Cambodia, Thailand, and Vietnam: "Ganja leaves and stalks are used extensively in the cuisine"[3] as well as medicinally. Recognized as an analgesic, in Cambodia cannabis is used to treat

> cholera, malaria, dysentery, anorexia and loss of memory;
> it relieves asthma and calms the nerves; suppresses polyps,
> coughing, dizziness and convulsions [4]; facilitates diges-
> tion and childbirth; it stimulates lactation, purifies the
> blood and cleans the bile; regulates the function of the
> heart, liver and lungs; eliminates intestinal parasites, de-
> congests the organism and is a treatment for paralysis.
> [Martin, in press]

In the form of an infusion, it is also used as an analgesic in Thailand folk medicine -- sun-dried leaves boiled in water are taken for migraines, "stiffness," and dizzy spells; infusions of ganja are also taken before meals and sleep as a relaxant. The therapeutic effects are recognized in the official pharmacopoeia as well as in folk usage.

In Cambodia, ganja is also taken to restore appetite and combined with other plants to facilitate digestion. Hemp cigarettes, smoked daily, will reduce polyps of the nose and relieve asthma. Elaborate prescriptions, based on as many as a dozen different plants, including hemp, are prepared as specifics for hemorrhoids, throat polyps, diarrhea, dysentery, and convulsions. Hemp preparations are also administered to facilitate contractions in difficult childbirth.

In Vietnam, cannabis is taken to alleviate loss of memory and mental confusion, to eliminate blood waste, and to treat gynecological and obstetrical problems: for example, cannabis is commonly taken for dysmenorrhea, and 21 kernels boiled in water may be given to the expectant mother to reset the neonate in normal position at birth. Allergies and rheumatism are treated by a preparation made by pulverizing roasted cannabis kernels in baby's urine; a small glass of the extract is taken three times a day. Pulverized kernels, when mixed with rice and water, "arrest the fall of hair." Cannabis also serves as a vermifuge to eliminate taenia (Martin, in press).

Traditionally used in indigenous Nepalese medical systems (especially Ayurvedic), as James Fisher, an anthropologist, reports:

> [Cannabis] is an ingredient in compounds used to treat diarrhoea,
> cholera, tetanus, rheumatism, and insomnia, among many other
> maladies. It is also employed as a cough suppressant, digestive

aid, stimulus to whet the appetite, soporific, aphrodisiac,
and antimalarial agent for hill people who move to the
plains. Cannabis is never prescribed alone but always in
a mixture with other herbs or ingredients. A compound
used in the treatment of diarrhoea and cholera, for example, contains some fifteen different ingredients, including dried ginger, black pepper, nut grass, sea salt,
black salt, opium, cannabis, and the ashes of a clam
shell. In these preparations cannabis is first washed in
a cloth with water seven times to remove impurities.
[Fisher, in press]

Cultivation of cannabis in southern Russia has been traced back to the
seventh century B.C., and hemp medications are reported to have been widely
used in folk medicine in Russia and Eastern Europe (Benet, in press). Inhalation of vapors was a variation in the method of treatment (probably stemming
from ancient Scythian use -- see Benet, in press, and Emboden, 1972); vapor
from hemp seeds thrown on hot stones was inhaled to alleviate toothache. It
was also used in liniment form; a mixture of hemp flowers, wax, and olive oil
was used to dress wounds in Poland, and oil from crushed hemp seeds was used
to treat jaundice and rheumatism in Russia. According to a report published
in 1934, cited by Benet, hemp has been successfully used in Soviet central
Asia to cure chronic alcoholism. Sweetmeats made of hemp are given to boys
before circumcision to reduce pain (Benet, in press). Therapeutic use in central Asia has also been reported as an antidepressant and to restore potency,
especially after venereal disease. Folk use in central Asia is considered to be
as high as or higher than its use in India.[5]

There is now also field data from Jamaica of the extensive medicinal
use of ganja (Rubin and Comitas, 1972, 1975). It is taken in the form of teas
and tonics and used as a liniment for a variety of ailments (some 30 were listed
in the project data).[6]   Ganja may be mixed with other folk plants for specific treatment, but traditional users eschew prescription medicines: even phensic
(an aspirin compound) is seldom used.

The medicinal plants of Jamaica include 160 species, distributed among
62 families, many of which have been incorporated into the folk pharmacopoeia.
Cannabis, however, is the principal folk medicinal, used for both prophylactic
and therapeutic purposes; even adamant non-smokers reported taking ganja medicinally and its use in this form crosscuts age, sex, and social class lines.

Ganja tea drinking, the most prevalent form of ganja consumption in
Jamaica, starts in early childhood in the rural areas and is administered in
gradually increased doses as the child gets older. It is given to prevent marasmus, help the child grow strong, and to "brainify" the child of school age:
rural nanas apply a ganja preparation (ganja and white rum) to the anterior
fontanelle of the neonate to insure these qualities at birth. A crude method
of vaporizing may also be used for children with respiratory infections: adults
blow ganja smoke at the sick child. Generally, Jamaican users point to the
beneficial behavioral as well as prophylactic and therapeutic effects of ganja

and contrast these with the potential deleterious effects of rum drinking.

William Partridge reports medicinal uses of cannabis in a Colombia municipio: "There is widespread belief in the efficacy of cannabis mixed with rum or aguardiente and applied to the skin for pains of joints and muscles." Another method of alleviating pain is to rub the crushed green leaves on the skin. In general, the "knowledge that cannabis can be used for treatment of pain is widespread." It is also taken for health maintenance; cases cited by Fabrega and Manning "involve men of advanced age who smoked all their lives and have enjoyed excellent health" (Partridge, in press).

In Brazil, the most common method of preparation for medicinal use is as a tea: "An infusion is taken to relieve rheumatism, 'female troubles,' colic and other common complaints. For toothache, marihuana is frequently packed into and around the aching tooth and left for a period of time during which it supposedly performs an analgesic function" (Hutchinson, in press).

Traditional uses of zamal (cannabis) in the island of Réunion (in the Indian Ocean) include the preparation of therapeutic infusions by local healers: "Boiled roots were used to reduce infants' vomiting" and an infusion of the leaves was used to reduce fever. However, rigorous anti-cannabis laws "have made the healers cautious in their choice of herbs" and zamal has been replaced by other plants. Traditional uses continue clandestinely, however, highlighting other folk uses of cannabis reported from various areas: for example, roots of zamal are planted in a field "particularly where squash is grown to rid the area of parasitic insects." And "in veterinary medicine, it is quite common to pulverize zamal leaves in the drinking water of chickens to prevent contagious and infectious diseases" (Benoist, in press). Antiparasitic and veterinary uses are also reported from other areas.

This is a swift sampling of the traditional medicinal uses of cannabis mentioned in the 1973 conference papers. The materials on folk medicinal uses are partly based on field data; for example, conference participants were asked to provide information about uses reported in each area, as well as any information available in regional reports. Neither the field reports nor the historical accounts provide any control data on observed effects or cures; they deal essentially with beliefs, both among healers and subjects, of the perceived effects of cannabis on a wide variety of ailments. These traditional beliefs are apparently bolstered by widespread pragmatic experience, and the subjective effects must be taken into consideration. "Is belief cure and belief kill," as one of our Jamaican subjects said: beliefs about the curative powers of cannabis are undoubtedly pervasive and there are numerous regional regularities in specific therapeutic folk practices.

There is also experimental evidence of the therapeutic qualities of cannabis from a medical source: the Medical Faculty of the Palacky University, Olomouc, Czechoslovakia. Through the courtesy of the Canadian Commission into the Non-Medical Use of Drugs, we received an English translation of a series of ten papers issued by a work group of the Medical Faculty, under the editorship of Professor Jan Kabelik of the Experimental Institute for Medical

Plants. The papers are summaries of lectures and discussions at a scientific conference held in December, 1954, one part of which was "dedicated exclusively to the medical and particularly to the antibiotic effects of hemp[7] (Kabelik, 1955: 2).

In the introduction to the collected papers, Professor Kabelik notes that their institute "discovered" 2,000 plants with antibiotic properties, including hemp 'which was till then not so recognized...we became especially interested in hemp because of its intensive effect and the stability of the antibiotic effects, which is at the same time strongly analgesic." He provides a historical summary of the therapeutic effects of cannabis covering a broad range of historical sources, and notes (Kabelik, 1955: 2, 3):

> After studying also the ancient herbaria and popular pharmacology and that of the primitive medicine men, I found that these admirable properties of hemp have been utilized since ancient times. It is interesting to observe that this very effective medical plant, which was well known in the early history and middle ages and was used till the end of the 19th century, became forgotton and abandoned -- without justification -- in the modern pharmacology... [8]

> Its high antibiotic effect was again discovered and confirmed in our institute...hemp extract proved itself valuable often when all modern antibiotic measures, including terramycin [and others] failed. [9]

The Olomouc papers indicate a great deal of sophistication about the botany and biochemistry as well as the history and folk uses of cannabis; the papers include reports on the pharmacology of cannabis constituents based on their laboratory studies, on the isolation of active substances by means of paper chromatography, on the development of effective preparations based on chemical and bacteriological tests. The results of experiments with different dosages of Cannabis sativa (var. indica) extracts on rats and guinea pigs to determine dosages for analgesic, anticonvulsive, and local anesthetic effects are also reported. Several papers on the antibacterial and therapeutic effects observed in experimental treatment in several medical departments are also included. A bibliographic list, dated December, 1972, cites other articles based on their research, but these were not available for review (see Appendix). The collected papers in the 1954 series are highly technical and the translations are rather stilted, but several brief summaries follow.

The stomatology section of the Medical Faculty reported that cannabis preparations were used experimentally in the treatment of herpes labialis and periodontal pain (ulcerous gingivitis). Over 500 cases were treated; as a result "spray and hemp salve applications became simply a regular method of treatment in our section." The report notes that "our therapeutic results have therefore an empiric character and require further verification in order that they can be generally applied and become of advantage to practical medical treatments" (Kabelik, 1955: 50, 51).

A paper by Dr. Hubacek covering results obtained by the university section on otorhinolaryngology (disease of the ear, nose, and larynx) reports that "the healing effect of cannabis in otorhinolaryngology...is remarkable [and] there were at no time [previously] achieved similar rapid successes" (Kabelik, 1955: 57).

Experiments with various cannabis preparations in the treatment of otitis media are reported, following poor results with the use of terramycin:

> The treatment of otitis [formerly] lasted several weeks and even months and years. The endeavour today is to propagate the therapy of chronic otitis with this most effective antibiotic [cannabis] in order that the patient can in shortest time return to his job and that he may be protected from all dangerous complications...Therefore, we again prepared the local antibiotic -- isolated extract from cannabis indica -- and began to test it on the chronic otitis media. In the case of 17 patients it was found that the microflora was sensitive to cannabis and in 5 cases it was not sensitive. [Kabelik, 1955: 58, 59]

Cures were also reported in three cases of chronic sinusitis and in cases of chronic tonsilopharyngitis treated by spray: "In 10 cases of cures the improvement was not only subjective but also objective." Dr. Hubacek also noted the treatment of two cases of rural patients with second-degree burns: "As I did not have any other therapeutic means in the case of a patient whose hand was burned by hot grease, I covered the burned area with 4% water solution of hemp extract on top of which I put the ointment. The patient stated that the pain disappeared shortly after the treatment and the hand healed" (Kabelik, 1955: 56, 57). This recalls the observation of treatment for burns by Rabelais previously cited.

The orthopedic department reported a "preliminary study" of treatment by local injections of cannabis solution of 14 patients with chronic specific fistulas. An analgesic effect was noted in certain cases, but further experimentation with the type of cannabis extract administered was to be undertaken for "definitive evaluation."

A paper was also presented on "The Importance of Hemp Seeds in the Therapy of Tuberculosis." Dr. Josef Sirek, the chief physician of a sanitorium, observed that therapeutic measures were very limited in their small, poorly equipped hospital. "However," he noted, "this role of the Cinderella was not completely without merit. Since we could not keep up with the avant-garde of modern physiotherapy [in the post-World War I period], we paid greater attention to the aspects which have been overlooked by others, especially in larger institutions" (Kabelik, 1955: 63). Dr. Sirek elaborates on the value of hygienic-dietetic treatment of tuberculosis with special dietetic formulas including oats:

> From the oat grains, the road leads directly to hemp seeds. Not so much because our forefathers have been eating hemp-seed

porridge and soups, but because the hemp seeds with their
contents of edestin and its richness in enzymes occupy the
leading place among the seeds generally. [Kabelik, 1955: 66]

And so we come full swing to "pot as health food."

The comparatively recent "discovery" of folk plants has stimulated research by pharmaceutical houses as well as the "back to nature" movement
among urban youth. Pharmaceutical houses have in the past offered grants to
anthropologists to bring back medicinally useful plants from the field. It is
interesting to note that the nineteenth-century Euro-American experimentation
with medicinal uses of cannabis was undertaken primarily by physicians rather
than by pharmaceutical laboratories. Originally introduced into Western
medicine by Dr. W. B. O'Shaughnessy, experimentation was undertaken by
Dr. J. J. Moreau de Tours and Dr. J. R. Reynolds, among others. Physicians
were in a position to test its use on a clinical basis. Medical use was even-
tually discontinued partly due to difficulties in standardizing dosage. The
"Cinderella" effect led the Czechoslovakians to "rediscover" cannabis and to
experiment with cannabis therapy; perhaps our reliance on synthetic preparations has been our deprivation. Now that field reports are available of its
traditional medical uses for specific ailments and dose-specific preparations
can be developed, perhaps the medical profession will reconsider the therapeutic uses of cannabis.

The range and diversity of its folk uses for analgesic and antibiotic
effects reported over time and space may lead to medical and pharmacological
skepticism; this is a healthy scientific approach which should not deter experimentation with its therapeutic potential. The recurrent controversy about cannabis, unfortunately, tends to publicize spectacular pathological findings frequently based on questionable methodology and to polarize the scientific community. The controversy even extends to the presumably "neutral" question of
the botanical classification of cannabis as a monotypic or polytypic genus
(Schultes, in press). The significance of cross-cultural findings may also be
clouded by sociocultural differences in expectations, use, and conditioned
reactions, that is, the "set and setting" effects.

Some scientists, having discovered "culture," are saying that such-
and-such an effect of cannabis may be "true in that culture but not in ours."
We have to be able to distinguish between subjective, perceived effects and
actual organic effects. The Jamaican findings, for example, indicate no
statistically significant differences between chronic cannabis smokers and non-
smokers on a broad range of medical, psychological, and psychiatric indices.
The one exception, and that is a trend, is the finding of functional hypoxia
among heavy long-term chronic smokers. EEG and ECG results, as well as the
results of neuropsychological tests, are not influenced by cultural factors or
by social class membership. There are indications of similar findings in other
societies. A report of a pilot study of the long-term effects of chronic cannabis use in Pakistan notes that "no significant abnormalities could be detected"
on medical examination of 70 male subjects who had smoked (and consumed)
cannabis for at least 20 years:

There was no impairment in work functions. Nothing abnormal was found in the neurological examinations.
Nothing very suggestive medically was discovered except
for the blood pressure and pulse. In all cases, the diastolic pressure rose and the pulse rate was increased [after
smoking charas (hashish)]. In no case was loss of libido
reported. Our study appears to show that cannabis does
not produce any serious long-term effects. [Kahn, Abbas, and
Jensen, in press]

Dr. Alvaro de Pinho, a Brazilian psychiatrist, reported that in a
study of 728 patients at the psychiatric hospital in Bahia, marihuana was not
a significant factor. Acute schizophrenic psychoses occurred in some young
people who were involved in youth movements and were known to have used
marihuana. Complete and rapid remission of the acute states occurred (de Pinho,
in press). Dr. B. R. Elejalde, a geneticist, reports that chromosomal studies
of regular marihuana users in Colombia do not reveal any abnormalities (Elejalde,
in press). There are recent reports from Jamaica that ganja is being taken to
combat cancer. 10

While the findings in two current multidisciplinary field studies of the
effects of long-term chronic smoking of cannabis -- Greece and Costa Rica --
have not as yet been published, there have been no advance reports of pathological findings. Multidisciplinary research on subjects in a natural rather
than a laboratory setting should be replicated in other societies.

One of the prevalent uses of cannabis reported in several areas is as
an energizer. This has been documented in the Jamaica study where ganja is
regularly smoked during breaks in agricultural field work and other manual
tasks. In Colombia, marihuana is smoked by day-laborers and peasants to reduce fatigue, increase fuerza, or force, and to give animo, or spirit, for
working (Partridge, in press). In Jamaica, where pragmatic rather than "psychedelic" reactions are anticipated and experienced, ganja teas are taken as
a health/energy maintenance program over an extended period by men who are
planning to go overseas on contract work. The energizing effect is given as
the principal motivation for use by Jamaican working-class males. This effect,
frequently reported by working-class users in other societies, should be examined
in cross-cultural contexts with reference to the "amotivational syndrome" attributed to marihuana use in the United States (Rubin and Comitas, 1975). 11

Further, it should be noted for this conference that cannabis is used
both as a "stimulant" and "sedative" in Jamaica; the desired effect is situa-
tionally determined -- smoked before breakfast or during work breaks, ganja
serves as an energizer; taken at bedtime, ganja assures a good night's sleep
and waking refreshed. Whether this is due to titration and/or to psychocultural
conditioning would have to be determined by periods of monitoring and/or detailed reporting by trained subjects. The data reported in the study is based
on extensive reports from clinical subjects and other long-term chronic smokers.

Alternately praised and attacked for its reputed attributes and effects, the traditional multipurpose uses of cannabis have endured over time and space despite legal sanctions. Therapeutic use of cannabis covers a broad range of similar ailments which have plagued our species: was this some esoteric ethnographic belief system, or was it pragmatic folk knowledge passed down through the ages by oral tradition?

Both sacred and secular in folk beliefs -- assuager, energizer, healer -- the folk fascination with this extraordinary plant should be well worth exploring for its therapeutic potential.

NOTES

[1] Francois Rabelais learned about cannabis cultivation on the estate of his father who "grew much hemp on his property" (Stearn, in press).

[2] The "fictionalized version of the plant (named) after his giant hero" Pantagruel (Grinspoon, 1971: 33).

[3] Cannabis sativa is known by many names in different world areas. Ganja, the Hindi term, is prevalent in areas where the plant, and possibly the complex surrounding its multipurpose uses, was diffused from India.

[4] O'Shaughnessy (1842) and other 19th-century Western physicians reported on the beneficial therapeutic effects of cannabis as an anticonvulsant. Reports which "suggest that marijuana may possess an anticonvulsant effect in human epilepsy" are cited in a recent article by Consroe, Wood, and Buchsbaum (1975).

[5] This information appears in a Russian publication, by L. V. Antzyferov, "Hashish in Central Asia," Journal of Socialist Health Care in Uzbekstan (1934).

[6] Some of the medicinal uses reported are for: aches/pains, arthritis, asthma, "blood pressure," breathing difficulties, constipation, chest pains, eardrops, "bad eyes," fever, "fits," gonorrhea (also taken as a prophylactic), "heart," headaches, indigestion, kidneys, malaria (with other "bush"), marasmus (in newborn), "bad skin," swellings and yaws. Poultices made of dried leaves of ganja ashes are used to treat open wounds/ulcers. Tea/tonic users may consume as much as the equivalent of 2-3 spliffs (ganja cigarettes) daily. Healing practices by Fundamentalist cult leaders include medication with folk herbals, of which ganja is a "secret" ingredient, although ganja use per se is proscribed.

[7] The term "hemp," generally associated with the use of cannabis for manufactured products, is a generic synonym for cannabis in Eastern Europe.

[8] As is well known, it was also extensively used in Western medicine during the nineteenth century and was included in the pharmacopoeia of the United States (extractum cannabis) from 1850 until 1942.

[9] Dr. Kabelik notes that "the male bushy types of hemp with big headed blooms" are suitable for hashish and seeds, "and especially for antibiotic properties." He adds, "It is interesting to note that in older times they considered that the hemp which carried seeds was the female type" (Kabelik, 1955: 7).

[10] Louis Harris has suggested that THC "may lead to new drugs to prevent transplant rejection and to combat cancer" (Newsweek, September 2, 1974). Dr. Sallan (Harvard University) has used THC effectively as an anti-emetic agent in cancer therapy (Philadelphia Inquirer, September 14, 1975), and Drs. Butler and Regelson have demonstrated the anti-depressant effects in delta-9-THC

in terminal cancer patients (New York Post, September 20, 1974).

[11]However, the full report of the study of chronic marihuana use by Dr. Jack
H. Mendelson (Harvard University), funded by the U. S. Army, which has now
been released, refutes the "amotivational" allegations: "No impairment in
motivation to work for money even when users smoked a large number of marijuana cigarettes" is one of the conclusions listed in the abstract. The Journal
notes that the Mendelson report "clearly substantiates many of the conclusions
drawn in the Jamaica-Ganja study." (The Journal, November 1, 1975, published by the Addiction Research Foundation, Toronto).

REFERENCES

Benet, S. Early diffusion of folk uses of hemp. In V. Rubin (Ed.), Cannabis and culture. The Hague: Mouton, 1975, in press.

Benoist, J. Réunion: Cannabis in a pluricultural and polyethnic society. In V. Rubin (Ed.), Cannabis and culture. The Hague: Mouton, 1975, in press.

Consroe, P. F., Wood, G. C., & Buchsbaum, H. Anticonvulsant nature of marihuana smoking. Journal of the American Medical Association, 1975, 234 (3), 306-307.

de Pinho, A. R. Social and medical aspects of the use of cannabis in Brazil. In V. Rubin (Ed.), Cannabis and culture. The Hague: Mouton, 1975, in press.

Elejalde, B. R. Marihuana and genetic studies in Colombia: The problem in the city and country. In V. Rubin (Ed.), Cannabis and culture. The Hague: Mouton, 1975, in press.

Emboden, W. A., Jr. Ritual use of Cannabis sativa L.: A historical-ethnographic survey. In P. Furst (Ed.), Flesh of the gods. New York: Praeger, 1972.

Fisher, J. Cannabis in Nepal: an overview. In V. Rubin (Ed.), Cannabis and culture. The Hague: Mouton, 1975, in press.

Great Britain. Indian Hemp Drugs Commission, 1893-1894. Marijuana report. Silver Springs, Md.: Thomas Jefferson, 1969.

Grinspoon, L. Marihuana reconsidered. Cambridge, Mass.: Harvard University Press, 1971.

Hutchinson, H. W. Patterns of marihuana use in Brazil. In V. Rubin (Ed.), Cannabis and culture. The Hague: Mouton, 1975, in press.

Kabelik, J. (Ed.). Hemp as medicine. Acta Universitatis Palackianae Olomucensis, 1955, 6(2), 27-114.

Khan, M. A., Abbas, A., & Jensen, K. Cannabis usage in Pakistan: a pilot study of long-term effects on social status and physical health. In V. Rubin (Ed.), Cannabis and culture. The Hague: Mouton, 1975, in press.

Li, H. The origin and use of cannabis in Eastern Asia: their linguistic-cultural implications. In V. Rubin (Ed.), Cannabis and culture. The Hague: Mouton, 1975, in press.

Martin, M. A. Ethnobotanical aspects of cannabis in Southeast Asia. In V. Rubin (Ed.), Cannabis and culture. The Hague: Mouton, 1975, in press.

Mikuriya, T. H. (Ed.). Marijuana medical papers 1839-1972. Oakland, Calif.: Medi-Comp Press, 1973.

O'Shaughnessy, W. B. On the preparation of the Indian hemp or gunjah (Cannabis indica): The effects on the animal system in health, and their utility in the treatment of tetanus and other convulsive diseases. Transactions of the Medical and Physical Society of Bombay, 1842, 8, 421-461.

Partridge, W. L. Cannabis and cultural groups in a Colombian municipio. In V. Rubin (Ed.), Cannabis and culture. The Hague: Mouton, 1975, in press.

Radosevic, A., Kupinic, M., & Grlic, L. Antibiotic activity of various types of cannabis resin. Nature, 1962, 195, 1007-1009.

Rubin, V. Cannabis and culture. The Hague: Mouton, 1975, in press.

Rubin, V. & Comitas, L. Effects of chronic smoking of cannabis in Jamaica. Report, 1972, Research Institute for the Study of Man, Contract No. HSM-42-70-97, National Institute of Mental Health.

Rubin, V. & Comitas, L. Ganja in Jamaica: A medical anthropological study of chronic marihuana use. The Hague: Mouton, 1975.

Schultes, R. E. Plant kingdom and hallucinogens. Bulletin on Narcotics, 1969, 21(3), 3-16.

Schultes, R. E. Man and marihuana. Natural History, 1973, 82, 59-68, 78, 82.

Schultes, R. E., Klein, W. M., Plowman, T., and Lockwood, T. E. Cannabis: An example of taxonomic neglect. In V. Rubin (Ed.) Cannabis and culture. The Hague: Mouton, 1975, in press.

Snyder, S. H. Uses of marijuana. New York: Oxford University Press, 1971.

Stearn, W. T. Typification of Cannabis sativa L. In V. Rubin (Ed.), Cannabis and culture. The Hague: Mouton, 1975, in press.

APPENDIX

A List of Documentation on Cannabis Problems Published by the Work Group on the Medical Faculty of the Palacky University, Olomouc, Czechoslovakia.

(Original in Czech; summary in English and German; Czech titles here omitted.)

1. Krejci, Z.: "The Antibiotic Effect of Cannabis indica," Dissertation, Masaryk University, Brno, 1950.

2. Krejci, Z.: "The Antibacterial Effect of Cannabis indica," Lekarske listy 1, 20, 500-503 (1952).

3. Kabelik, J.: "Hemp – its History – Traditional and Popular Application," Acta Univ. Olomuc. Fac. Med. 6, 31-41 (1955).

4. Krejci, Z. "The Antibacterial Effect of Cannabis indica." Acta Univ. Olomuc. Fac. Med. 6, 43-57 (1955).

5. Krejci, Z., Santavy, F.: "Isolation of Other Substances from the Leaves of the Indian Hemp," Acta Univ. Olomuc. Fac. Med. 6, 59-66 (1955).

6. Klabusay, L., Lenfeld, J.: "Pharmacodynamic Effect of Substances Isolated from Cannabis indica," Acta Univ. Olomuc, Fac. Med. 6, 67-72 (1955).

7. Soldan, J.: "Therapeutical Results in Stomatology after Application of Substances Obtained from Cannabis indica," Acta Univ. Olomuc. Fac. Med. 6, 73-78 (1955).

8. Simek, J., et al: "Application of the Cannabis indica Extract in Preserving Stomatology," Acta Univ. Olomuc. Fac. Med. 6, 79-82 (1955).

9. Hubacek, J.: "Study on the Effect of Cannabis indica in Oto-Rhino-Laryngology," Acta Univ. Olomuc. Fac. Med. 6, 83-86 (1955).

10. Navratil, J.: "Effectiveness of Cannabis indica on Chronic Otitis Media," Acta Univ. Olomuc. Fac. Med. 6, 87-89 (1955).

11. Procek, J.: "Preliminary Study on the Local Effect of Cannabis indica: A Remedy for Specific Fistulas," Acta Univ. Olomuc. Fac. Med. 6, 91-92 (1955).

12. Sirek, J.: "Importance of Hempseeds in the Tuberculosis Therapy," Acta Univ. Olomuc Fac. Med. 6, 93-108 (1955).

13. Krejci, Z., Heczko, P.: "On the Treatment of the Papilla Rhagadae in Suckling Puerperial Mothers and on the Prevention of Mastitis Caused by Staphylococci," Acta Univ. Olomuc. Fac. Med. 14, 277-282 (1958).

14. Krejci, Z., Horak, M., Santavy, F.: "Constitution of the Cannabidiol Acid and of an Acid of the M. P. 133°C Isolated from Cannabis sativa L.," Acta Univ. Olomuc. Fac. Med. 16, 9-17 (1958).

15. Kabelik, J.: "Hanf (Cannabis sativa) - antibiotishes Heilmittel."
      1. Mitteilung: Hanf in der Alt - und Volksmedizin. Die Pharmazie 12, 439 (1957).

16. Krejci, Z.: "Hanf (Cannabis sativa) - antibiotishes Heilmittel."
      2. Mitteilung: Methodik und Ergebnisse der bakteriologishen Untersuchung und vorlaufige klinishe Erfahrugen. Die Pharmazie 13, Heft 3, 155-166 (1958).

17. Krejci, Z., Horak, M., Santavy, F.: "Hanf (Cannabis sativa) - antibiotishes Heilmittel." 3. Mitteilung: Isolierung und Konstitution zweier aus Cannabis sativa gewonnener sauren. Die Pharmazie 14, Heft 6, 349-355 (1959).

18. Kabelik, J., Krejci, Z., Santavy, F.: "Hemp as a Medicament," Bullet. on Narcotics 12, No. 3, 5-19 (1960).
      1. Part - Kabelik, J.: "Treatment with Cannabis in Ancient Folk and Official Medicine up to the beginning of the 20th Century," Pp 5-8.

      2. Part - Santavy, F., Krejci, Z.: "A Brief Survey of the Methods of Isolation and the Physical and Clinical Properties and Structure of the Isolated Antibacterial Substances," Pp 8-12.

      3. Part - Krejci, Z.: "Methods and Results of the Bacteriological Experiments," Pp 12-19.

      4. Part - Krejci, Z.: "Survey of Clinical Experiences," Pp 19-22.

19. Krejci, Z.: "To the Problem of Substances with Antibacterial and Hashish Effect in Hemp," Cas. lek. ces. 43, 1351-1354 (1961).

20. Krejci, Z.: "Antibacterial Substances of Cannabis Used in the Prevention and Therapy of Infections," Dissertation, 259 Pp (1961).

21. Krejci, Z., Vybiral, L.: "Thin Layer (Aluminum Oxide) Chromatographic Isolation of Biologically Active Substances from Cannabis sativa L. and the Biological Detection of Antibacterially Active Substances," Scr. Med. Brno 35, 71-72 (1962).

22. Santavy, F.: "Notes on the Structure of Cannabidiol Compounds (Absolute Configuration)," Acta Univ. Olomuc. Fac. Med. 35, 5-9 (1964).

23. Krejci, Z.: "Applications de la chromatographie sur couches minces
     a l'analyse du cannabis," United Nations Document ST (SOA) SER.
     S/13, 1-15 (1965).

24. Krejci, Z.: "L'analyse du hachiche et du chanvre indien a l'aide de
     la chromatographie sur couche mince," Acta Univ. Olomuc. Fac.
     Med. 43, 111-124 (1966).

25. Krejci, Z.: "Micro-method of Thin-layer Chromatography Adapted for
     the Analysis of Cannabis," United Nations ST (SOA) SER.S/16 (1967).

26. Krejci, Z.: "Changes with Maturation in the Amounts of Biologically
     Interesting Substances of Cannabis," The Botany and Chemistry of
     Cannabis, J. A. Churchill, London (1970).

27. Hrbek, J., Krejci, Z., Komenda, J., Siroka, L., Navratil, J.: "In-
     fluence of Smoking Hashish on Higher Nervous Activity in Man,"
     (Symposium on the Chemistry and Biological Activity of Cannabis),
     Acta Pharmaceutica Suecica 8, 689-690 (1971).

28. Navritil, J., Medek, A., Hrbek, J., Krejci, Z., Komenda, S.,
     Dvorak, M.: "The Effect of Cannabis on the Conditioned Alimentary
     Motor Reflexes in Cats," Activitas Nervosa Superior 14/2, 109 (1972).

29. Hrbek, J., Komenda, S., Siroka, L., Krejci, Z., Navratil, J., Medek,
     A.: "Acute Effect of THC (4, 18, 16 mg) on Verbal Associations,"
     Activitas Nervosa Superior 14/2, 107-108 (1972).

30. Hrbek, J., Komenda, S., Krejci, Z., Siroka, A., Navratil, J.: "On
     the Effect of Some Drugs on the Higher Nervous Activity in Man.
     Tetrahydrocannabinol (4, 8, 16 mg)" Acta Univ. Olomuc. Fac. Med.
     (1972).

CHAPTER 2

PROSTAGLANDINS AND CANNABIS -- IV: A BIOCHEMICAL BASIS

FOR THERAPEUTIC APPLICATIONS

Sumner Burstein

Worcester Foundation for Experimental Biology

Shrewsbury, Massachusetts

NOTE: The preparation of this paper was supported by
a grant from the National Institute on Drug Abuse
(DA-01170). The results on cell culture were obtained
by Ms. Sheila Hunter and the prostaglandin radioimmunoassays were performed by the Herschel Laboratory of the
Worcester Foundation.

INTRODUCTION

A great deal has been published on the chemistry and pharmacology
of cannabis * (Mechoulam, 1973); however, relatively little is known about
the biochemical effects of this drug. Several reports have been made of
effects on the biosynthesis of biogenic amines (Paton and Pertwee, 1973)
and a number of metabolic studies have been done (Burstein, 1973). To
date, however, no thesis as to the mode of action of cannabis on the
molecular level has been made.

A comparison of the pharmacological profile of cannabis with other
drugs led Paton to conclude: "It would have amounted to a modest substitute for aspirin in the days before aspirin was available" (Paton, Pertwee and
Temple, 1972). Vane (1973) has suggested that the inhibition of prostaglandin
(PG) biosynthesis by aspirin and other anti-inflammatory drugs is responsible
for the beneficial effects of these compounds. Considerable support has
been gained for this theory especially since the fundamental role of PG synthesis in the physiological responses of a wide variety of tissues has been
demonstrated (Horton, 1969).

---

* The term cannabis is meant to include not only the plant and derived
drugs, but also metabolites and related compounds.

Some time ago, based on the above observations we tested delta-1-tetrahydrocannabinol (THC) as an inhibitor of PG synthesis (Burstein and Raz, 1972). We found that it did, in fact, reduce the conversion of the precursor arachidonic acid to PGE2 in an ovine seminal vesicle preparation (Figure 1). The experimental design was similar to that used by others and showed a potency for THC similar to that for aspirin (ID_{50} THC $= 318\,\mu M$; ID_{50} aspirin $= 46.7\,\mu M$).

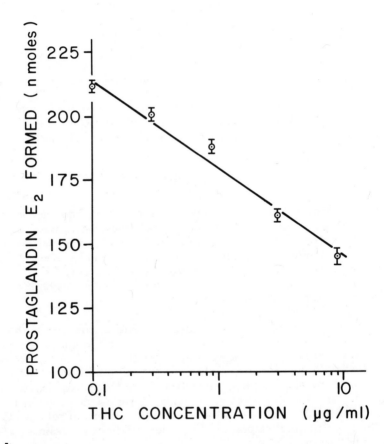

Figure 1.

The effect of various concentrations of THC on the conversion of arachidonic acid to PGE2 by ovine seminal vesicles. Each point represents the mean of two determinations (Burstein and Raz, 1972).

We have recently extended these studies to include several of the naturally occurring cannabinoids using a similar system, namely, bovine seminal vesicle microsomes with 8,11,14-eicosatrienoic acid as the precursor (Burstein, Levin and Varanelli, 1973). These results (Table 1) showed that PG inhibition is a general property of these cannabinoids and could be attributed to the olivetyl portion common to all of the structures. It seemed that the terpene portion served to moderate the effect in varying degrees.

Table 1

Inhibition of PGE$_1$ Synthesis by
Some of the Natural Cannabinoids

| Substance | ID_{50}* | | | |
	(μg/ml)	(M x 10^{-4})	Correlation	Psychoactivity
Cannabinol	22	0.70	0.96	–
Cannabidiolic acid	43	1.20	0.99	–
Delta-8-THC	64	2.04	0.72	+
Cannabidiol	69	2.20	0.74	–
Cannabichromene	83	2.64	0.79	–
Delta-9-THC	100	3.18	0.86	+
Crude marihuana extract	173	–	0.47	+
Cannabicyclol	>100	>3.18	–	–
Olivetol	18	1.0	–	–

* These values represent the average of at least two experiments in which inhibition was measured at 1, 10, and 100 μg/ml of inhibitor in triplicate. The results were evaluated by a computer generated linear plot of PG synthesized vs log concentration of inhibitor. Correlation refers to the degree of fit of the experimental values to the resulting line (Burstein, Levin and Varanelli, 1973).

Some of our findings have recently been confirmed and extended by Crowshaw and Hardman (1974) utilizing a rabbit renal medulla preparation. They showed that while PGE_2 synthesis was reduced by delta-1-THC, $PGF_{2\alpha}$ synthesis was stimulated. 7-OH-delta-1-THC, 7-OH-delta-6-THC, and DMHP also behaved in a similar fashion. It has been generally observed that drugs such as indomethacin seem to inhibit both PGE and PGF production, suggesting that the cannabinoids may be unique in their bimodal response.

It is believed that the PG's interact with cyclic-AMP in mediating hormone and drug action on the cellular level (Hittelman and Butcher, 1973). Figure 2 summarizes these proposed interactions and indicates the points at which various drugs are believed to act. Kelly and Butcher (1973) have reported that delta-1-THC can antagonize the effects of PGE_1 (and epinephrine) on c-AMP levels in WI-38 fibroblasts derived from human lung. It is not known at this time whether or not this effect of THC is related to our observations on PG synthetase.

PG - cAMP INTERACTIONS

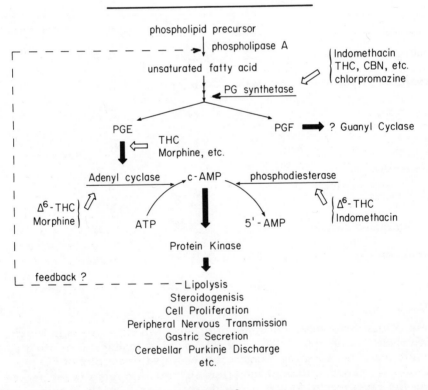

Figure 2

Sofia, Knobloch, and Vassar (1973) have studied the anti-edema properties of several cannabinoids and their findings lend strong support to our
theory. They found that THC, CBD, and CBN were all effective in reducing
carrageenan-induced edema in the rat paw. Moreover, they reported that
olivetol was also active, showing that a similar structure-activity relationship
exists for both PG inhibition and anti-inflammatory effects.

The anticonvulsant activity of THC, CBD, and CBN has been reported
by Karler, Cely, and Turkanis (1973, 1974). While this property may not be
related to PG synthesis, the involvement of PG's in motor function (Coceani,
1974) and the fact that non-psychoactive cannabinoids are also effective suggests a possible relationship.

One of the more striking clinical effects of THC not related to mood
alteration is its ability to lower intraocular pressure (Hepler and Frank, 1971;
Frank, Hepler, Epps, Ungerleider, and Szara, 1972). This has led to the suggestion that it may be useful in treating glaucoma. The involvement of increased PG synthesis in raising intraocular pressure has been demonstrated by
Podos, Becker, and Kass (1973). Green and Podos (1974) also showed that
prior treatment of the rabbits with delta-1-THC blocked the adverse effects
of arachidonic acid but not that of PGE_2. These findings suggest to us that
other cannabinoids in addition to THC which are effective PG synthetase
blockers might be useful agents for relieving elevated intraocular pressure.

Bronchodilation by cannabis in normal subjects has been reported by
two laboratories (Tashkin, Shapiro, and Frank, 1973; Vachon, Fitzgerald,
Solliday, Gould, and Gaensler, 1973). Since it is well known that the PG's
have profound effects on respiratory smooth muscle (Cuthbert, 1973), the implication can be made that the action of cannabis is mediated by altered PG
release. This explanation is complicated by the fact that E and F series of
PG's can have opposite effects on the lung (Horton, 1969). However, Crowshaw and Hardman (1974) have found a bimodal response for THC on renal
medulla synthetase (noted above) which may also be the case in lung tissue.
We have also seen a similar effect in cell cultures (see Table 4 below) so that
this point will obviously have to be established by further study.

In contrast to the above reports showing bronchodilation, Davies,
Radcliffe, Seaton, and Graham (1975) found that delta-1-THC (10 mg oral)
gave no significant effect. The authors pointed out that the previous studies
involved experienced cannabis users while their subjects claimed no prior use.
Moreover, the other studies included higher doses of THC and there was the
possibility of the presence of other cannabinoids. An interesting correlate to
these lung effects has been reported by Kaymakcalan, Ercan, and Turker (1975).
They gave evidence for the release of PG's from the perfused guinea-pig lung
by delta-1-THC; however, the precise nature of the product(s) was not
ascertained.

Endocrine-related effects for cannabis have been observed in men by
Kolodny, Masters, Kolodner, and Toro (1974). A 44 percent lowering of
plasma testosterone was found in subjects who smoked marihuana regularly.

Interestingly, we have observed a dramatic drop in the plasma testosterone of mice after the administration of modest amounts of CBN but not with THC (Bartke and Burstein, unpublished). Once again, this may or may not involve PG's; however, the data are suggestive.

Delta-1-THC has been shown to suppress the LH surge in rats and to reduce ovulation (Nir, Ayalon, Tsafriri, Cordova, and Lindner, 1973). The latter effect was also exhibited by indomethacin (Tsafriri, Lindner, Zor, and Lamprecht, 1972), implicating PG synthesis. The possibility is therefore raised that other cannabinoids may be effective antifertility agents.

Hollister (1971) has proposed that THC may be a useful hypotensive agent if the mental effects could be avoided. The cardiovascular-renal effects of the PG's have been extensively studied and shown to be of major importance (Lee, 1974). This again suggests a possible use for non-psychoactive cannabinoids which affect PG synthesis.

The reports cited above strongly suggest that the mode of some of the actions of cannabis may be mediated by alteration of prostaglandin production in the body. On the molecular level, it has been shown that many cannabinoids inhibit the in vitro synthesis of PG's. This effect parallels that of therapeutically useful drugs such as aspirin, indomethacin, and chlorpromazine (Krupp and Wesp, 1975).

Pharmacological observations such as the anti-edema properties of cannabis provide further analogies to the above comparison with "established" PG inhibitors. The opposing effects of THC and PGE on intraocular pressure suggest an immediate application for a non-psychoactive cannabinoid in medicine.

It therefore seemed quite worthwhile to extend our initial findings on the interaction between cannabis and PG biosynthesis to provide a biochemical basis for further in vivo and clinical studies on therapeutic applications of cannabis.

THE SUBCELLULAR APPROACH

The PG synthetase system has not been isolated to date; however, several tissues are particularly rich in this enzyme complex and the "microsomal" fractions of these have been used to study the effects of certain drugs on PG synthesis. The best-known example is the use of seminal vesicle preparations to demonstrate activity for a variety of anti-inflammatory agents (Robinson and Vane, 1974).

The procedure involves the exposure of the synthetase to the PG precursor (usually arachidonic acid) followed by either a chemical or biological assay for the prostaglandins. In the presence of a number of therapeutic drugs, there is a marked decrease in the activity of the enzyme system which has been correlated to some degree with anti-inflammatory activity. More recently,

Krupp and Wesp (1975) have shown that psychotropic drugs such as chlorpromazine and chlorimipramine also inhibit PG synthetase in vitro, demonstrating
that other types of agents are active in this system.

Some time ago we reported that delta-1-THC was effective in reducing
the conversion of arachidonic acid to PG's by the animal vesicle preparation.
Radio-labeled precursor was used, and the products were analyzed by separation
on thin layer chromatography. The analytical technique was validated by
independently measuring the PGE formed using radioimmunoassay (Table 2)
as well as gas chromatography (Burstein and Raz, 1972). This approach has
proved useful in identifying substances which are PG synthetase inhibitors,
and we have applied this technique in two somewhat different situations.

First, we have assayed most of the major naturally occurring cannabinoids for inhibitory activity (Burstein et al, 1973). Surprisingly, delta-1-THC
was not the most active as it has been in a number of other biological systems.
While delta-1-THC was less potent than aspirin, cannabinol was equally effective (Table 1). Some interesting structure-activity relationships were also uncovered. The common feature of all the cannabinoids is the alkyl resorcinol
moiety, and indeed when olivetal was tested, it was as active as CBN. By
contrast, terpenoids resembling the other half of the cannabinoid structure
such as limonene and p-cymene were without any activity.

A second application of this method has been more recently made in
the isolation of inhibitors from crude extracts of cannabis. The role of the
volatile oil fraction from the plant has not been extensively studied with respect to possible pharmacological effects. We found that there are at least

Table 2

Comparison of Methods of Analysis for
Microsomal PG Synthetase*

Conditions	PGE$_1$ Produced (μg/incubation)	
	TLC-Analysis	R.I.A.
Blank Control	0.35, 0.64	0.13, 0.17
1 mg Enzyme	3.3 , 2.9	2.4 , 2.3
5 mg Enzyme	8.0 , 8.3	5.6 , 5.1
5 mg + Indomethacin (0.3 μg)	2.7 , 3.4	2.6 , 2.4
10 mg Enzyme	11.2 , 12.2	14.3 , 12.5

* The preparation of the enzyme and the tlc analysis were done
as previously reported (Burstein et al, 1973). R.I.A. was
performed by the Herschel Laboratory, Worcester Foundation.

two highly inhibitor substances present (Table 3) and have identified one of
these an eugenol (Burstein, Varanelli, and Slade, 1975). Interestingly, eugenol
is also present in nutmeg (Myristica fragrans) which has been used as a mood-
altering drug. Eugenol has also been employed as a mild local anesthetic in
dentistry.

Table 3

Inhibition of Prostaglandin E_1 Biosynthesis by

Essential Oil Constituents of Cannabis sativa and Related Substances

Substance	Occurrence		ID_{50} [a] ($\mu g/ml$)
Fraction 1	C. sativa		2.3
Fraction 5	C. sativa		[b]
Eugenol	C. sativa	M. fragrans	5.6
Safrole		M. fragrans	47
Myristicin		M. fragrans	170
Methoxy eugenol		M. fragrans	2.6
Borneol	C. sativa		>100
Fenchyl alcohol	C. sativa		>100
Linalool	C. sativa	M. fragrans	NI[c]
α-Terpineol	C. sativa	M. fragrans	NI
Limonene	C. sativa	M. fragrans	NI
p-Cymene	C. sativa	M. fragrans	NI
Carvacrol			4.1
2-Cymidine	C. sativa		12.5
β-Carophyllene	C. sativa		910
delta-1-THC	C. sativa		100
Cannabigerol	C. sativa		95

[a] ID_{50} = dose which causes 50% inhibition.

[b] Fraction 5 was a mixture; therefore, an ID_{50} could not be calculated.
However, it appears to be of the same order of activity as fraction 1.

[c] NI = non-inhibitory.

Source: Burstein, Varanelli, and Slade, 1975.

While this subcellular approach to the study of the relationship of prostaglandins and cannabis offers the advantage of simplicity, the very valid question of relevance is raised. The major support for its continued use is the correlation of the results obtained with those from anti-inflammatory agents.

CELL CULTURE SYSTEMS AS A MODEL

Cells in culture are assuming greater importance in studies on drug action due to improved methodology and the availability of a variety of cell lines. A relevant example is the current use of neuroblastoma cultures in examining various problems in neurobiology (Haffke and Seeds, 1975). Of particular interest are the reports on the effects of morphine and other opiates on c-AMP metabolism in these cells (Sharma, Nirenberg, and Klee, 1975; Traber, Fischer, Latzin, and Hambrecht, 1975). For example, it was shown that morphine can reduce the stimulation of adenyl cyclase by PGE, and it was suggested that opiate dependence could be explained with such a mechanism. Similar effects have also been demonstrated using subcellular systems, showing there is a correlation between these types of models (Collier, Francis, and McDonald-Gibson, 1975).

Delta-1-THC was shown by Kelly and Butcher (1973) to have a profound effect on adenyl cyclase similar to that of morphine described above. They used WI-38 fibroblasts derived from human lung, a well-established line which has been widely used in a variety of studies. Both PGE_1 and epinephrine elevated the levels of c-AMP in these cells and both effects could be effectively blocked by the prior addition of delta-1-THC (3.2 μM). Aside from the intrinsic value of these observations, their results indicate that cell culture models may be useful in studying the action(s) of the cannabinoids.

We have begun to explore the possibility of using cell culture to study the effects of the cannabinoids on PG release. Initially, as noted above, we attempted to adapt the labeled precursor method to this type of system. While there was a good uptake of the precursor by the cells, the major products were none of the well-known PG's.

As an alternate method, we are now using radioimmunoassay to monitor the levels of PG's produced from endogenous precursors (Caldwell, Burstein, Brock, and Speroff, 1971; Stylos, Burstein, Rosenfield, Ritzi, and Watson, 1973; Stylos, Howard, Ritzi, and Skarmes, 1974). The assay we have does not distinguish the PG_1 from the PG_2 series; however, at this stage, it is not crucial to have those individual values. The measurements obtained reflect the steady state levels of PG's, that is, the amount being synthesized minus the amount which is metabolized, and reflect what is probably the situation in vivo.

Thus far, we have applied this method to a study of the effects of eugenol and THC on PG synthesis in primary monolayer cultures of mouse mammary epithelial cells (Table 4). Our results show that eugenol does reduce the

Table 4

Inhibition of Prostaglandin Production[a] in

Mouse Mammary Cell Culture Media

	Drug (mg/ml x 10^{-5})	PGE (ng/ml)	PGF (ng/ml)
Control[b]	--	$0.44 + 0.24$	$2.36 + 0.23$
Eugenol	0.25	$0.49 + 0.02$	$0.33 + 0.07$
"	2.5	< 0.2	0.5
"	2.5	< 0.2	1.08
Collagen[c]	--	7.29	22.7
Collagen + Eugenol	0.25	$4.82 + 0.90$	2.17
"	2.5	$0.48 + 0.06$	0.60
Naproxen	0.20	$0.28 + 0.32$	4.83
Control[b]	--	$1.19 + 0.11$	$3.85 + 0.40$
Delta-1-THC	0.50	$0.60 + 0.10$	$3.27 + 0.68$
"	5.0	$0.77 + 0.31$	$3.30 + 0.44$
"	5.0	$3.87 + 0.29$	$8.37 + 0.12$

[a] Estimated by radioimmunoassay. Values are the mean $\pm$ S. E. of three experiments; other values represent the average of duplicates.

[b] Confluent monolayers of C3H tumor cells.

[c] Sigma, bovine achilles tendon, 270μg/ml.

Source: Burstein and Hunter, unpublished.

basal levels of PGE and is also capable of reversing the stimulatory effect of collagen on both PGE and PGF synthesis. The basal level of PGF seems to be affected in a more complex fashion, and this will have to be studied in more detail. In general, these results agree with those we obtained on eugenol in the subcellular preparation, described above.

The effects of delta-1-THC on these cells also suggest a fairly complex relationship between drug concentration and PG levels. At lower concentrations, both PGE and PGF levels are depressed to different degrees, while at 50×10^{-5} mg/ml, both are stimulated two- to three-fold over basal levels. There is also a striking difference between the dosages needed to inhibit PG levels here and in the seminal vesicle preparation where the ID_{50} for THC was about 0.1 mg/ml.

It is interesting to note that the differential effects on PGE and PGF production seen here with both eugenol and THC could not have been easily obtained with the isolated enzyme preparation. Another point which becomes obvious in looking at the cell culture data is that the ratios of E to F are significantly altered in the presence of the various agents shown in Table 4. The significance of this observation is not certain; however, if the E and F prostaglandins are responsible for different physiological effects the results of such changes could be profound.

CONCLUSIONS

There is considerable circumstantial evidence that some if not all of the actions of cannabis are mediated by a prostaglandin-cyclic nucleotide system. This includes clinical, pharmacological, and biochemical observations using a wide variety of models and techniques. The diversity of actions apparently mediated by the prostaglandins would seem to coincide with the range of cannabis activities, lending support to the possible connection of the two. This fact, however, makes it difficult to obtain conclusive experimental results to either prove or disprove the theory.

Experiments with subcellular preparations have pointed to the possibility that prostaglandins are indeed involved. What is now needed are data from better models involving more complex systems. Cell culture may be the answer, and we have presented evidence that cannabis action on PG release can be studied in such models. These models would be useful in exploring therapeutic applications by allowing structure-activity relationships, toxic effects, tolerance development, and the like to be examined under controlled laboratory conditions.

REFERENCES

Bartke, & Burstein, S. Unpublished research.

Burstein, S. H. Labeling and metabolism of the tetrahydrocannabinols. In R. Mechoulam (Ed.), Marihuana. New York: Academic Press, 1973.

Burstein, S. & Hunter, S. Unpublished research.

Burstein, S. & Raz, A. Inhibition of prostaglandin E_2 biosynthesis by delta-1-tetrahydrocannabinol. Prostaglandins, 1972, 2, 369-374.

Burstein, S., Levin, E., & Varanelli, C. Prostaglandins and cannabis -- II: Inhibition of biosynthesis by the naturally occurring cannabinoids. Biochemical Pharmacology, 1973, 22, 2905-2910.

Burstein, S., Varanelli, C., & Slade, L. T. Prostaglandins and cannabis -- III: Inhibition of biosynthesis by essential oil components of marihuana. Biochemical Pharmacology, 1975, 24, 1053-1054.

Caldwell, B., Burstein, S., Brock, W., & Speroff, L. RIA of the F PGs. Journal of Clinical Endocrinology and Metabolism, 1971, 33, 171.

Coceani, F. Prostaglandins and the central nervous system. Archives of Internal Medicine, 1974, 133, 119-129.

Collier, H. O. J., Francis, D. L., McDonald-Gibson, W. J., Roy, A. C., & Saeed, S. A. Prostaglandins, cyclic AMP and the mechanism of opiate dependence. Life Sciences, 1975, 17, 85-90.

Crowshaw, K., & Hardman, H. F. Effect of delta-9-THC on PG synthesis and the relationship of this effect to the hypothermic response in mice. Federation Proceedings, 1974, 33, Abstr. #1847.

Cuthbert, M. F. Prostaglandins and respiratory smooth muscle. In M. F. Cuthbert (Ed.), The prostaglandins. Philadelphia: Lippincott, 1973.

Davies, B. H., Radcliffe, S., Seaton, A., & Graham, J. D. P. A trial of oral delta-1-THC in reversible airways obstruction. Thorax, 1975, 30, 80-85.

Frank, I. R., Hepler, R. S., Epps, L., Ungerleider, J. T., & Szara, S. Marihuana and delta-9-tetrahydrocannabinol: Effects on intraocular pressure in young adults. Fifth International Congress on Pharmacology, 1972, Abstr. 426.

Green, K., & Podos, S. M. Antagonism of arachidonic acid-induced ocular effects by delta-1-THC. Investigative Ophthalmology, 1974, 13, 422-429.

Haffke, S., & Seeds, N. W. Neuroblastoma: The E. coli of neurobiology. Life Sciences, 1975, 16, 1649.

Hollister, L. E. Marihuana in man: Three years later. Science, 1971, 172, 21-28.

Hepler, R. S., & Frank, I. R. Marihuana smoking and intraocular pressure. Journal of the American Medical Association, 1971, 217(10), 1392.

Hittelman, K. J., & Butcher, R. W. Cyclic AMP and the mechanism of action of prostaglandins. In M. F. Cuthbert (Ed.), The prostaglandins. Philadelphia: Lippincott, 1973.

Horton, E. Hypotheses on the physiological roles of prostaglandins. Physiological Reviews, 1969, 49, 122-161.

Karler, R., Cely, W., & Turkanis, S. A. The anticonvulsant activity of CBD and CBN. Life Sciences, 1973, 13, 1527-1531.

Karler, R., Cely, W., & Turkanis, S. A. A study of the relative anticonvulsant and toxic activities of delta-9-THC and its congeners. Research Communications in Chemical Pathology and Pharmacology, 1974, 7, 353-358.

Kaymakcalan, S., Ercan, Z. S., & Turker, R. K. The evidence of the release of prostaglandin-like material from rabbit kidney and guinea-pig lung by delta-1-THC. Journal of Pharmacy and Pharmacology, 1975, 27, 564-568.

Kelly, L. A., & Butcher, R. W. The effects of delta-1-THC on cyclic AMP levels in WI-38 fibroblasts. Biochimica Biophysica Acta, 1973, 320, 540-544.

Kolodny, R. C., Masters, W. H., Kolodner, R. M., & Toro, G. Depression of plasma testosterone levels after chronic intensive marihuana use. New England Journal of Medicine, 1974, 290, 872-874.

Krupp, P., & Wesp, M. Inhibition of prostaglandin synthetase by psychotropic drugs. Experientia, 1975, 31, 330-331.

Lee, J. B. Cardiovascular-renal effects of PGs. Archives of Internal Medicine, 1974, 133, 56-76.

Mechoulam, R. (Ed.) Marihuana: Chemistry, pharmacology and metabolism. New York: Academic Press, 1973.

Nir, I., Ayalon, D., Tsafriri, A., Cordova, T., & Lindner, H. R. Suppression of the cyclic surge of LH secretion and of ovulation in the rat by delta-1-THC. Nature, 1973, 243, 470-471.

Paton, W. D. M., & Pertwee, R. G. The pharmacology of cannabis in animals. In R. Mechoulam (Ed.), Marihuana. New York: Academic Press, 1973.

Paton, W. D. M., Pertwee, R. G., & Temple, D. The general pharmacology of cannabinoids. In W. D. M. Paton & J. Crown (Eds.), Cannabis and its derivatives. London: Oxford, 1972, 65.

Podos, S. M., Becker, B., & Kass, M. A. PG synthesis, inhibition and intraocular pressure. Investigative Ophthalmology, 1973, 12, 426.

Robinson, H. J., & Vane, J. R. (Eds.) Prostaglandin Synthetase Inhibitors. New York: Raven Press, 1974.

Sharma, S. K., Nirenberg, M., & Klee, W. A. Morphine receptors as regulators of adenylate cyclase activity. Proceedings of the National Academy of Sciences, 1975, 72, 590-594.

Sofia, R. D., Knobloch, L. C., & Vassar, H. B. The anti-edema activity of various naturally occurring cannabinoids. Research Communications in Chemical Pathology and Pharmacology, 1973, 6, 909-918.

Sofia, R. D., Nalepa, S. D., Harakal, J. J., & Vassar, H. B. Anti-edema and analgesic properties of delta-9-THC. Journal of Pharmacology and Experimental Therapeutics, 1973, 186, 646-655.

Stylos, W., Burstein, S., Rosenfeld, J., Ritzi, E., & Watson, D. RIA for the initial metabolites of the F PGs. Prostaglandins, 1973, 4, 553-565.

Stylos, W., Howard, L., Ritzi, E., & Skarmes, R. The preparation and characterization of PGE$_1$ antiserum. Prostaglandins, 1974, 6, 1-13.

Tashkin, D. P., Shapiro, B. J., & Frank, I. M. Acute pulmonary physiologic effects of smoked marijuana and oral delta-9-THC in healthy young men. New England Journal of Medicine, 1973, 289, 336-341.

Traber, J., Fischer, K., Latzin, S., & Hamprecht, B. Morphine antagonizes action of prostaglandin in neuroblastoma and neuroblastoma X glioma hybrid cells. Nature, 1975, 253, 120-122.

Tsafriri, A., Lindner, H. R., Zor, N., & Lamprecht, S. A. Physiological role of PGs in the induction of ovulation. Prostaglandins, 1972, 2, 1-10.

Vachon, L., Fitzgerald, M. X., Solliday, N. H., Gould, I. A., & Gaensler, E. A. Single dose effect of marihuana smoke. New England Journal of Medicine, 1973, 288, 985-989.

Vane, J. R. Inhibition of prostaglandin biosynthesis as the mechanism of action of aspirin like drugs. Advances in Biosciences, 1973, 9, 395-411.

CHAPTER 3

ON THE THERAPEUTIC POSSIBILITIES OF SOME CANNABINOIDS

R. Mechoulam
N. Lander
S. Dikstein

Hebrew University School of Pharmacy
Jerusalem, Israel

E. A. Carlini

Departamento de Psicobiologia, Escola Paulista de Medicina
Sao Paolo, Brazil

M. Blumenthal

Department of Ophthalmology
Central Hospital of the Negev, Ben-Gurion University
Beersheva, Israel

INTRODUCTION

Cannabis has been used as a therapeutic agent since ancient times. Li (1974) and Rosenthal (1971) have described its use by the ancient Chinese and in medieval Arab society. Walton (1938) and more recently Mikuriya (1973) have summarized the medical use of cannabis in Europe during the nineteenth and early twentieth century. In spite of the very promising and rather non-toxic effects of the drug, its use rapidly declined due to the notorious variability of crude cannabis preparations. The advances made since the determination of the structure of cannabidiol in 1963, the isolation in pure form and structure elucidation of delta-1-THC in 1964, and the development of various synthetic routes during the middle sixties (Mechoulam, 1973) have clarified the chemistry and pharmacology of the cannabinoids and have made possible initiation of research into the use of pure natural or synthetic cannabinoids as drugs.

The potential medical uses of cannabinoids are legion. A partial list, based on recent pharmacological or clinical evidence (either recent or nineteenth century), should include the following conditions:

Anorexia	Asthma	Nausea
Pain	Peptic Ulcer	Alcoholism
Glaucoma	Epilepsy	Depression
Migraine	Anxiety	Inflammation
Hypertension	Insomnia	Cancer

Obviously, one of the major goals in any pharmaceutical program will be not only to find new potent compounds, but to separate the various activities. This situation recalls the prostaglandin field.

In the present lecture, we intend to present ongoing work in a few areas being carried out in collaboration by several groups. Not all authors have participated in every part of this work. Hence the names of the workers responsible for a particular aspect are indicated in the subtitles within the lecture.

ANTICONVULSANT ACTIVITY OF OXYGENATED CANNABIDIOL DERIVATIVES*

(Carlini, Lander, Mechoulam)

Ibn al-Badri, in a treatise on hashish written around 1464 and preserved in manuscript form, tells that the poet Ali ben Makki visited the epileptic Zahir-ad-din Muhammed, the son of the Chamberlain of the Caliphate Council in Baghdad, and gave the reluctant Zahir-ad-din hashish as medication. It cured him completely but he could not be without the drug ever after (Rosenthal, 1971).

During the nineteenth century, several medical publications reported observations or experimental evidence on the anti-convulsive action of cannabis (O'Shaughnessy, 1842; Shaw, 1843; Reynolds, 1890). More recent work has indeed confirmed the action of cannabinoids of the THC-type (Loewe and Goodman, 1947; Garriott, Forney, Hughes, and Richard, 1968; Bogan, Steele, and Freedman, 1973, and ref. therein). Due to the psychotropic activity of such compounds, their clinical use in epilepsy seems unwarranted.

The observation (Carlini, Leite, Tannhauser, and Berardi, 1973; Isquierdo, Orsingher, and Berardi, 1973; Karler, Cely, and Turkanis, 1973) that cannabidiol, which has no THC-like psychotropic activity, possesses anticonvulsant activity, has increased the pharmaceutical potential in this area. It seemed of interest to initiate an investigation on the structure-activity relationships of cannabidiol-type compounds.

---

* And there is nothing new under the sun. Ecclesiastes 1:9.

We have synthesized several new oxygenated cannabidiol derivatives. Protection against maximal electroshock convulsions, potentiation of pentobarbital sleeping time, and reduction of spontaneous motor activity were the effects measured.

The four compounds shown in Figure 1 were synthesized. Their syntheses are described in Schemes 1 and 2 (Figure 2).

Pentobarbital Sleeping Time

Male albino mice were injected i.p. with the appropriate dose of the drug, followed an hour later by 50 mg/kg of sodium pentobarbital. The interval of time to lose and recover the righting reflex was recorded. Cannabidiol, as well as compounds I–IV, were equally potent in potentiating barbiturate sleeping time at doses ranging from 6.25 to 100 mg/kg. In none of the experiments were statistically significant differences found among the compounds; that is, they did not differ in potency. Compound I was toxic: about one-third of the animals died within 24 hours after administration of 100 mg/kg. The other compounds caused no deaths at this dose level.

Spontaneous Motor Activity

Male albino mice were injected i.p. with the substances under study. At fixed periods, they were introduced into cages with photocells. The number of crossings of the light beam were recorded.

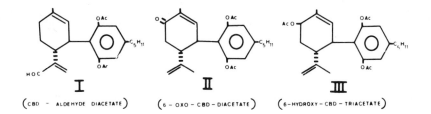

Figure 1

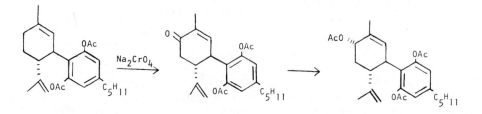

Scheme   I

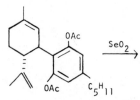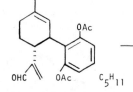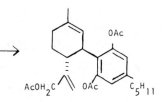

Scheme   II

Figure 2

Only CBD and IV significantly (Student t test) decreased spontaneous motor activity at 12.5 to 25 mg/kg, while compounds I, II, and III caused no significant reduction. This separation of activity is of interest and should be further pursued.

Transcorneal Electroshock

Male albino rats received a transcorneal electroshock of 35 ma, 0.2 sec. duration. The times of flexion and extension of posterior limbs were measured to the nearest second. One hour later, the animals were injected i.p. with the drug under study and the electroshock was applied 1, 2, 4, 8, and 24 hours after the injection.

CBD as well as compounds II, III, and IV at 100 and 200 mg/kg possess an anticonvulsant effect which reaches its peak about 1-2 hr after injection. CBD and II are the most active compounds, while I caused the death of 50 percent of the animals, the rest showing ptosis, hypothermia, and flaccidity.

Discussion

Our results extend previous reports that CBD potentiates barbiturate sleeping time and protects mice against electroconvulsive shock (Karler, Cely, and Turkanis, 1973; Paton and Pertwee, 1973) to 4 other CBD derivatives, namely cannabidiol aldehyde-diacetate (I), 6-oxo-CBD-diacetate (II), 6-hydroxy-CBD-triacetate (III), and 9-hydroxy-CBD-triacetate (IV). Compound I was very toxic. Compound IV had about the same activity as CBD in increasing pentobarbital sleeping time and in decreasing spontaneous motor activity, both at doses below the anticonvulsant ones. However, at 200 mg/kg, IV seems to be less active than CBD in protecting mice against electroshock. Of the two remaining compounds, 6-oxo-CBD-diacetate (II) seems to be the most promising. At 6.25-100 mg/kg dose, it was equally active as compounds CBD, I, III, and IV in potentiating barbiturate sleeping time. Furthermore, compound II yielded anticonvulsant protection to mice similar to that of CBD, both with a peak effect at 1-2 hr after injection, and with a good dose-response curve. On the other hand, at doses of 12.5 and 25 mg/kg, compound II did not interfere with the spontaneous motor activity of the mice. Thus, if one considers the decrease of spontaneous motor activity as a side effect concerning anticonvulsant activity, then compound II would be the drug of choice for further study. However, CBD and II were anticonvulsant only in large doses (100 and 200 mg/kg) when compared, for instance, with diphenyl-hydantoin, which is active at 5-10 mg/kg dosage in this method.

We hope to be able to find compounds in this series which are active at lower doses and for more prolonged periods of time.

A detailed chemical report (together with other material) will be presented elsewhere (Lander, Ben-Zvi, Mechoulam, Martin, Nordqvist, and

Agurell, 1975); the detailed pharmacological paper is in press (Carlini, Mechoulam, and Lander, 1975).

ANTIGLAUCOMATIC ACTIVITY

(Dikstein, Blumenthal, Mechoulam)

Smoking cannabis can lead to a significant fall in intraocular pressure (IOP) in man (Hepler, Frank, and Ungerleider, 1972). Green and Peterson (1973) have investigated this phenomenon in rabbits which have normal ocular pressure.

We wish now to report some preliminary experiments with cannabinoids on rabbits with stable glaucoma induced by α-chymotrypsin injection into the eye.

The Method

Rabbits were anesthetized with intravenous nembutal 30 mg/kg. Four percent pilocarpine was used to induce miosis of one eye. To the same eye, 75 units of α-chymotrypsin (Quimotrase) in 0.05 ml saline was injected into the posterior chamber through a 27-gauge needle.

After about 10 days, the injected eye developed buphthalmus, and in most of the eyes, posterior dislocation of the lens and optic disc involvement was seen. Stable glaucoma was established after 4 weeks, at which time the angle structures almost disappeared. We used only those rabbits which had IOP between 35-60 mm Hg.

The overall rate of success is about 25 percent, and preliminary pathology indicates changes in the angle outflow channels. Measurement of the aqueous pressure was carried out after tranquilizing the rabbits by injecting 15 mg/kg Rumpun[R] (Bayer) intravenously. Pressure was measured by Schiotz Tonometer, using a 10 gm weight and special rabbit calibration tables (Best, Pola, Galin, and Blumenthal, 1970).

The drug to be tested was applied in 1/2 ml saline solution or suspension into the conjunctival sack for 1 minute. Four percent pilocarpine hydrochloride and 1 percent epinephrine bitartarate (Eppy) were used as stock solutions and diluted to the proper concentration by saline immediately before being used.

Standardization

Since pressure did not return to the original level in every case, we measured half-time of recovery, that is, the time until half of the total pressure drop was recovered. Figure 3 shows the dose-response curves of pilocarpine and epinephrine. We wish to remark that at the highest concentration used (2% pilocarpine and 1% epinephrine), the IOP sometimes remained constantly low (up to one month). It can be seen that in equal concentrations epinephrine is 2-4 times longer-acting than pilocarpine. If we compare activity on the basis of concentrations which cause lowering of the aqueous pressure for a specific identical time, then epinephrine is at least 100 times more active than pilocarpine. For comparative purposes, we determined the smallest concentration (in steps of 10-fold) causing one-half recovery time of about 12 hours.

Results

Cannabidiol was found to be ineffective at 1 percent concentration, while cannabinol acetate at the same concentration showed some effects. However, (-)-delta-6-THC at 0.001 percent concentration showed activity comparable to that of pilocarpine at the same concentration. We observed no effect on the pupilla.

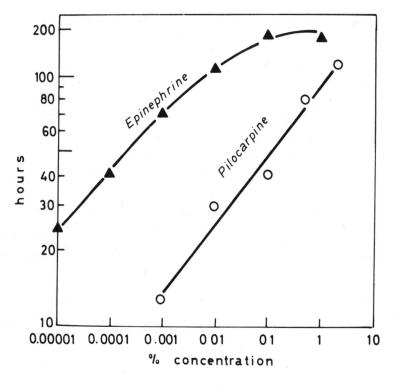

Figure 3

Judging by the above, obviously very limited number of compounds tested, the antiglaucoma effect follows the structure activity relationships recorded for the cannabinoids in the central nervous system. Indeed, the (3S, 4S) unnatural (+)-delta-6-THC showed no activity at 0.01 percent concentration.

A much more extensive list of compounds will have to be studied before drawing conclusions as to the feasibility of separation psychotropic and anti-glaucoma effects.

Antiglaucoma drugs (as drops) are usually self-administered. Hence, commercialization of an antiglaucoma cannabinoid drug which still shows "marihuana type" effects (even only on per os illegal consumption!) will be subject to considerable practical difficulties. In any case, the relevancy of our animal model to the glaucomatic human patient will first have to be established.

Neurotransmitters and Cannabis

Do the effects of cannabinoids on neurotransmitters relate to their pharmacologic actions in vivo? The influence of several cannabinoids on biogenic amines have been examined but the results are inconsistent (Paton and Pertwee, 1973). In a recent publication, Banerjee, Snyder, and Mechoulam (1975) have shown that there is a certain correlation between neurotransmitter uptake inhibition in vitro with "THC-like" pharmacologic potency. Thus, delta-1-THC, delta-6-THC, and their 7-hydroxy metabolites are potent inhibitors of the uptake of norepinephrine (NE) and serotonin (5-HT) in hypothalamic preparations of synaptosomes and of dopamine (DA) in the corpus striatum; γ-aminobutyric acid (GABA) uptake into cerebral cortical preparations is also inhibited. Blocking of the free phenolic group essentially abolishes both CNS effects and neurotransmitter uptake. The acidic metabolite, delta-6-THC-7-oic acid as well as cannabinol, are also inactive. Cannabidiol, however, is an important exception. It has the same affinities for 5-HT, NE and GABA uptake as delta-1-THC, yet it shows no "THC-like" effects in humans. We would like to speculate that the anticonvulsive action of cannabidiol is due to its inhibition of GABA uptake. This suggestion follows current views on the relationship between epilepsy and GABA (Meldrum, 1975). In any case, if a correlation exists between 5-HT, NE and GABA uptake, and CNS effects, it is certainly not a simple one. The recognition of this possible polytypic behavior points the need to investigate other cannabinoids which have no "THC-like" properties. Cannabigerol, for example, only slightly reduces affinity for the 5-HT and NE uptake systems, as compared to delta-1-THC or delta-6-THC, but is more potent than these two compounds on GABA uptake. It causes no "THC-like" effects on rhesus monkeys. Maybe a more detailed analysis of the pharmacologic profile of cannabigerol will reveal its hidden potential. One should keep in mind, however, that numerous effects caused by cannabinoids can be best explained by a cholinergic mechanism (Drew and Miller, 1974).

THC is considered to lack activity against monoamine oxidase (MAO) (Paton and Pertwee, 1973). However, recently Schurr and Livne (1975) have shown that delta-1-THC and hashish extract exhibit a preincubation-dependent inhibition of MAO activity, while cannabidiol was ineffective. An intriguing tissue selectivity was observed: while MAO from porcine <u>brain</u> mitochondria is strongly affected by THC (especially when the substrate is benzylamine; less so with tyramine), MAO of porcine <u>liver</u> mitochondria is not affected by either delta-1-THC, cannabidiol, or hashish extract with either benzylamine or tyramine as a substrate.

The existence of isoenzyme MAO's has been extensively documented in recent years and some selective inhibitors of the different isoenzymes are known (Biel and Bopp, 1974). The latter authors have commented that "Although it is not clear which form of MAO, which substrate or which inhibitor may be associated with depression and antidepressant activity, further investigations along this line may provide the insight necessary to develop a MAO inhibitor with useful therapeutic properties in depression as well as with a decreased propensity for causing side effects."

Further work by the same group (Schurr and Livne, 1975) has indicated that certain cannabinoids, such as 6-oxo-cannabidiol diacetate, are even more potent than THC as MAO inhibitors. Their selectivity is yet unknown. However, the therapeutic potential of the cannabinoids in this field is obvious, and undoubtedly considerable amount of work will continue to be invested in this area.

REFERENCES

Banerjee, S. P., Snyder, S. H., & Mechoulam, R. Cannabinoids: Influence on neurotransmitter uptake in rat brain synaptosomes. Journal of Pharmacology and Experimental Therapeutics, 1975, 194, 74-81.

Best, M., Pola, R., Galin, M. A., & Blumenthal, M. Tonometric calibration for the rabbit eye. Archives of Opthalmology, 1970, 84, 200-205.

Biel, J. H. & Bopp, B. Antidepressant Drugs. In M. Gordon (Ed.) Psychopharmacological Agents. Vol. III, New York: Academic Press, 1974.

Bogan, W. D., Steele, R. A., & Freedman, D. X. Delta-9-tetrahydrocannabinol effect on audiogenic seizure susceptibility. Psychopharmacologia, 1973, 29, 101-106.

Carlini, E. A., Leite, J. R., Tannhauser, M., & Berardi, A. C. Cannabidiol and Cannabis sativa extract protect mice and rats against convulsive agents. Journal of Pharmacy and Pharmacology, 1973, 25, 664-665.

Carlini, E. A., Mechoulam, R., & Lander, N. Anticonvulsant activity of four oxygenated cannabidiol derivatives. Research Communications in Chemical Pathology and Pharmacology, 1975 (in press).

Drew, W. G. & Miller, L. L. Cannabis: Neural mechanisms and behavior -- a theoretical review. Pharmacology, 1974, 11, 12-32.

Garriott, J. C., Forney, R. B., Hughes, F. W., & Richard, A. B. Pharmacologic properties of some cannabis related compounds. Archives Internationales de Pharmacodynamie et de Therapie, 1968, 171, 425-434.

Green, K. & Pederson, J. E. Effect of delta-1-tetrahydrocannabinol on aqueous dynamics and ciliary body permeability in the rabbit. Experimental Eye Research, 1973, 15, 499-507.

Hepler, R. S., Frank, I. M., & Ungerleider, J. T. Pupillary constriction after marijuana smoking. American Journal of Ophthalmology, 1972, 74, 1185-90.

Izquierdo, I., Orsingher, O. A., & Berardi, A. C. Effect of cannabidiol and other Cannabis sativa compounds on hippocampal seizure discharges. Psychopharmacologia, 1973, 28, 95-102.

Karler, R., Cely, W., & Turkanis, A. The anticonvulsant activity of cannabidiol and cannabinol. Life Sciences, 1973, 13, 1527-1531.

Lander, N., Ben-Zvi, Z., Mechoulam, R., Martin, B., Nordqvist, M., & Agurell, S. Total syntheses of cannabidiol and delta-1-tetrahydrocannabinol metabolites. Journal of the Chemical Society, Perkin Transactions II, 1975 (in press).

Li, H. C. An archeological and historical account of Cannabis in China. Journal of Economic Botany, 1974, 28, 437-448.

Loewe, S. & Goodman, L. S. Anticonvulsant action of marihuana active substances. Federations Proceedings, 1947, 6, 352.

Mechoulam, R. (Ed.) Marijuana chemistry, pharmacology, metabolism and clinical effects. New York: Academic Press, 1973.

Meldrum, B. S. Epilepsy and GABA mediated inhibition. International Review of Neurobiology, 1975, 17, 1-36.

Mikuriya, T. H. (Ed.) Marijuana: Medical Papers 1839-1972. Oakland, Calif.: Medi-Comp Press, 1973.

O'Shaughnessy, W. B. On the preparations of the Indian hemp or gunjah. Transactions of the Medical and Physical Society of Bombay, 1842, 421-461.

Paton, W. D. M. & Pertwee, R. G. Effects of cannabis and certain of its constituents on pentobarbitone sleeping time and phenazone metabolism. British Journal of Pharmacology, 1972, 44, 250-261.

Paton, W. D. M. & Pertwee, R. G. The pharmacology of cannabis in animals. In R. Mechoulam (Ed.), Marijuana chemistry, pharmacology, metabolism and clinical effects. New York: Academic Press, 1973.

Reynolds, J. R. Therapeutic uses and toxic effects of Cannabis indica. Lancet I. 1890, 637-638.

Rosenthal, F. The herb hashish versus medieval Muslim society. Leiden: E. J. Brill, 1971.

Schurr, A. & Livne, A. Differential inhibition of mitochondrial monoamine oxidase from brain by hashish components. Biochemical Pharmacology, 1975 (in press).

Schurr, A., Livne, A., & Mechoulam, R., unpublished results.

Shaw, J. On the use of Cannabis indica in tetanus, in hydrophobia and in cholera. Madras Quarterly Medical Journal, 1843, 5, 74-80.

Walton, R. P. Marihuana. America's new drug problem. Philadelphia: Lippincott, 1938.

Ophthalmic Effects

CHAPTER 4

OCULAR EFFECTS OF DELTA-9-TETRAHYDROCANNABINOL

Keith Green

Departments of Ophthalmology and Physiology
Medical College of Georgia
Augusta, Georgia

Keun Kim

Department of Ophthalmology
Medical College of Georgia
Augusta, Georgia

Karen Bowman

Department of Ophthalmology
Medical College of Georgia
Augusta, Georgia

NOTE: This work was supported in part by Public Health
Service Research Grants EY 01413, from the National
Eye Institute, and DA 01214 from the National Institute
on Drug Abuse. We thank Dr. Monique Braude for making
the tetrahydrocannabinol available for use in this study.

Glaucoma is responsible for 14% of all new reported blindness cases
(Kahn and Moorhead, 1973), and thus represents a significant clinical problem
which must be treated either medically or surgically. Various medications
are currently available, but only a few are widely used and the addition of
another highly effective drug to the ophthalmological armamentarium would
provide a greater choice for medical therapy.

Since the initial reports (Hepler and Frank, 1971; Hepler, Frank and Ungerleider, 1973) of a significant decrease in intraocular pressure (IOP) following the smoking of a marihuana cigarette, the potential use of marihuana as a therapeutic agent in glaucoma has been obvious. More extensive studies in man (Hepler, Frank and Petrus, 1975) have further shown that repeated smoking always caused a 20% to 30% fall in IOP lasting for 4 to 5 hours, and that no tolerance to its use developed. No cumulative effects were observed in the subjects during repeated smoking and the ocular findings were minimal. The only persistent findings were a decrease in tear secretion, a reduction in ocular pulse pressure (determined during tonography), and dilation of the conjunctival vessels. Obviously, smoking is neither a satisfactory nor consistent method of administering a drug and a topical form of application for potential therapeutic use in ophthalmology should be sought (Green, 1975). Several of the derivatives of tetrahydrocannabinol (THC – the active extract of marihuana) are active in reducing the IOP when given topically in sesame oil (Green and Bowman, 1975). The potential therapeutic value was, therefore, established; yet much remained to be determined, and more remains to be known, concerning the ocular effects of THC.

We have described the fall in rabbit IOP following the intravenous administration of THC (Green and Pederson, 1973) and, a year ago, we reported (Green and Bowman, 1975) that delta-9-tetrahydrocannabinol (THC) showed some interaction with the adrenergic innervation system of the eye. Specifically, an alpha-adrenergic blocking agent, phentolamine, was found to partially inhibit the intraocular pressure-reducing effect of THC. Further studies have been made on the interaction between various sympathetic blocking agents (Green and Kim, 1975a), the procedure of surgical denervation, prostaglandin synthetase inhibitors, and THC in the eye which reveal that the ocular THC effect is mediated through the adrenergic nervous system. Initial data has also been obtained on the ocular penetration of THC from various potential ophthalmic vehicles. It is important to keep in mind that aqueous humor formation in the rabbit is greatly affected by beta-adrenergic agonists but alpha-agonists have little effect, whereas C_{tot}, or total outflow facility (vide infra) is primarily affected by alpha-adrenergic agonists and beta-agonists have little effect (Chiou and Zimmerman, 1975; Green and Kim, 1975a).

The extended studies on the interaction between adrenergic blocking agents and THC revealed that both alpha- and beta-adrenergic antagonists interfered with the normal rabbit ocular response to THC. The different blockers appeared to act in slightly different ways, however. The antagonists employed were the alpha-antagonists phentolamine and phenoxybenzamine, and the beta-antagonists propranolol and sotalol, which all evoked changes in both IOP and total outflow facility (C_{tot}, a measure of the ease with which fluid leaves the eye). All antagonists reduced the fall in IOP induced by THC by about 50%, except for sotalol which completely abolished the IOP fall. Only the alpha-antagonists strongly inhibit the THC-induced increase in C_{tot}. The beta-antagonist inhibition of C_{tot} indicates that THC acts by increasing C_{tr} per se (or true outflow facility; total outflow facility is the sum of two pathways, C_{tr} and C_{ps}, the former through Schlemm's canal and episcleral vessels and the latter back through the ciliary processes). The alpha-adrenergic antagonists may inhibit a THC-induced effect on vaso-constriction of afferent episcleral plexus vessels which are involved in aqueous humor drainage and undergo change to regulate C_{tr}.

The net result of these studies (Green and Kim, 1975a) was to demon-strate that THC acts in the normal eye primarily by vasodilating the efferent blood vessels of the rabbit uvea by beta-adrenergic stimulation, and reducing the capillary pressure within the ciliary processes which further creates an IOP fall. The vasodilatory action is consistent with the known effect on con-junctival blood vessels (Hepler, Frank and Ungerleider, 1972). THC could, therefore, have a dual role on both afferent and efferent vessels by stimula-tion at some point along the neuronal pathway. Since the blockers act, for the most part, at the receptor sites rather than at other points along the nerve axis, then the above data suggests that THC produces some of its action peripherally by stimulation of alpha- and beta-adrenergic receptor sites. Of course, THC could be acting alone to produce some effects, and yet also be stimulating the release of norepinephrine from the nerve terminals in the iris which would aid in increasing C_{tot} and lowering IOP. The latter two effects are well known ocular responses to norepinephrine, and this drug could also cause vasoconstriction of the afferent uveal vessels. This explanation would mean that the primary effect of THC would be on the beta-receptors and the secondary effect caused either by release of norepinephrine, or release of the negative feedback of norepinephrine release usually modulated by pro-staglandin since THC is a prostaglandin synthetase inhibitor (Burstein and Raz, 1972; Green and Podos, 1974).

In order to further examine other possible interactions in detail we performed experiments in THC-treated rabbits, using agents which blocked transmission in sympathetic ganglia and surgical sympathetic denervation, as well as a prostaglandin synthetase inhibitor, indomethacin (Green and Kim, 1975b). The ganglionic blocker, hexamethonium chloride, was used at a concentration of 1 mg/kg, which caused a small fall in IOP and a minor fall in the mean systemic blood pressure together with an increase in C_{tot} (Table 1). It is immediately obvious (Figure 1) that hexamethonium chloride is successful in partially blocking the THC-induced fall in IOP but has little effect on the THC-induced C_{tot} increase (Table 1) which was 80% of the normal THC-induced increase. The beta-agonist action of THC is revealed by the IOP fall, although this is only to 30% of that evoked in a normal eye by THC. Ganglionic blockade, therefore, causes a 70% reduction in the THC lowering of IOP, suggesting that THC acts centrally to influence peri-pheral sites. In these animals, norepinephrine is still present in the nerve terminals and could still be released by THC to change C_{tot}, possibly by in-hibiting the negative feedback of prostaglandin (formed in response to nore-pinephrine at the nerve terminal) which modulates norepinephrine release (Hedqvist and Brundin, 1969; Hedqvist and Von Euler, 1972; Neufeld and Page, 1975). The experiments with the ganglionic blocker, therefore, indi-cate that THC has peripheral effects on alpha- and beta-adrenergic receptor

Table 1

$\dfrac{IOP_0 - IOP_{60}}{IOP_0} \times 100$				$\dfrac{C_{tot\,60} - C_{tot\,0}}{C_{tot\,60}} \times 100$			
THC	THC + gangx	C-6	THC + C-6	THC	THC + gangx	C-6	THC + C-6
25.23	6.94 (6)	8.98 (4)	17.39 (4)	24.89	14.13 (6)	15.25 (4)	34.67 (4)
19.52	5.83 (4)	(THC = 8.41)			9.60	(THC = 19.42)	
29.13 *	5.58 (4)				+ 15.59		
28.00	7.48 (4)						

Change in intraocular pressure and total outflow facility caused by delta-9-tetrahydrocannabinol alone and in combination with adrenergic blocking procedures. Gangx, ganglionectomized; C-6, hexamethonium chloride (1 mg/kg body weight)
$(IOP_0 - IOP_{60}/IOP_0) \times 100$ value is obtained by taking IOP_0 as the time that THC was injected, irrespective of the time relative to any other procedure. For example, with C-6, IOP_0 is 30 minutes after C-6 injection, but for ganglionectomy IOP_0 is the intraocular pressure at a time after the initial stabilization. A similar description applies to C_{tot}. All data for THC and THC + gangx were obtained in paired eyes.

*, data from paired eyes in other experiments where, beyond 60 minutes after THC injection, another procedure was followed; comparable data from other similar experiments.

+,

Values in parentheses are numbers of experimental eyes.

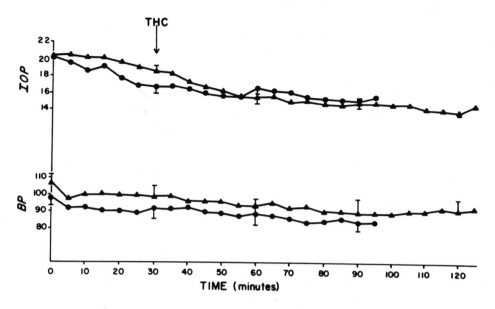

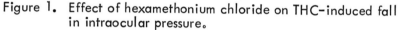

Figure 1. Effect of hexamethonium chloride on THC-induced fall
in intraocular pressure.

IOP and BP are in mm Hg. Hexamethonium chloride was
injected at 0 time. ●, hexamethonium chloride alone;
▲, hexamethonium chloride plus THC.

sites (Table 2), as well as a central effect. Of course, it may be that the
changes evoked by the ganglionic blocker are so great as to mask much of
the effect that THC may have in these animals. This is possible because of
the effect on systemic blood pressure; thus, to avoid this type of problem,
animals were utilized which had been subjected to a unilateral superior
cervical ganglionectomy.

The surgical procedure was performed under urethane anesthesia at
least 14 days before testing with THC. At 10 days post-ganglionectomy the
animals were tested for adrenergic supersensitivity by placing one 50 μl drop
of 0.1% or 1% norepinephrine onto each eye. The normal eye shows no
pupil dilatation whereas the experimental eye shows a marked mydriasis within
10 minutes (the mydriasis is more pronounced with 1% norepinephrine). At
least 4 days were allowed for all exogenous norepinephrine to be either
metabolized or lost from the eye. It is known (Roth and Richardson, 1969)
that the adrenergic nerves of the iris degenerate completely within 14 days
after ganglionectomy, thus there are no norepinephrine reserves in the eye
which could be potentially released by THC. Under these circumstances any
effect of THC would be the result of direct THC-adrenergic receptor interactions or central effects.

Table 2

Drug(s)	Effect	Interpretation
Alpha-agonist*	$IOP=$ $C_{tot}\uparrow$	Alpha-agonist acts primarily on outflow facility
Beta-agonist*	$IOP\downarrow$ $C_{tot}=$	Beta-agonist acts primarily on aqueous humor formation
THC	$IOP\downarrow$ $C_{tot}\uparrow$	Beta-stimulation; vasodilation of efferent uveal vessels, lowers capillary pressure. Alpha-stimulation, increase in outflow facility
THC + indomethacin	$IOP\downarrow 1/5$ $C_{tot}=$	Indomethacin appears to act as alpha-antagonist
THC + alpha-antagonist	$IOP\downarrow 1/2$ $C_{tot}=$	THC is alpha-agonist or stimulates release of NE (by inhibition of PG or directly), also has beta-agonist action
THC + beta-antagonist	$IOP=$ $C_{tot}\uparrow$	THC acts as beta-stimulator, also has alpha-agonist action
THC + C-6	$IOP\downarrow 2/3$ $C_{tot}\uparrow 1\ 1/3$	THC could release NE or inhibit PG negative feedback on NE release. Must also be a ganglionic or preganglionic effect for full expression of IOP fall
C-6	$IOP\downarrow 1/3$ $C_{tot}\uparrow 1/2$	
THC + ganglionectomy	$IOP\downarrow 1/3$ $C_{tot}\uparrow 1/3$	THC cannot release NE, thus is pure alpha-agonist. Beta-stimulation decreases IOP by 1/3 of normal. Must be central effect since ganglionic section and blockade decrease THC effect

Presentation of progression of interpretation of data obtained with various adrenergic blocking procedures. $\downarrow$ decrease; $\uparrow$ increase; =, no change. Increase or decrease has designation of approximate change in parameter relative to full THC-alone induced change.
*, from Chiou and Zimmerman, 1975.

THC was injected into the animals and IOP, C_{tot}, and mean systemic blood pressure (BP) measured. In the normally innervated eye the THC-response was normal, a reduction in IOP (C_{tot} was measured in only one eye of each pair – the denervated eye), but in the ganglionectomized eye the response was severely reduced (Figure 2). The IOP did fall by about 30% of normal throughout the experimental time period and C_{tot} increased by about 30% of the normal THC-induced rise (Table 1). In these animals there is no norepinephrine in the nerve terminals, thus any effect on C_{tot} must be due to the direct alpha-agonist action of THC. The beta-stimulatory effect of THC is revealed by the IOP reduction but for both C_{tot} and IOP the response is only one third of normal. The effect on C_{tot} can be interpreted as a pure alpha-agonist effect (Table 1 and 2). The absence of the full expression of THC on IOP in the ganglionectomized animal and the animal subjected to ganglionic blockade strongly suggests that there is a central effect of THC which would exert an effect on the IOP. Experiments with indomethacin, a prostaglandin synthetase inhibitor (applied topically as a 0.1% solution, 4 drops every 5 minutes about 1 hour prior to THC) reveal an almost complete inhibition of the THC-induced increase in C_{tot} and a partial decrease in IOP (30% compared to THC alone). Indomethacin, therefore, appears to act as an alpha-adrenergic antagonist, leaving only the beta-adrenergic agonist action of THC revealed as a fall in IOP.

Further experiments in ganglionectomized animals consisted of intra-venous infusions of prostaglandin E_2 (PGE$_2$) to determine if the presence of PGE$_2$ evoked the full ocular THC response, or the topical application of 0.1% norepinephrine, or a combination of the two drugs. PGE$_2$ infused at a rate which caused only a 1 or 2 mm Hg rise in IOP of a normal eye had a similar, transient effect on the IOP of a denervated eye of a THC-treated animal, but no further lowering of IOP was found. Topical norepinephrine caused an IOP fall in the normal denervated eye which was expected due to the adrenergic supersensitivity. In the presence of THC, however, the IOP reduction is 34% greater in the denervated eye at 60 minutes after topical norepinephrine than after norepinephrine in a non THC-treated animal. This result indicates that, in the normally innervated eye, both THC and norepine-phrine are needed for the full revelation of the THC effect.

It would appear, therefore, that THC acts in the eye by having a direct effect on both alpha- and beta-receptors per se. The increase in C_{tot} can be explained by a direct effect on alpha-receptors which regulate outflow as well as vasodilatory beta-effect on the efferent blood vessels of the anterior uvea. It appears that THC also mediates, in some synergistic manner, nor-epinephrine release from the nerve terminal. Possibly the role of THC as a PG-synthetase inhibitor (Burstein and Raz, 1972; Burstein, Levin and Varanelli, 1973; Green and Podos, 1974) could play a role. If the concept of Hedqvist (Hedqvist and Von Euler, 1972) is correct, norepinephrine causes the release of PG, which in turn modulates further norepinephrine release; it is possible that THC interferes with this process by blocking PG formation, enabling more norepinephrine to be released.

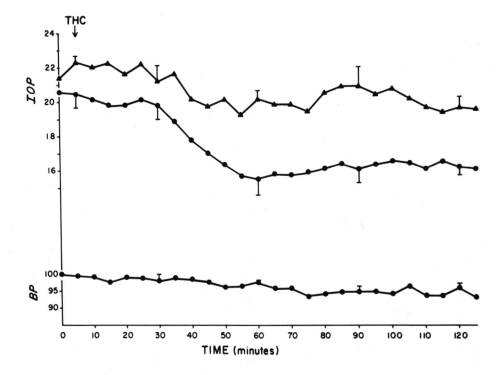

Figure 2.   Effect of unilateral superior cervical ganglionectomy
on THC-induced fall in intraocular pressure.
IOP and BP are in mm Hg. ●, normal eye;
▲, ganglionectomized eye.

It appears, therefore, that the effects of THC are modulated in the eye by the adrenergic nervous system (Table 2). The complete understanding of this complex interaction requires further pharmacological testing. It would be interesting to know if any marihuana smokers in the studies made thus far in man had a unilateral pre- or post-ganglionic Horner's syndrome, which is a natural ganglionectomy caused by paralysis of the cervical sympathetic nerve. In terms of therapy, however, these results suggest that THC does indeed act in the eye by interaction at both the adrenergic receptor and nerve ending. Possibly, these effects reflect behavior of THC in the rest of the body, and the eye acts as a "window" on systemic effects.

More recent experiments have been concerned with penetration of delta-9-THC into the ocular fluids and tissues following topical application of the drug (Bigger, Green and Bowman, unpublished observations). Fifty μl of either light or heavy mineral oil, sesame oil, or a 10% Tween 80-isotonic saline solution were added to the eye of a rabbit. The solutions were made to contain 1 mg delta-9-THC (0.2 mg ^{14}C-labeled and 0.8 mg non-labeled) per ml of solution. At 1, 2, 4, and 6 hours after instillation of the vehicle plus drug 150 μl of aqueous humor, the cornea, lens, and iris-ciliary body were removed from the eye (at 4 and 6 hours the lens was not taken), weighed wet, digested and counted in a liquid scintillation counter.

Some of the results are shown, for iris and aqueous humor, in Figure 3 A and B and illustrate the decided superiority of heavy and light mineral oil and the Tween-80-saline solution over sesame oil in providing a higher concentration of delta-9-THC to the intraocular fluids and tissues. Both corneal and aqueous humor concentrations (Figure 3 B) are higher with light or heavy mineral oil and each is slightly higher than Tween-80-saline, and a similar relationship is true for the iris concentration of delta-9-THC (Figure 3 A). The corneal concentrations were high and showed a 50% decrease during the 6-hour experiment, but again the order of superiority was that seen in other tissues. Florescein staining of the cornea was examined by instillation of a fluorescein solution onto the cornea at 2 and 5 hours after drug instillation, followed by washing with saline. This procedure highlights areas where the corneal epithelium is damaged, since the dye can be readily visualized under a blue light. The Tween-80-saline solution was by far the most damaging to the cornea, since fluorescein was widespread over the surface in a rather diffuse pattern at 2 hours. The other solutions did not produce any degree of staining greater than that normally seen in the rabbit cornea. At 6 hours, the Tween-80 eyes were clear, and some light, diffuse punctate staining was apparent with heavy mineral oil.

The dose delivered to the anterior chamber of the eye (Figure 3 B), where presumably THC can produce its effects is about the same as that delivered by the smoking of one marihuana cigarette (Galanter, Wyatt, Lemberger, Weingartner, Vaughn and Roth, 1972), at least from 0.1% solution. Higher concentrations have not been tested, but presumably the dose would be proportionate up to some maximum value, which would depend upon the ease of THC release from the vehicle, corneal THC permeability,

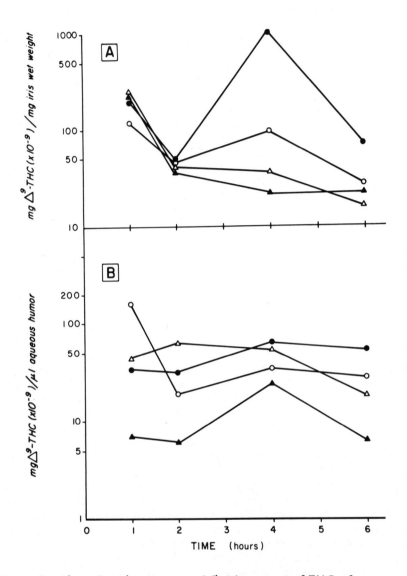

Figure 3. Plot of ocular tissue and fluid content of THC after
topical application of a 0.1% solution.
A, iris concentration of delta-9-THC, μg/mg tissue wet
weight.
B, aqueous humor concentration of delta-9-THC, μg/ 1
aqueous humor. •, heavy mineral oil; o, light mineral oil;
▲, sesame oil; Δ, 10% Tween-80 saline solution.

and the relative efficiency of using a higher concentration drop in the face of washing off the eye by the tears.

There is somewhat of a correlation between the physiological effect and the penetration data, since a comparison of the IOP-reducing effects revealed that heavy mineral oil was superior to sesame oil. This correlates well with the intraocular penetration of the drug (Figure 3 and Table 1). The nature of the response, up to a 25% or 30% fall in IOP, is fairly readily detectable.

We have also examined the relationship of dose to effect in the eye and attempted to relate this to the reduction in IOP caused by a drop of THC applied to one eye only. We find that even after THC is applied to one eye there is a pressure fall in both eyes. Albeit the fall in the second eye is both smaller and later in onset, this does illustrate systemic absorption of the drug by the orbital tissues. Whether this is true in man where totally different tear film kinetics prevail is a question to be answered by further study.

Similarly, there does not appear to be a steep dose-response curve to THC in the rabbit eye since small topical doses also evoke a response but the increase in response increases only gradually as the dose is increased substantially.

There are more than the obvious differences between man and rabbit, not the least of which is tear film kinetics. The difference in the blink rate of man and rabbit is great since man blinks about 5 times per minute but the rabbit blinks only 3 to 5 times per hour. This major difference leads, of course, to vastly different penetration rates for drugs, but the same qualitative relationship must be determined in man under carefully controlled conditions.

Our ocular penetration studies have only employed delta-9-THC thus far, and until many other labeled cannabinoids are available, then we must test other compounds physiologically (IOP, C_{tot}, BP, and the like) to determine their relative efficacy and presence or absence of systemic side effects. Agents which have little or no central nervous system effects are high in priority, for these could cause a few side effects but still act locally. The local or peripheral effects would need to be enhanced, however, since the central effect is responsible for a significant proportion of the IOP fall. High local concentrations may be achieved which would not present systemic problems after absorption. The vehicle for THC delivery is very important, too, since it must satisfy the requirements of THC solubility, shelf stability, neutral pH, and release of the drug into the eye following topical instillation.

A multidisciplinary approach must be employed with biochemists, pharmacologists, pharmacists, physiologists, and ophthalmologists working in a systematic manner to answer many of the questions raised by the work already undertaken. There is a great need for further study of these compounds and the ophthalmologist should not only be aware of the clinical effects of these drugs but of their potential therapeutic value.

Preclinical and clinical studies to date indicate that the fall in IOP caused by THC is equally as good as most drugs commonly used in ophthalmology today. This effect probably represents one of the most potentially valuable therapeutic uses of THC and deserves intensive investigation. If clinical trials indicate no long-term effects (and the diversity of opinion which exists on this point makes this, at best, uncertain at this time, although most studies have been made using doses higher than those predicted for topical application), then it is entirely possible that some form of topical cannabinoid would be made available for clinical use. One would hope that the reputation which the drug has obtained in society would not be responsible for a prejudice to be present against its use, should the point be reached where cannabinoids are available for opthalmic use.

References

Burstein, S., & Raz, A. Inhibition of prostaglandin E_2 biosynthesis by delta-1-tetrahydrocannabinol. Prostaglandins, 1972, 2, 369-374.

Burstein, S., Levin, E., & Varanelli, C. Prostaglandins and cannabis. II. Inhibition of biosynthesis by the naturally occurring cannabinoids. Biochemical Pharmacology, 1973, 22, 2905-2910.

Chiou, C. Y., & Zimmerman, T.J. Ocular hypotensive effects of autonomic drugs. Investigative Ophthalmology, 1975, 14, 416-417.

Galanter, M., Wyatt, R. J., Lemberger, L., Weingartner, H., Vaughan, T. B., & Roth, W. T. Effects on humans of delta-9-tetrahydrocannabinol administered by smoking. Science, 1972, 176, 932-936.

Green, K. Marihuana and the eye. Investigative Ophthalmology, 1975, 14, 261-263.

Green, K., & Bowman, K. Effect of marihuana derivatives on intraocular pressure in the rabbit. In M. Braude & S. Szara (Eds.), Pharmacology of Cannabis. New York: Raven Press, 1975, in press.

Green, K., & Kim, K. Interaction of adrenergic blocking agents with prostaglandin E_2 and tetrahydrocannabinol in the eye. Investigative Ophthalmology, 1975, 14. (a)

Green, K., & Kim, K. Mediation of ocular tetrahydrocannabinol effects by adrenergic nervous system. Investigative Ophthalmology, 1975, submitted for publication. (b)

Green, K., & Pederson, J.E. Effect of delta-1-tetrahydrocannabinol on aqueous dynamics and ciliary body permeability in the rabbit. Experimental Eye Research, 1973, 15, 499-507.

Hedqvist, P., & Brundin, J. Inhibition of prostaglandin E_1 of norepinephrine release and of effector response to nerve stimulation in the cat spleen. Life Sciences, 1969, 8, 389-395.

Hedqvist, P., & Von Euler, V. S. Prostaglandin controls neuromuscular transmission in guinea-pig vas deferens. Nature New Biology, 1972, 236, 113-114.

Hepler, R. S., & Frank, I. M. Marihuana smoking and intraocular pressure. Journal of the American Medical Association, 1971, 217, 1392.

Hepler, R. S., Frank, I. M., & Ungerleider, J. T. Pupillary constriction after marihuana smoking. American Journal of Ophthalmology, 1972, 74, 1185-1190.

Hepler, R. S., Frank, I. M., & Petrus, R. Ocular effects of marihuana. In M. Braude & S. Szara (Eds.), Pharmacology of Cannabis. New York: Raven Press, 1975, in press.

Kahn, H. A., & Moorhead, H. B. Statistics on blindness in the model reporting area, 1969-1970. Washington, D.C.: U.S. Department of Health, Education and Welfare, Pub. No. (NIH) 73-427.

Neufeld, A. H., & Page, E. D. Regulation of adrenergic neuromuscular transmission in the rabbit iris. Experimental Eye Research, 1975, 20, 549-562.

Roth, C. D., & Richardson, K. C. Electron microscopical studies on axonal degeneration in the rat iris following ganglionectomy. American Journal of Anatomy, 1969, 124, 341-349.

CHAPTER 5

EXPERIENCES WITH ADMINISTRATION OF MARIHUANA TO GLAUCOMA
PATIENTS

Robert S. Hepler
Robert J. Petrus

University of California
Los Angeles, California

INTRODUCTION

In 1971 Hepler and Frank reported reduction in intraocular pressure
occurring after healthy young adults smoked marihuana. These initial observations led to additional studies designed to compare the pressure-
reducing effects of placebo, smoked marihuana, and injected THC.
Consistent, statistically-significant pressure reduction was observed in
double-blind studies. Drop in intraocular pressure (IOP) was also observed in hospitalized subjects observed repeatedly for 12-hour periods.
Additional hospitalized subjects were permitted to smoke marihuana ad
libitum during a 5 1/2-hour period and comparisons were made between
the pressure-reducing effects of smoking varying numbers of marihuana
cigarettes. It was observed, for instance, that a subject smoking 22
cigarettes had only a slight further decrease in IOP as compared with a
subject who smoked only 2 cigarettes. Hospitalized subjects observed for
a total of 35 days, and other subjects observed for a total of 94 days,
continued during these periods of prolonged chronic use of marihuana to
show decrease in IOP with each period of intoxication. The results of
these various investigations were reported at the International Conference
on the Pharmacology of Cannabis, Savannah, Georgia, on December 4,
1974 (Hepler, Frank and Petrus, 1974). Graphical representation of
the data is given in Figures 1-4. Publications by Shapiro (1974), Green
and Podos (1974), and Purnell and Gregg (1975), among others, have confirmed the apparent IOP-reducing effect of marihuana and cannabinoids.

% CHANGE

INTRAOCULAR PRESSURE

SMOKED		30 min	180 min
Placebo	N=86	7%	10%
1% THC	N=44	29	22
2% THC	N=44	25	17
4% THC	N=48	34	22
INGESTED			
5 mgm THC	N=40	14	15
10 mgm THC	N=40	23	18
20 mgm THC	N=40	24	23

Figure 1.

INTRAOCULAR PRESSURE

SUBJECTS INTOXICATED AT 3:30 PM

	8:00 AM	10:00 AM	12:00 AM	2:00 PM	4:00 PM	5:00 PM	6:00 PM	7:00 PM	8:00 PM	9:00 PM
P	13.71	13.88	13.96	13.58	13.08	12.58	12.85	12.79	12.92	12.83
1%	13.73	13.54	13.42	13.42	11.92	11.31	11.17	11.09	11.65	11.96
2%	13.92	13.80	13.72	13.30	11.18	10.35	10.42	10.67	11.53	11.77

Placebo   N=6

1% Marijuana N=13

2% Marijuana N=15

Figure 2.

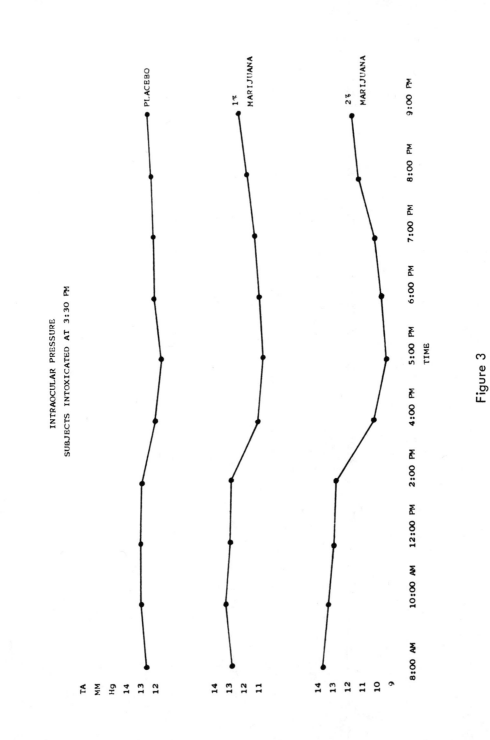

Figure 3

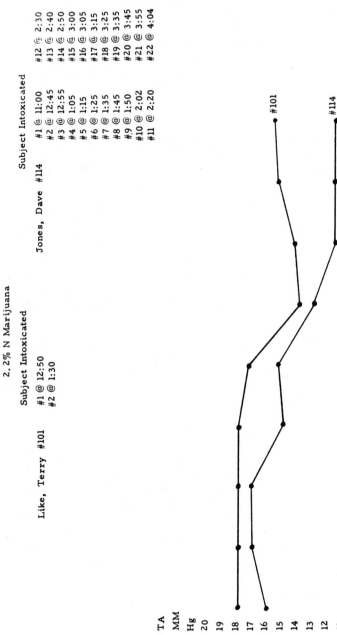

Figure 4

Glaucoma is the second most common cause of blindness in the United States. All of the various types of glaucoma have in common the features of abnormally elevated IOP, which over a variable period of time damages the optic nerve through mechanisms not entirely understood. It appears at present that elevated IOP interferes with normal blood supply to the optic nerve, which consequently leads to a characteristic form of optic nerve atrophy. At first peripheral vision is lost, followed in the later stages by loss of central vision as well. Vision once lost to glaucomatous optic atrophy can never be regained, hence the need for effective control of IOP.

Conventional therapy of open-angle glaucoma, which encompasses approximately 90% of all cases of glaucoma, utilizes miotic drops, epinephrine drops, and carbonic anhydrase inhibiting substances taken orally to reduce ocular secretion of aqueous. Filtering surgical procedures are reserved as last-resort measures, since they have a high incidence of failure to control glaucoma and they have a significant incidence of serious complications. The various medications used in treatment of glaucoma have side effects of visual alteration, ocular discomfort, and possible induction of cataracts. Carbonic anhydrase inhibitors often induce deterioration in appetite and feeling of well-being, and can induce serious side effects such as gastric ulcer and renal stone formation. Above all, even with the use of all presently-available forms of medical therapy there are many patients whose IOPs are not controllable, who therefore lose vision and may become blind.

The data presented in this chapter is the result of effort to determine the IOP-lowering effect, hence potential therapeutic usefulness, of marihuana administered to patients with chronic simple (open-angle) glaucoma.

EXPERIMENTAL METHODS

Patients with glaucoma were recruited by newspaper advertisement, by word of mouth, and from the author's private practice. The advertisements outlined the requirements for good general health, absence of any physical potential for becoming pregnant in the case of female subjects, absence of cardiac or respiratory disorders, and absence of use of medications which could have autonomic side effects. An interviewer experienced in glaucoma telephoned potential candidates to learn the details of their glaucoma history. Each patient's ophthalmologist was contacted to learn more about the ophthalmological history, and to obtain permission for participation of the patient in the study. In the case of some subjects, the responsible ophthalmologist was asked to approve brief changes in the patient's customary therapeutic regimen during the experimental sessions.

Potential subjects came to the research suite for a total of four sessions. In the first session a detailed ophthalmological examination, a physical and psychiatric screening evaluation, and laboratory studies were performed in order to demonstrate good general health. Any patients who might have an element of narrow-angle glaucoma were excluded. The first

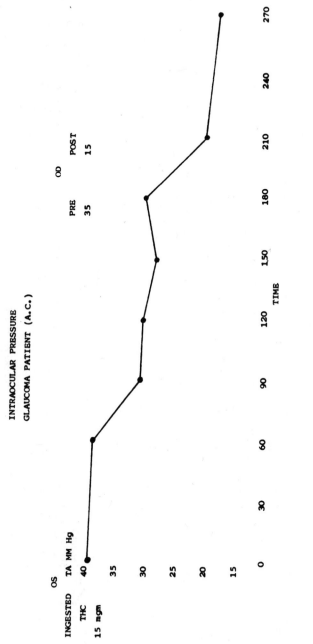

Figure 5

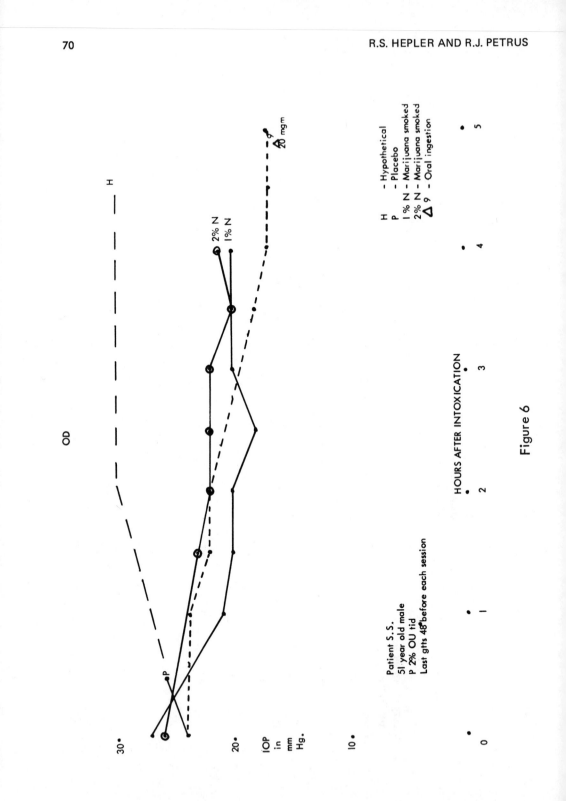

Figure 6

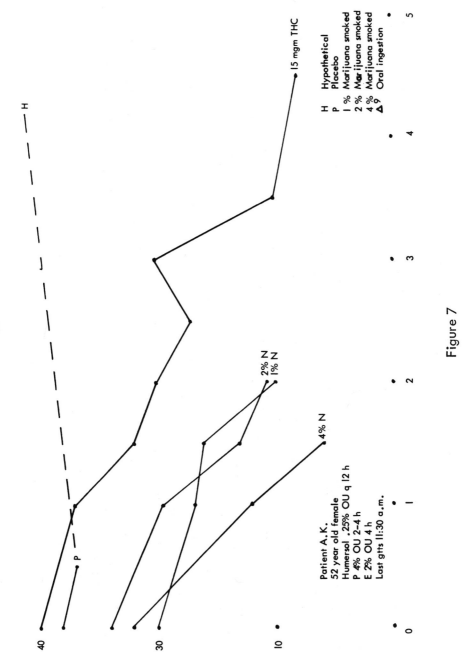

Figure 7

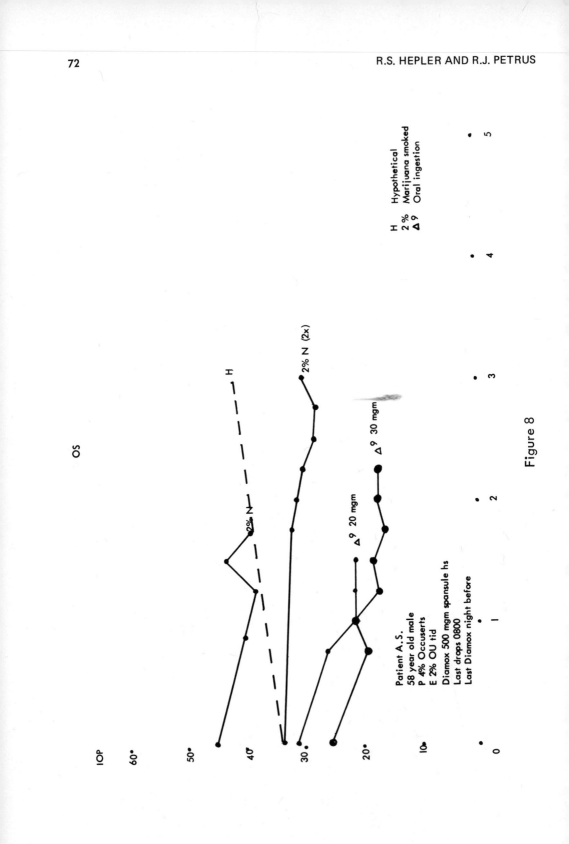

Figure 8

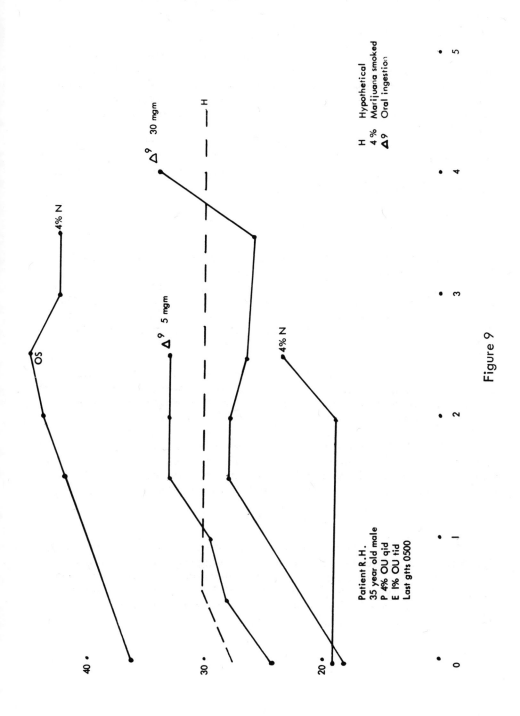

Figure 9

experimental session concluded with a trial smoking of placebo with consequent IOP measurements in order to familiarize the subject with procedures
to be used in the subsequent sessions.

The experimental sessions were planned at a minimum of one-week
intervals. Patients with mild to moderate glaucoma were asked to discontinue their customary medication usage 24-48 hours before each of the
experimental sessions, while patients with severe or uncontrolled glaucoma
were instructed to continue use of their medications up through the time they
reported to the research suite. Marihuana was smoked or THC administered
orally at each of the three experimental sessions, during which the subjects
were retained for approximately 4 hours in comfortable and relaxing surround-
ings. Repeated measurements of IOP were made by the same examiner, using
the same Goldmann applanation tonometer.

RESULTS

Most, but not all, subjects demonstrated an impressive decrease in
IOP which is best illustrated by representative examples shown in Figures
5-8. Figure 9 reflects unexplained failure to achieve IOP reduction, which
has been observed in 2 of a series of 12 extensively studied subjects. Due
to technical difficulties encountered with some of the subjects it was not
always possible to extend the observations after intoxication to a full 4
hours.

The extent of variation in severity of glaucoma, in the nature of
medications being used (these are indicated at the bottom left corner of each
figure), and in other variables encountered in work using human subjects
makes it difficult to generalize and to summarize the data obtained,
particularly while the numbers of subjects is still small. On each figure
there is plotted a hypothetical curve (indicated H) which reflects what an
experienced observer of glaucoma patients might expect the level of IOP to
be in each subject. Although not a true placebo in the customary sense,
this estimation gives a basis against which to compare the observed IOPs.

CONCLUSIONS

Patients with proven glaucoma frequently, although not invariably,
demonstrate substantial decrease in IOP following smoking of marihuana or
ingestion of THC. The pressure-reducing effects appear to be additive to
the effects of conventional glaucoma medications, hence providing a basis
for continued interest in the possible therapeutic effects of marihuana in
the treatment of chronic simple glaucoma.

REFERENCES

Green, K., & Podos, S. M. Antagonism of arachidonic acid–induced ocular effects by delta–tetrahydrocannabinol. Investigative Ophthalmology, June 1974.

Hepler, R. S., & Frank, I. R. Marijuana smoking and intraocular pressure. JAMA, 1971, 217, 1392.

Hepler, R. S., Frank, I. R., & Petrus, R. J. Ocular effects of marijuana smoking. International Conference on the Pharmacology of Cannabis, Savannah, Georgia, December 4, 1974, in press.

Purnell, W. D., & Gregg, J. M. Delta-9-Tetrahydrocannabinol, euphoria and intraocular pressure in man. Annals of Ophthalmology, July 1975.

Shapiro, D. The ocular manifestations of the cannabinols. Ophthalmologica, 1974, 168, 366–369.

CHAPTER 6

THE EFFECT OF DELTA-9-TETRAHYDROCANNABINOL ON INTRAOCULAR
PRESSURE IN HUMANS

Paul Cooler

Department of Ophthalmology
University of North Carolina School of Medicine
Chapel Hill, North Carolina, and
McPherson Hospital
Durham, North Carolina

John M. Gregg

Department of Oral Surgery
University of North Carolina School of Medicine
Chapel Hill, North Carolina

NOTE: This investigation was supported by National
Institute of Health research grant #DEO2668 from the
National Institute of Dental Research and by National
Institute of Health grant #RRO5333 from the Division
of Research Facilities and Resources.

One of the physiologic effects of marihuana, which was noted as
early as 1971, is its ability to lower intraocular pressure (Hepler and Frank,
1971). This has been documented in at least one controlled study in human
subjects with normal intraocular pressures (Hepler, Frank and Ungerleider,
1972). In addition, Purnell and Gregg (1975) at the University of North
Carolina have reported a decrease in intraocular pressure in two subjects
when given intravenous delta-9-tetrahydrocannabinol, the active component of marihuana. The purpose of this study is to describe further the
effects of intravenous delta-9-tetrahydrocannabinol on intraocular pressure
in subjects with normal intraocular pressures.

Delta-9-tetrahydrocannabinol is considered one of the most psychoactive components of marihuana. Some workers feel that its metabolite,

77

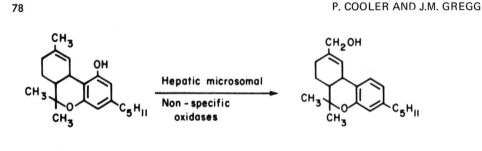

Figure 1.   Chemical Structure of Psychoactive Marihuana Compounds.

11 hydroxy-tetrahydrocannabinol, is the active form. Both are polycyclic hydrocarbons with phenol rings (Figure 1). There is a close similarity to estradiol, which may be of significance in that there has appeared in the literature a report in which three chronic marihuana users developed gyne-comastia while using the drug and who had otherwise normal secondary sex characteristics and normal endocrine evaluations (Harmon and Aliapoulios, 1972).

MATERIALS AND METHODS

Ten healthy paid male volunteers between the ages of 20 and 30 were selectively recruited. A screening battery of tests including liver function studies was performed to insure all participants were in good health. The Minnesota Multiphasic Personality Inventory was also administered. Prior drug experience was elicited and all subjects reported previous exposure to marihuana with 3 reporting casual use at the time of the study.

Four preparations were used in a double blind fashion: delta-9-tetrahydrocannabinol 0.044 mg/kg of body weight or 3.0 mgm average total dose; delta-9-tetrahydrocannabinol 0.022 mg/kg of body weight or 1.5 mgm average total dose; diazepam sodium (Valium) 0.157 mg/kg of body weight or 10 mgm average total dose; and placebo, which was human serum albumin. The delta-9-tetrahydrocannabinol was solubilized in human serum albumin after the method of Perez-Reyez, Timmons, and Lipton (1972). In a double blind fashion 1 of the 4 preparations was given intravenously as a preoperative medication 15 minutes prior to a third molar extraction on four different occasions. The arm was draped and the drug in-jected via an indwelling catheter to mask the time of injection.

Baseline intraocular pressures were measured by Schiotz and Mackay-Marg tonometers prior to administration of the drug. Intraocular pressures were then measured at 30-minute intervals thereafter until the pressures began to return to the baseline level and at 24 hours.

RESULTS

At the higher dosage, delta-9-tetrahydrocannabinol lowered the intraocular pressure in all 9 subjects given the higher dose (Figure 2). At the lower dosage level intraocular pressure decreased in 9 of 10 subjects. Diazepam sodium lowered the intraocular pressure in 6 subjects and placebo in 3.

Patient	Age	↑Δ⁹-THC	↓Δ⁹-THC	Diazepam	Placebo
J.S.	22	30	24	8	0
R.B.	28	15	15	15	0
G.B.	22	51	36	0	6
D.G.	24	51	51	16	0
M.B.	24	41	22	0	0
R.P.	27		41	15	6
C.C.	20	42	30	18	0
J.C.	24	30	35	0	0
J.L.	24	35	8	29	8
B.B.	24	41	30	0	0
Range		15-51%	8-51%	0-29%	0-8%
Average		37%	29%	10%	2%

Figure 2.   Intraocular Pressure Decrease Expressed as Percent of Baseline Normal.

The average decrease in intraocular pressure for the 10 subjects showed a dose-related response: 37% with the high dose, 29% with the low, 10% with diazepam sodium, and 2% with placebo. However, there was a great variability in response as indicated by the range, 15% to 51% with the high dose and 8% to 51% with the low dose.

The peak activity occurred between 30 and 90 minutes. The average time interval for peak activity was 60 minutes for both strengths. The exact duration of peak activity was not determined in this study but was less than 90 minutes post-drug injection (Figure 3).

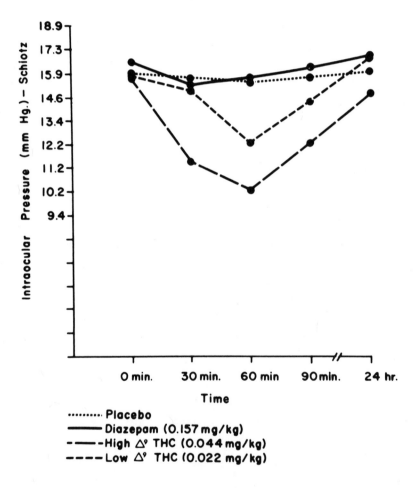

Figure 3.   Average Intraocular Pressure vs Time.

Vital signs were monitored throughout the study by means of a continuous polygraph system and arm and chest leads (Figure 4). The compiled data show no statistically significant change in respirations or blood pressure. However, 2 of the subjects when given the higher dose and 1 when given the low dose experienced a marked decrease in blood pressure in the range of 80/40 with concomitant pre-syncopal symptoms. The subject who became so hypotensive with the lower dosage level was not given the higher dose.

The change in heart rate was both more pronounced and more consistent. Six of the 10 subjects experienced an increase in heart rate which ranged from 95 to 142 beats per minute with the higher dosage level. This represented an average percentage increase in heart rate of 24% with a range of increase from 22% to 65%. None experienced a bradycardia.

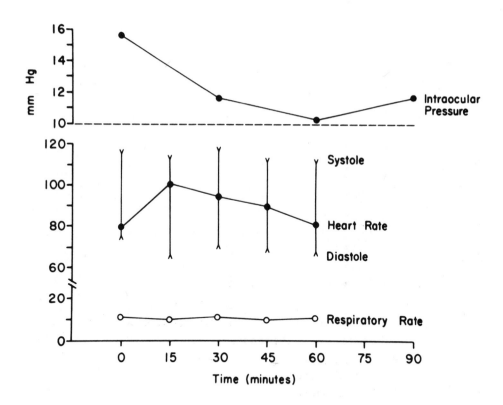

Figure 4. Effect of Delta-9-Tetrahydrocannabinol (0.044 mg/kg body weight) on Intraocular Pressure, Blood Pressure, Pulse and Respiratory Rate.

Only 1 subject experienced EKG changes during the administration of the delta-9-tetrahydrocannabinol. This was in an individual with a resting heart rate of 55 with 3 to 5 premature ventricular contractions per minute. These were completely abolished by both dosage levels.

The analgesic and anti-anxiety properties of these preparations were also studied. Analgesia was measured by both cutaneous stimulation with a galvanic current and periosteal stimulation with a pressure algometer, a strain-gauge type device. Our testing showed no appreciable analgesic properties with either cutaneous or periosteal stimulation (Figures 5 and 6).

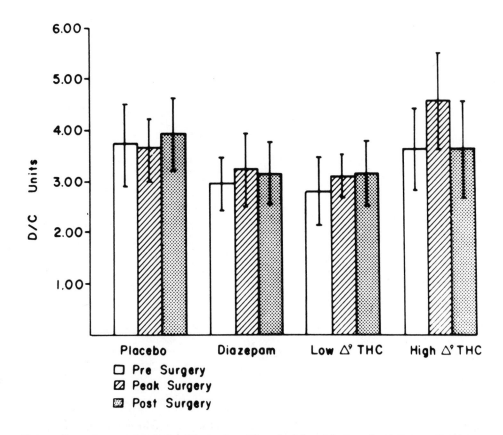

Figure 5. Cutaneous Pain Detection Thresholds with Surgical Premedicants Including Delta-9-Tetrahydrocannabinol.

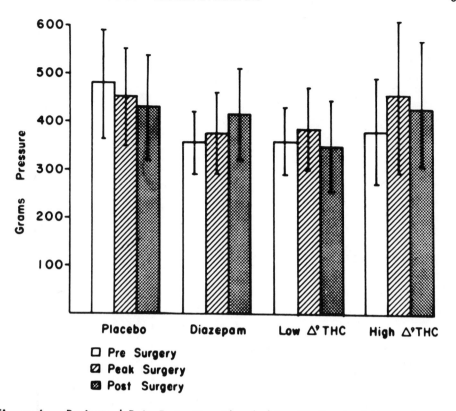

Figure 6. Periosteal Pain Detection Thresholds with Surgical Premedicants Including Delta-9-Tetrahydrocannabinol.

The anti-anxiety properties of these preparations were also tested (Figure 7). This was done by the Spielberger scoring system, a check-list of questions concerning the subject's emotional state, which was presented to him before and during surgery. The anxiety level during surgery increased only slightly with placebo, decreased slightly with diazepam sodium, but increased markedly with both strengths of delta-9-tetrahydrocannabinol.

Since delta-9-tetrahydrocannabinol does have psychotropic effects, an attempt was made to get some measure of these by asking the subject to describe his euphoric or dysphoric state and attempt to quantitate this feeling at regular intervals. Despite the pleasant feeling frequently described by marihuana users, each of our subjects reported intervals of dysphoria or an unpleasant sensation following administration of delta-9-tetrahydrocannabinol which was not described with diazepam sodium or placebo. The degree of unpleasantness correlated with the measured degree of anxiety which existed prior to each experiment. Figure 8 lists the subjective effects described by the 10 subjects.

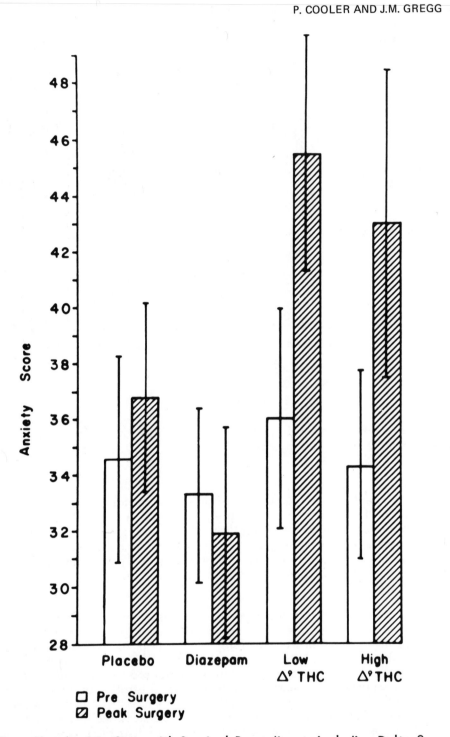

Figure 7. Anxiety State with Surgical Premedicants Including Delta-9-Tetrahydrocannabinol.

I. Depersonalization
    Temporal-Spacial Alterations
    Body Perception Distortions
    Perception Distortions (Illusions)

II. Euphoria-Stimulation
     Drowsiness
     Body Heaviness
     Body Coldness
     Dizziness
     Perceptions Distortions
     Elation, Laughing
     Well-being, Relaxation

III. Dysphoria
      (Anxious-Depressive)
      Panic
      Anxiety
      Paranoia
      Visceral Dysfunction
      Nausea
      Depression
      Flashbacks
      Hallucinations

Figure 8. Subjective Syndromes with Delta-9-Tetrahydrocannabinol.

DISCUSSION

The mechanism of action of delta-9-tetrahydrocannabinol in lowering intraocular pressure is still speculative. However, at present it appears most likely to affect the production of aqueous. Green and Pederson (1973) at the Wilmer Institute in a study with rabbits demonstrated a decrease in intraocular pressure and an increase in heart rate very similar to our findings. They also measured a decrease in secretion of aqueous to one-fourth normal range in in vitro preparations. It is not clear if this represents a direct effect on the active transport mechanism or an epinephrine-like effect on the ciliary body circulatory system.

Work by Beaconsfield, Ginsburg, and Rainsbury (1972) supports the latter mechanism. He has shown that the tachycardia produced by marihuana can be blocked by the beta-adrenergic blocker, propanolol. This would suggest a mechanism similar to a beta-adrenergic substance or epinephrine-like compound.

Another study employing intravenous delta-9-tetrahydrocannabinol in humans further suggests a mechanism of action similar to that of a beta-adrenergic substance (Malit, Johnstone, Bourke, Kulp, Klein and Smith, 1975). Although dosage levels used in this study were three to four times those we used, their findings with regard to the effects on respirations, heart rate, and anxiety are quite similar to ours. This study also cites recent work (Jones, 1971; Meyer and associates, 1971) demonstrating the influence of expectations and environment on the psychological effects of delta-9-tetrahydrocannabinol, which may help explain the anxiety experienced by our subjects in a rather austere laboratory setting.

SUMMARY

The effects of intravenous delta-9-tetrahydrocannabinol on intraocular pressure, blood pressure, pulse, and respirations were studied in 10 healthy subjects. In addition, the analgesic and anti-anxiety properties were also monitored. Diazepam sodium and human serum albumin as placebo were used as control substances.

Delta-9-tetrahydrocannabinol lowered normal intraocular pressures 15% to 50% in all subjects at dosage levels of 1.5 to 3.0 mgm. It also had a moderate cardio-acceleratory effect in all subjects with no significant effect on blood pressure in 8 of 10 subjects. Two experienced marked hypotension. No effect was demonstrated on respirations. No analgesic properties by cutaneous or periosteal stimulation were demonstrated. Anxiety level increased with both strengths of delta-9-tetrahydrocannabinol. All patients experienced periods of dysphoria with both strengths which were not noted with diazepam sodium or placebo.

References

Beaconsfield, P., Ginsburg, J., & Rainsbury, R. Marijuana smoking: Cardiovascular effects in man and possible mechanism. New England Journal of Medicine, 1972, 287, 209-219.

Green, K., & Pederson, J. E. Effect of delta-9-tetrahydrocannabinol on aqueous dynamics and ciliary body permeability in the rabbit. Experimental Eye Research, 1973, 15, 499-507.

Harmon, J., & Aliapoulios, M. A. (Letter) New England Journal of Medicine, 1972, 287, 936.

Hepler, R. S., & Frank, I. M. (Letter) Journal of the American Medical Association, 1971, 217, 1392.

Hepler, R. S., Frank, I. M., & Ungerleider, J. T. Pupillary constriction after marijuana smoking. American Journal of Ophthalmology, 1972, 74, 1185-1190.

Jones, R. T. Marijuana-induced "high": Influence of expectation, setting and previous drug experience. Pharmacology Review, 1971, 23, 359-369.

Malit, L. A., Johnstone, T. W., Bourke, D. I., Kulp, R. A., Klein, V., & Smith, T. C. Intravenous delta-9-tetrahydrocannabinol: Effects on ventilatory control and cardiovascular dynamics. Anesthesiology, 1975, 42, 666-673.

Meyer, R. E., Pillard, R. C., Shapiro, L. M., et al. Administration of marijuana to heavy and casual marijuana users. American Journal of Psychiatry, 1971, 128, 198-204.

Perez-Reyez, M., Timmons, M.D., Lipton, M. A., et al. Intravenous injection in man of delta-9-tetrahydrocannabinol. Science, 1972, 177, 633-635.

Purnell, W. D., & Gregg, J. M. Delta-9-tetrahydrocannabinol, euphoria and intraocular pressure in man. Annals of Ophthalmology, 1975, 7, 921-923.

DISCUSSION

Hepler: I'd like to ask this of Dr. Cooler. What happened to the intraocular pressures of those two subjects who became excessively hypotensive?

Cooler: They were within the range of what we recorded in the paper.

Hepler: But were they toward the lower end of that range? It would be interesting to know whether they had a particular marked ocular hypotensive effect.

Cooler: If I recall, one became severely hypotensive.

Hepler: Some people experienced in glaucoma who have known in a peripheral way the work that is being discussed here have said, "Well, if you get any effect at all, it is only because you are lowering blood pressure." Of course, we all know the reasons why that isn't a valid explanation; but, those two subjects would be interesting. We do not have the experience of seeing either tachycardia in the older patients that I have used or a fall in blood pressure. The drug is being administered differently, but if one is concerned, for instance, in any possible therapeutic use in older individuals being compromised by their cardiac status, I maintain that, at least the way we administer it, we did not get indications of any problem.

Cooler: I would be a little bit afraid to give it to older people in marginal health. You mentioned a THC-induced increase in variability of intraocular pressure. I would like to ask a question. Has any subject experienced dysphoria in the lab setting? Do your subjects describe a pleasant feeling or unpleasant feeling?

Tashkin: It depends on what we are doing in the laboratory. If we have the subjects stick in a group, carousing around in the corridors, they

89

experience a pleasant feeling. It can be a matter of setting. A laboratory need not be austere.

Rosenberg: The majority of patients we studied experienced a euphoric feeling, but there were 3 cases (out of 35) who had an acute state marked by fear that lasted for two or three hours. I think, apart from those 3, about 10 percent had a dysphoric, quite frightening experience; the rest had a quite pleasant experience.

Cooler: We noted a pattern to this. They would feel very unpleasant for a while, and then they would feel very good, and then very bad.

Harris: I don't know what everybody is so surprised about. This is the pharmacology of the substance. It produces a mixed depressant effect on a whole variety of systems; it's got a curve which goes up and down and, depending on the time when you measure it, you are likely to see either euphoria or dysphoria, depending on the dose. The peculiar nature of this compound is extremely complex -- it's not just a simple depressant of the nervous system as Valium is; it doesn't behave in the same way. And that is what's so fascinating and so interesting about it. We used to think it was because we had bad stuff. We thought we were going to solve all our problems by getting pure synthetic delta-9-THC. But that didn't solve the problem. It's still the same, a very complex drug. It's not surprising at all that you see these variations.

Cohen: I would like to add that some work at UCLA indicates that marihuana produces an increase in hypnotizability, which means an increase in suggestability -- which might increase the effect of setting on the individual's emotional response.

Hepler: Out of roughly 16 intoxications of older people in a very benign supportive setting, we have had roughly 3 negative, dysphoric responses.

Turkanis: I want to address my question to Dr. Green. You mentioned several times in your talk that the rabbit was markedly different from the human. Would the mechanism for lowering intraocular pressure in humans be different from that in rabbits because of basic differences in physiologic mechanism in the formation of fluid?

Green: The basic mechanisms of fluid formation in man and rabbit are probably the same in regard to the physiology. The major difference is in their pharmacologic response to drugs. My interpretation of the action of THC would bear remarkably on that difference.

Turkanis: I have one other question. What success have people had in using topical preparations in humans?

Green: We are in the process of trying to do that. A member of our department has had an award from the National Eye Institute to do exactly

that -- put topical preparations on the eye. But we are running into problems -- or he is running into problems. I am merely acting as the preclinical
consultant. The FDA wants to know if the vehicle is causing any damage.
The concerns are with the vehicle; they don't seem to be concerned with the
THC.

Hepler: About topical ophthalmic preparations: there is much difficulty in getting approval for medication applied topically to the eye in this
country. In Europe there are many useful drugs marketed which are not available in this country and never will be. The reasons why we are not putting
new formulations of drops in people's eyes are twofold: the problem of getting
approval plus the medical-legal problem. Imagine if one of the subjects went
ahead and developed a cataract a few years later, not necessarily related to
the drops that were put in, but you can imagine what some sharp lawyer would
make out of that.

Cohen: I would like to ask whether aspirin reduces intraocular pressure.

Green: I have used 600 mg. aspirin p.r. in a rabbit and it doesn't
do anything to intraocular pressure.

Harris: Dr. Green, you postulate that there is a beta-blocking activity
with THC, and that seems to go directly opposite to what we know of our ability
to block the cardiac effect.

Green: No, it's an alpha and a beta agonist.

Harris: That doesn't make sense from the pharmacology point either.

Lemberger: With all respect to Dr. Green, I think you throw in these
terms -- alpha agonist, beta agonist, antagonist -- around too loosely because,
first of all, in no other system are these compounds known to have these effects:
"alpha agonist," "beta agonist." An alpha agonist is something that will act
directly on an alpha receptor site, and I think using those terms is not clarifying,
it's just making it more complex.

Green: When we look at the actions of delta-9-THC on these various
components, the only conclusion that I can reach is that we must have the
direct actions on receptors.

Lemberger: In any other system, this is not true. If it were an alpha
agonist, for example, you would expect an elevation of blood pressure rather
than a decrease in blood pressure. The beta-stimulant effect that it has on
the heart is not due to the compound per se, because if you were to take an
isolated heart and add the compound, you would expect to see an increase in
heart rate. This is not the case. THC is not an alpha or a beta stimulant.

Green: We don't know how it's actually acting but it is a sympathomimetic.

Harris: I think we are getting into semantics, because you are using terms that to us as pharmacologists have rather specific meanings.

Lemberger: How did you give it, by slow infusion?

Cooler: By slow infusion. Over five minutes.

Braude: What percentage of eugenol is in the marihuana?

Mechoulam: Quite a lot. It depends on each particular sample, on what kind of marihuana, how it is harvested. Sometimes there are huge amounts of monoterpenes and other small molecules, and the particular smell that we get is not due to any one component. It is a combination of about thirty components, and sometimes eugenol is pretty high on the list.

Rubin: The point that Dr. Mechoulam makes is extremely important. You have to know what you are researching with. Everybody has been using Cannabis sativa as a product. I am not even sure that it is Cannabis sativa any more.

Mechoulam: I would like to make a comment on Dr. Rubin's very interesting paper. It seems that the antimicrobial substances are present as acids. We have tested both the acids and the neutral components. The acids -- all of them -- are strongly antibiotic, and this is not so surprising.

Miller: Animals become tolerant to the effects of THC over time; what implications might this have for using cannabinoids therapeutically?

Hepler: The eye pressure drop continues to occur -- it does not show tolerance -- over a period of 94 days. Subjects show it every day.

Karler: I think Perez-Reyes claims that tolerance does not develop to psychological effects. When he gave the drug intravenously, he found that there was no difference in the dose he had to give individuals who were chronic smokers two years or longer.

Harris: I think that those studies have been really cleared up by Dr. Jones' work and the work of Dr. Cohen's laboratory where they have been exposing individuals to very large doses for long periods of time.

Jones: Well, I don't want to talk about my work specifically. The tolerance to every other drug I can think of is a dose-related phenomenon. If Perez-Reyes, for example, had brought in people who used one shot of bourbon a day for two years, I don't think he would demonstrate a tolerance for alcohol. His data is not inconsistent with ours. We happen to give bigger doses more frequently and we get a very dramatic tolerance in four days if we give, say, 10 mgs. of THC every 4 hours.

Tashkin: I am not going to present these data this afternoon, so I might as well report it now. I am involved with Dr. Cohen at UCLA, and we have given subjects 5 to 10 mgs. of delta-9-THC daily, and after 27 days there is no change in the magnitude of acute physiological effects. Subsequently, we had subjects smoke an average of 100 mgs. of THC per day, and after 47 days, we did demonstrate considerable tolerance. So it does appear that dose does affect tolerance. However, after 47 days, the subjects felt just as high after a given dose of THC, which happened to be 20 mgs, as they had felt at the outset.

Jones: I just want to make another comment about the tolerance issue. The issue is not does tolerance develop, yes or no. It is: Does tolerance develop within the particular system we are interested in? For example, tolerance may develop for the intraocular pressure drops but not for bronchial changes, and so on.

Szara: In one particular study, the subjects reported after the first cigarette in the morning there seemed to be no tolerance, but after the second cigarette the high was lower, and after the sixth cigarette there was almost no psychological effect or high reported on the same day. But overnight, again, the tolerance disappeared, and in the morning there was again a high.

Jones: There is another drug that does that, and one that many tobacco smokers are familiar with. Your physiologic changes in response to your first cigarette in the morning will be dramatically different from your last cigarette in the day.

Vachon: I would like to ask a question of Dr. Hepler. THC is known for having vasodilatory activity, and I was wondering if it would have the same activity on the retina.

Hepler: I just happen to have looked at the retinal vessels, which is an admittedly imprecise way to answer your question. You don't see any change in the calibre of the retinal vessels. We have photographed the ocular fundus before and after and studied the slide photographs. We don't see any changes. But there could be significant change going on that we simply would not see manifested by change in the calibre of those vessels.

Harris: Again, the vascular effects are quite complicated. It is not just a simple vasodilation because while some vascular beds are dilated, other vascular beds are constricted. So the overall picture, most of the time as we see it in man, even with fairly large doses, is a relatively small and negligible change in the overall blood pressure, but this is not to say that there aren't very dramatic vascular alterations going on.

Neu: I want to ask Dr. Hepler if he gave patients THC without continuing the medication they were on, and whether or not the reduction in intraocular pressure is potentiated.

Hepler: The greatest pressure drops we saw were in orally administered THC. I am thinking of two particular patients. One was continued on his medication, and another was a mild glaucoma patient who was two days off her therapy. They both showed very profound drops.

Neu: Did you ever give them the THC in addition to the drug at the same time and study what happened?

Hepler: That first patient was unlike all the others in that he had a new device, a soft lens sitting down inside the cul-de-sac giving continuous release of a miotic. So he was unlike all the others in that he had continued conventional glaucoma medication to which we added THC.

Cohen: Does that really answer the question? Was there a potentiating effect?

Hepler: I don't think we can answer that. We just see a profound additional effect.

Sallan: I would like to comment on tolerance and also ask a question of the ophthalmologists. We have been using oral delta-9-THC as an antiemetic and we found that tolerance was a real bugaboo. Certain individuals and not others, for reasons that we can't explain at all, would respond initially and after a second, third, and fourth dose of THC might subsequently lose both their ability to become high and concomitantly lose their antiemetic effect. Others get high and sustain an antiemetic effect with repeated doses, some with as many as 40 or 50 different exposures. The question I have is in regard to duration of therapeutic responses in lowering intraocular pressure. I notice in one graph that you showed, Dr. Cooler, the heart rate was already going down, but intraocular pressure was going down as well. I wonder if you can correlate the duration of decreased intraocular pressure with the other pharmacologic responses to the THC.

Cooler: Dr. Hepler asked that question, too, and I cannot answer it. I know that in the individual case that he asked about, it was found that there was no correlation.

Hepler: There is a gap in our knowledge. After about five hours -- between five hours and 25 hours, we really don't have any information. It's one of the things we need to fill in. The only hospitalized patients we have used gave us such totally bizarre results that I am in a state of confusion.

Pulmonary and Preanesthetic Effects

CHAPTER 7

BRONCHIAL EFFECTS OF AEROSOLIZED DELTA-9-

TETRAHYDROCANNABINOL

Donald P. Tashkin
Bertrand J. Shapiro
Sheldon Reiss
James L. Olsen
Jon W. Lodge

Department of Medicine
U.C.L.A. School of Medicine
Los Angeles, California
and Division of Pharmaceutics
University of North Carolina School of Pharmacy
Chapel Hill, North Carolina

NOTE: This research was supported by Contract No. HSM 42-71-89 from the National Institute on Drug Abuse.

INTRODUCTION

Previous studies have demonstrated that the smoking of marihuana or ingestion of its principal psychoactive ingredient, delta-9-tetrahydrocannabinol (delta-9-THC), causes acute bronchodilatation both in healthy young men (Vachon, Fitzgerald, Solliday, 1973; Tashkin, Shapiro and Frank, 1973) and in patients with either chronic, stable bronchial asthma (Tashkin, Shapiro and Frank, 1974) or experimentally-induced bronchospasm (Tashkin, Shapiro, Lee, 1975). The mechanism of THC-induced bronchodilatation has been shown not to be due to a sympathomimetic or atropine-like effect (Shapiro, Tashkin and Frank, 1973), suggesting that cannabinoid compounds may have unique therapeutic utility since they appear to relax bronchial smooth muscle by a mechanism different from that of currently available bronchodilator agents. Smoking would not appear to be a satisfactory route of administration of cannabinoid compounds for possible therapeutic purposes, however, in view of previous findings of depressed alveolar macrophage bacteriocidal activity following acute exposure to cannabis smoke (Cutting, Watson, Goodenough, Simmons,

Laguara and Huber, 1974) and of mild but significant impairment in bronchial dynamics after heavy subacute marihuana smoking (Tashkin, Shapiro, Lee, and Harper, forthcoming), presumably due to a chronic irritant effect of the smoke (Henderson, Tennant and Guerry, 1972). Oral delta-9-THC, although capable of causing significant, prolonged bronchodilatation in man (Tashkin et al., 1973; Tashkin et al., 1974), is also not suitable for therapeutic use because of unwanted psychotropic and cardiovascular effects. Inhalation of pure delta-9-THC as an aerosol might have less irritating effects on the airways than the smoked plant material and might also have advantages over ingestion of delta-9-THC by producing more bronchodilatation by topical action while minimizing systemic physiological effects.

The present study was a pilot study to evaluate the cardio-pulmonary and psychotropic effects in healthy males of different doses of delta-9-THC administered by inhalation as an aerosol and to compare these effects with those produced by smoking or ingestion of comparable quantities of delta-9-THC.

MATERIAL AND METHODS

Seven young male experienced marihuana smokers ranging in age from 22 to 33 years and without evidence of significant medical, pulmonary, or psychiatric disease were recruited for study. After informed consent, subjects were studied on 7 days separated by at least 48 hours. On the first study day, a medical, psychiatric, and drug-use history, detailed questionnaire of respiratory symptoms, physical examination, 12-lead electrocardiogram, and battery of pulmonary function tests were administered. The latter included spirometry with calculation of forced vital capacity (FVC), forced expired volume in one second (FEV_1), maximal mid-expiratory flow rate (MMEFR), single-breath diffusing capacity for carbon monoxide (DL_{CO}), closing volume (CV) (Anthonisen, Danson, Robertson, 1969-70), and whole-body plethysmographic measurements of airway resistance (R_{aw}), thoracic gas volume (V_{tg}), and specific airway conductance ($SG_{aw}-1/R_{aw}/V_{tg}$) (DuBois, Botelho and Comroe, 1956; DuBois, Botelho, Bedell, 1956; Briscoe and DuBois, 1958). Spirometric and plethysmographic measurements were repeated 5, 15, 30, 60, 90, and 120 minutes after inhalation of a standard therapeutic dose of isoproterenol (1250 micrograms) delivered via an intermittent-positive-pressure breathing device for comparison with results of subsequent administration of delta-9-THC by aerosol, smoking, and ingestion.

During the remaining six study days, subjects inhaled 0, 5, 10, or 20 mg synthetic delta-9-THC as an aerosol, smoked a cigarette containing 900 mg of marihuana assayed at 2.2% delta-9-THC, or ingested 20 mg synthetic delta-9-THC dissolved in sesame oil within a gelatin capsule. The order in which the different test preparations were administered was randomized in a cross-over fashion and administration of the aerosolized preparations was double-blinded. The latter consisted of delta-9-THC dissolved in normal alcohol, difluorodichloromethane and tetrafluorodichloroethane (propellants), and sorobitan trioleate (detacifier) within a 15-ml capacity container fitted with 67 microliter metered dose value (Emson Research, Inc., 118 Burr Court, Bridgeport, Conn. 06605) (Olson, Lodge, Shapiro and Tashkin, forthcoming). Four aerosol preparations were employed: one did not contain delta-9-THC (placebo), and the other 3 delivered 0.5 mg, 1 mg, and 2 mg delta-9-THC per actuation, respectively. On the days when subjects were scheduled to receive aerosol preparations, they exhaled to residual volume, wrapped their lips around the mouth piece of the nebulizer, inspired deeply while activating the nebulizer, and held their breath for several seconds. This procedure was repeated 10 times at 30-second intervals so that subjects inhaled a total dose of 0, 5, 10, or 20 mg delta-9-THC, depending on which aerosol preparation was used.

On each test day subjects were studied beginning at approximately 9 AM after an overnight fast and after having refrained from cannabis or other drug use for over 12 hours. Measurements consisted of systolic and diastolic blood pressure, heart rate, respiratory rate, FVC, FEV_1, and MMEFR (spirometry), and R_{aw}, V_{tg}, and SG_{aw} (plethysmography). In addition, a catheter was inserted into a peripheral vein to permit analyses of 10 cc samples of blood for delta-9-THC and metabolites using a radio-immunoassay technique (Gross, Soares, Wing and Schuster, 1975). Two sets of control measurements 15 minutes apart were obtained prior to admini-stration of the scheduled drug preparation and measurements and blood sampling were repeated at 5, 15, 30, 60, 90, and 120 min and hourly thereafter up to 6 hours after drug administration. In addition, at each measurement period subjects were asked to rate their "high" on a scale of 0-7, the latter repre-senting the maximum "high" they had ever experienced in the past. They were also asked to indicate whether or not they experienced any other unusual reactions following drug administration, such as dryness of the mouth or throat, throat or bronchial irritation, cough, discomfort in the chest, nausea, and the like.

CALCULATIONS

For each subject during each study day and for each measured variable, control measurements were averaged. At each time interval following drug administration post-drug measurements were calculated as **percent** changes from the mean control values. For each drug and dose level, control values for each variable and percent changes from control values at each time interval were averaged. Significance of the changes at each time interval following each test preparation was determined by comparing the percent change following that preparation with the percent change following placebo at the same time interval, using Student's t-test for paired data. A P value < 0.05 was considered significant (2-tailed test).

RESULTS

Anthropomorphic, historical, and baseline pulmonary function data are indicated in Table 1. All subjects smoked marihuana at least occasionally, no subject smoked hashish more than occasionally, and 5 subjects did not smoke tobacco. All subjects had normal baseline lung function except for one subject (D.O.) who had a borderline reduction in diffusing capacity.

Neither aerosolized, oral, nor smoked delta-9-THC resulted in any detectable changes in systolic, diastolic, or mean blood pressure, respiratory rate, or forced vital capacity. Spirometric flow rates (FEV$_1$ and MMEFR) improved significantly 15 min to 2 hours following smoked marihuana and 15 min to 3 hours following all doses of aerosolized delta-9-THC but not following either placebo aerosol or oral THC. These increases in flow rates were significantly greater than the changes following placebo aerosol. Following smoked marihuana and 5, 10, and 20 mg aerosolized delta-9-THC, peak increases in FEV$_1$ were 6.1 ± 1.8 S.E., 5.0 ± 1.5, 6.4 ± 2.0, and 6.7 ± 1.9 percent, respectively, and peak increases in MMEFR were 14.8 ± 4.2, 14.6 ± 3.8, 15.1 ± 6.4, and 17.7 ± 6.2 percent, respectively. The magnitude of these mean changes in FEV$_1$ is slightly greater than that reported following therapeutic doses of isoproterenol (Watanabe, Renzetti, Begin and Bigler, 1974). No significant differences were observed between increases in spirometric flow rates following different doses of aerosolized delta-9-THC or between aerosolized THC and smoked marihuana.

The changes in specific airway conductance at various times following different doses of aerosolized THC and 1250 micrograms isoproterenol are shown in Figure 1. Small but significant mean changes in SG$_{aw}$ (9-21%) were noted at 1 to 5 hours after placebo aerosol compared with baseline pre-drug values. Following 5-20 mg of aerosolized delta-9-THC, SG$_{aw}$ rose immediately and remained significantly elevated above baseline values for 5-6 hrs and above placebo values for 1-2 hrs. The peak mean increase in SG$_{aw}$ after 20 mg aerosolized delta-9-THC ($49.3 \pm 8.6\%$) was noted one hour after inhalation and was significantly greater than the rise in SG$_{aw}$ observed at 1 hour after inhalation of 5 mg delta-9-THC. At all other times the changes in SG$_{aw}$ following each dose of aerosolized delta-9-THC were not significantly different from one another, although the mean changes following 20 mg delta-9-THC were generally higher than those following the other doses. The mean increases in SG$_{aw}$ after isoproterenol were comparable to those following aerosolized THC at 5-15 min but less than those following THC at subsequent time intervals.

Comparison of the changes in SG$_{aw}$ following smoked, aerosolized, and oral THC (20 mg) is shown in Figure 2. After both smoked and aerosolized THC, SG$_{aw}$ increased immediately and remained significantly elevated above values after oral THC for one hour. SG$_{aw}$ increased significantly one hour after ingestion of THC and remained elevated for six hours. After one hour the changes in SG$_{aw}$ following smoked marihuana decreased progressively and were significantly less than the changes following aerosolized and oral THC at 3-6 hrs.

Table 1. Anthropomorphic, Historical, and Baseline Pulmonary Function Data

Subject	Age Yr	Hgt In	FVC % Pred.[a]	FEV % Pred.	FEF25-75 %Pred.	SGaw[c] L/Sec/cmH2O/L	DLCO % Pred.	Observed CV %VC	Predicted CV[b] %VC	Smoking History[d] Marihuana	Tobacco	Hash
DL	22	73	100	118	124	.148	118	0	16	C	A	B
MG	24	74	115	114	97	.34	126	8	18	D	A	A
MGr	22	73	122	130	134	.163	144	0	16	B	A	A
RH	23	72	127	134	119	.158	113	10.5	17	F	A	A
AJ	21	71	106	114	101	.142	125	0	17	C	B	B
TS	33	71	109	98	72	.179	112	12	22	D	C	A
DO	25	67	103	101	88	.128	78	6.5	18	E	A	B
Mean	24.3	71.6	111.7	115.6	105.0	0.150	116.7					
± SE	1.5	0.9	3.8	5.1	8.2	0.007	7.6					

a. Predicted values based on regression equation of Morris, Koski, and Johnson (1971) and Cotes (1965).

b. Upper limits of predicted values based on regression equation of Buist and Ross (1973).

c. Normal values >12 L/sec/cm H_2O/L based on data from our laboratory.

d. Legend:

Tobacco: A never, B < 1/2 pack/day, C 1/2-1 pack/day.
Marihuana or Hashish: A never, B occasionally, C 1-2 x/week, D 4-6 x/week, E daily, F several x/day.

EFFECT OF AEROSOLIZED Δ⁹-THC ON SPECIFIC AIRWAY CONDUCTANCE (N=7)

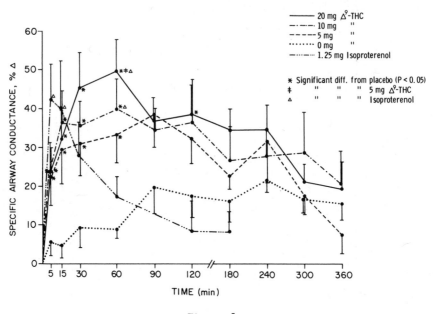

Figure 1

COMPARISON OF EFFECTS OF AEROSOLIZED, SMOKED AND ORAL Δ⁹-THC (20 mg)
ON SPECIFIC AIRWAY CONDUCTANCE (N=7)

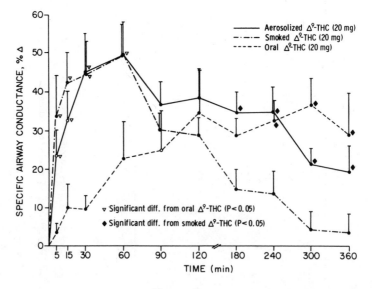

Figure 2

The effects of different doses of aerosolized THC and isoproterenol on heart rate are shown in Figure 3. Following placebo aerosol, heart rate did not change except at 30 and 120 min when heart rate decreased slightly but significantly。 Aerosolized THC resulted in significant increases in heart rate, peak increases (9-16%) occurring at 5 to 30 min after inhalation. Heart rate returned to values not significantly different from placebo 30 min after 5 mg and 90-120 min after 10-20 mg THC; a late rise in heart rate (16%) was noted 6 hrs after 20 mg of THC。 A dose response effect was noted in that pulse increments following 20 mg THC were significantly greater than those following 5 mg THC at 15-90 min。 Heart rate did not increase significantly at any time following isoproterenol。

Comparison of the changes in heart rate following 20 mg aerosolized, smoked, and oral THC is shown in Figure 4. After oral THC, heart rate did not change。 After smoked marihuana, heart rate increased immediately by an increment (44 $\pm$ 7 %) significantly greater than the change following both oral and inhaled THC (20 mg). The changes following both smoked and aerosolized THC were significantly greater than those following oral THC over the first 30 min after drug administration。

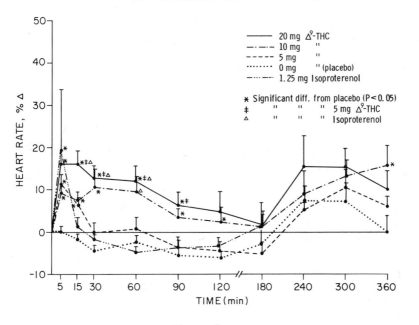

Figure 3

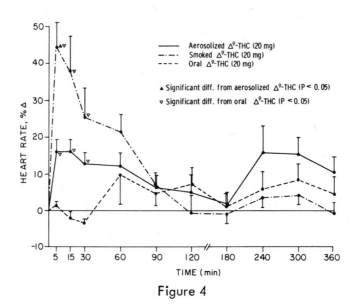

COMPARISON OF EFFECTS OF AEROSOLIZED, SMOKED AND ORAL Δ⁹-THC (20mg)
ON HEART RATE (N=7)

Figure 4

Effects of aerosolized THC on subjective "high" are shown in Figure 5.
No significant "high" was experienced after placebo aerosol. Although a
slight "high" was reported after 5 mg THC, this was not significant compared
with placebo aerosol. A modest but significant "high" compared with placebo
was noted at 5-30 min after 10 mg THC. After 20 mg THC, a significantly
greater "high" compared with 5 and 10 mg THC was observed over 15-120
min after inhalation of the aerosol.

Comparison of the effects of aerosolized, smoked, and oral THC on
the level of "high" is shown in Figure 6. From 5-15 min after smoked THC
a significantly greater "high" was experienced compared with aerosolized
THC. For 5-30 min, the "high" following both smoked and aerosolized THC
was significant compared with the oral route of administration. Subsequently,
the intoxicating effects of THC administered by all three routes were comparable.

Aside from a pleasant feeling of intoxication and slight dryness of the
throat following smoking, no other side effects were reported after smoked
marihuana or oral THC. No adverse side effects of aerosolized THC were
volunteered by 3 of the 7 subjects on direct questioning. Reported side
effects included slight to moderate throat irritation 5-15 min after aerosol
inhalation in 2 subjects, slight chest discomfort 5-60 min after aerosolization
of THC in 3 subjects, slight cough 5 min after aerosolization in 1 subject,
and moderate nausea and increased salivation 5-15 min after aerosol administration in 1 subject. Only 1 subject reported side effects after placebo aerosol
(moderate throat irritation). Most reported side effects were of a
magnitude after all doses of aerosolized THC.

EFFECT OF AEROSOLIZED Δ^9-THC ON LEVEL OF "HIGH" (N=7)

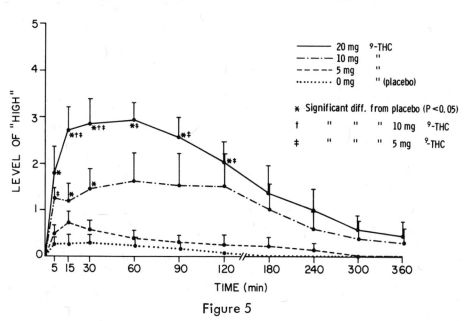

Figure 5

COMPARISON OF EFFECTS OF AEROSOLIZED, SMOKED AND ORAL Δ^9-THC (20 mg)
ON LEVEL OF "HIGH" (N=7)

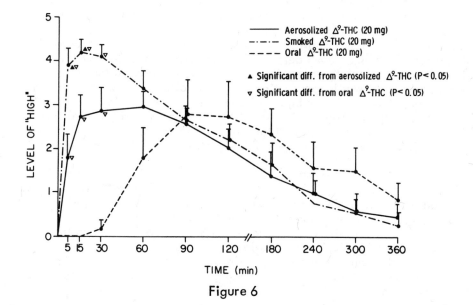

Figure 6

Blood levels of THC and metabolites following aerosolization of different doses of delta-9-THC and the smoking and ingestion of 20 mg of delta-9-THC will be reported separately.

DISCUSSION

The development of significant physiological changes following inhalation of aerosolized delta-9-THC without appreciable adverse side effects indicates that THC can be effectively administered by this route. The finding of cardiac and psychological as well as bronchial effects indicates that the administered THC was systemically absorbed after inhalation of the aerosol. Systemic absorption of THC most likely occurred at least partially from the respiratory tract and/or oropharyngeal cavity since systemic effects were noted almost immediately following aerosolization of the drug compared with the delay in onset of psychophysiological effects following ingestion of orally administered THC. On the other hand, some aerosolized THC may have been absorbed across the gut following swallowing of pharyngeally deposited aerosol since cardiac effects tended to be greater 2-6 hrs after aerosolized THC compared with effects noted over the same time period after smoking the same quantity of THC. This possibility is supported by previous findings indicating gastro-intestinal absorption of a major fraction of nebulized, radio-labeled isoproterenol (Lyons, Ayres, Dworetzky, Failliers, Harris, Dollery and Gandevia, 1973). The relatively short duration of systemic effects following nebulized isoproterenol, in contrast to aerosolized THC, is probably due to the rapid conversion of isoproterenol to inactive metabolites following absorption (Lyons et al., 1973) in contrast to the metabolism of delta-9-THC to active compounds (Lemberger, Axelrod and Kopin, 1971).

In the small number of subjects studied, the significant changes in SG_{aw}, heart rate, and "high" after aerosolized THC appeared to be somewhat related to the dose of inhaled drug. It is of interest that the smallest dose of aerosolized THC (5 mg) resulted in a peak bronchodilator effect approximating 80% of that following 20 mg delta-9-THC and comparable to that following 1250 micrograms isoproterenol. In addition, the bronchodilator effect of 5 mg delta-9-THC was longer lasting than that following isoproterenol (5 hr vs. 30 min). Moreover, the bronchodilatation following 5 mg of aerosolized THC was accompanied by only a modest (11%), short-lived (15 min) increase in heart rate and no significant "high" in contrast to significant pulse and psychological changes lasting up to 2 hours after 10 or 20 mg aerosolized THC.

Comparison of a comparable dose of THC administered by smoking, aerosolization, and ingestion revealed a comparable speed of onset and peak bronchodilator effect of the aerosolized and smoked drug in contrast to a slower onset and smaller peak bronchodilatation after oral THC. The duration of bronchodilatation following aerosolized THC was comparable to that following oral THC but longer than that following smoked marihuana. The pulse increments and "high" were greater following smoked marihuana compared with aerosolized THC and greater following the latter compared with oral THC over at least the first 30 min following drug administration.

These findings suggest possible therapeutic advantages of aerosolized THC, particularly in lower doses (5-10 mg), over both the smoked and oral routes of administration with respect to a greater speed of onset and/or duration of bronchodilatation and lesser cardiac and central nervous system effects. After studies to ascertain the safety of long-term administration of aerosolized THC to healthy individuals, additional studies would be of definite interest to determine the bronchial and systemic effects of lower doses of aerosolized THC in subjects with bronchospastic disorders.

REFERENCES

Anthonisen, N. R., Danson, J., Robertson, P. O., & Ross, W. R. D. Airway closure as a function of age. Resp. Physiol., 1969-70, 8, 59-65.

Buist, A. S. & Ross, B. B. Predicted values for closing volumes using a modified single breath nitrogen test. Am. Rev. Resp. Dis., 1973, 107, 744-752.

Briscoe, W. A. & DuBois, A. B. The relationship between airway resistance, airway conductance and lung volume in subjects of different age and body size. J. Clin. Invest., 1958, 37, 1279-1285.

Cotes, J.E. Lung function. Philadelphia, F. A. Davis, 375, 1965.

Cutting, M., Watson, A., Goodenough, G., Simmons, G., Laguara, R., & Huber, G. The effect of exposure to marijuana smoke on the bactericidal activity of pulmonary alveolar macrophages. Clin. Res., 1974, 21, 501A.

DuBois, A.B., Botelho, S. Y., Bedell, G. N., Marshall, R., & Comroe, J. H. A rapid plethysmographic method for measuring thoracic gas volume: A comparison with a nitrogen washout method for measuring functional residual capacity in normal subjects. J. Clin. Invest., 1956, 35, 322-326.

DuBois, A. B., Botelho, S. Y., & Comroe, J. H., Jr. A new method for measuring airway resistance in man using a body plethysmograph: Values in normal subjects and in patients with respiratory disease. J. Clin. Invest., 1956, 35, 327-335.

Gross, S. J., Soares, J. R., Wing, S.-L.R., & Schuster, R. E. Marijuana metabolites measured by a radioimmune technique. Nature, 1975, 252, 581-588.

Henderson, R. L., Tennant, F. S., & Guerry, R. Respiratory manifestations of hashish smoking. Arch. Otolaryng., 1972, 95, 248-251.

Lemberger, L., Axelrod, J., & Kopin, K. J. Metabolism and disposition of delta-9-tetrahydrocannabinol in man. Pharmacol. Rev., 1971, 23, 371.

Lyons, H. A., Ayres, S. M., Dworetzky, M., Failliers, C. S., Harris, M. C., Dollery, C. T., & Gandevia, B. Symposium on isoproterenol therapy in asthma. Ann Allerg., 1973, 31, 1.

Morris, J. F., Koski, A., & Johnson, L. C. Spirometric standards for healthy non-smoking adults. Am. Rev. Resp. Dis., 1971, 103, 57-67.

Olsen, J. L., Lodge, J. W., Shapiro, B. J., & Tashkin, D. P. An inhalation aerosol of delta-9-tetrahydrocannabinol. _J. Pharmacy and Pharmacol._, forthcoming.

Shapiro, B. J., Tashkin, D. P., & Frank, I. M. Mechanism of increased specific airway conductance with marijuana smoking in healthy young men. _Ann. Intern. Med._, 1973, _78_, 832.

Tashkin, D. P., Shapiro, B. J., & Frank, I. M. Acute physiological effects of smoked marijuana and oral delta-9-tetrahydrocannabinol in healthy young men. _N. Eng. J. Med._, 1973, _289_, 336-341.

Tashkin, D. P., Shapiro, B. J., & Frank, I. M. Acute effects of smoked marijuana and oral delta-9-tetrahydrocannabinol on specific airway conductance in asthmatic subjects. _Am. Rev. Resp. Dis._, 1974, _109_, 420-428.

Tashkin, D. P., Shapiro, B. J., Lee, Y. E., & Harper, C. Subacute effects of heavy marijuana smoking on pulmonary function in healthy males. _N. Eng. J. Med._, forthcoming.

Tashkin, D. P., Shapiro, B. J., Lee, Y. E., & Harper, C. E. Effects of smoked marijuana in experimentally-induced asthma. _Am. Rev. Resp. Dis._, 1975, _112_, 377-386.

Vachon, L., Fitzgerald, M. X., Solliday, N. H., Gould, I. A., Gaensler, E. Single-dose effect of marijuana smoke: Bronchial dynamics and respiratory-center sensitivity in normal subjects. _N. Eng. J. Med._, 1973, _288_, 985.

Watanabe, S., Renzetti, A. D., Jr., Begin, R., & Bigler, A. H. Airway responsiveness to a bronchodilator aerosol. 1. Normal human subjects. _Amer. Rev. Resp. Dis._, 1974, _109_, 530-537.

CHAPTER 8

AIRWAYS RESPONSE TO AEROSOLIZED DELTA-9-TETRAHYDRO-

CANNABINOL: PRELIMINARY REPORT

L. Vachon
A. Robins
E. A. Gaensler

Boston University School of Medicine
Boston, Massachusetts

NOTE: We wish to thank Dr. L. Woodland of A. D.
Little Co. who performed the biochemical analysis and
prepared the THC solutions.

Studies in the past three years have established a bronchodilator action
for smoked marihuana in normal (Vachon, Fitzgerald, Solliday, Gould, and
Gaensler, 1973; Tashkin, Shapiro, and Frank, 1974) and asthmatic (Tashkin,
Shapiro, and Frank, 1973; Vachon, Mikus, Morrisey, Fitzgerald, and Gaensler,
1976) subjects. Additionally, delta-9-tetrahydrocannabinol (THC) the principal active ingredient of marihuana (Gaoni and Mechoulam, 1964) has been
shown to have a bronchodilator effect in normal subjects (Tashkin et al, 1974)
and asthmatic subjects who were asymptomatic (Tashkin et al, 1973) or who
had experimentally induced bronchospasm (Tashkin, Shapiro, Lee, and Harper, 1975).

The mechanism of action is not clearly understood and may involve
one or more pathways: hystaminic, cholinergic, adrenergic, and prostaglandin
regulation.

Smoking and ingestion are not satisfactory methods of administration
for the study of the effects of THC on the pulmonary function in health and
disease. The total dose which it is necessary to administer produces unwanted
effects on the cardiovascular and central nervous systems. Tachycardia has
been the most consistent response to marihuana (Clark, 1975). The alteration
of mood and psychomotor functions constitute the major reason for its widespread social use. For therapeutic purposes, the desired bronchodilator action
must be separated from the other effects of THC. The biochemical approach
is to synthesize analogue compounds. An alternative method, which we

111

describe in this report, is to improve the therapeutic effectiveness by delivering the drug locally to allow the use of a much smaller total dose. The topical administration of adrenergic drugs by inhaled aerosols can produce maximal bronchial effects with minimal systemic effects, especially cardiovascular (Lovejoy, 1960) when the aerosol particles are in the micronic range. The presumed effect is to saturate the receptor sites on the bronchi while limiting the amount of drug available for systemic absorption.

MATERIALS, METHODS, AND SUBJECTS

The vehicle we have chosen is propylene glycol and water in a ratio of 9:1. This is capable of holding in clear solution up to 4.5 g of THC/100 ml. There is an inverse relationship between the amount of water and the concentration of THC in the solution; this is further influenced by temperature as it is necessary to preserve the solution at 4°C but to bring it up to room temperature for actual usage (see Figure 1).

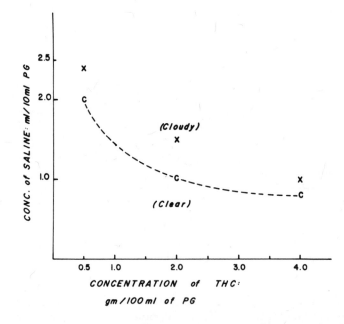

Figure 1. Temperature effect. The concentrations of THC in the propylene-glycol/water solutions above the dotted line would remain cloudy when they were brought up to room temperature after refrigeration at 4°C. The points absorbed are indicated by an "X." The concentration of THC in propyleneglycol/water solutions below the dotted line were clear upon return to room temperature. The points observed are indicated by a "C."

For the delivery of the aerosol, we found that an ultrasonic generator is not suitable because of the high viscosity of the vehicle. An effective instrument is the Dautrebande D-30 aerosol generator (Dautrebande, 1962). This is a cascade-type generator which operates continuously on compressed air. Progressively smaller particles are precipitated until only micronic size particles can escape in the gas stream. A short length of plastic tubing forms the mouthpiece. Two holes in the tubing (each less than 1 cm^2) allow the aerosol to escape when the subject is not inhaling and allow ambient air to enter the inspired stream when the flow of inhalation exceeds the maximum flow of the instrument. The D-30 is reported to generate an aerosol with particles having a mean diameter ranging between 0.5 and 2.5 microns, from a solution of 50 percent propylene glycol and 50 percent water. With our solution, the instrument produced particles with a mean diameter of 2 microns and with none above 5 microns.

The amount of THC actually offered for inhalation depends on the concentration in the solution, on the amount of the solution which is aerosolized, and on the volume of aerosol which is inhaled. In a preliminary step, we initially tested a concentration of 2 percent THC. It produced substantial decreases in airway resistance. However, this was accompanied by tachycardia and a sensation of "high." Additionally, the subjects objected to the harshness of the inhaled aerosol. A more diluted solution, 0.5 percent THC, was found usually ineffective. The mean of these concentrations, 1.25 percent, appeared to have an effect on airway resistance with few other side effects. This concentration, 1.25 g THC/100 ml, was used in this study.

The total dose delivered can be estimated. The D-30 delivers 0.0024 ml of solution per liter of aerosol measured at the mouthpiece. The total of 4 average vital capacity inhalations, described below, equaled about 22 liter (ATPS); this volume contains 0.053 ml of the solution. With a concentration of 1.25 percent of THC in the solution, the maximum dose available for inhalation is therefore 0.66 mg of THC. This is an overestimate of the actual dose as it requires the assumption that only gas containing the aerosol was inhaled. In fact, the relatively slow inhalation of 5.5 L (ATPS)/15 seconds represented a mean flow rate of 22 L/min which exceeds the flow rate of the instrument: 16.5 L/min at 7 psig. Air which did not contain the aerosol was drawn in through the side holes of the mouthpiece. The ratio of these flow rates is a reasonable, if theoretical, correction factor: (16.5/22) x .66 mg = .5 mg of THC approximately.

For comparison purposes, the vehicle alone, that is, propylene glycol and water in solution of 9:1, was administered using the D-30 nebulizer. Isoproterenol, a known bronchodilator, was also administered but from a standard Medihaler-Iso device. A dose of 0.075 mg of isoproterenol sulfate is reportedly delivered with each depression of the valve; the subjects received four doses, for a total of 0.3 mg. Each substance was administered on a separate day in a previously randomized order.

The technique of administration was the same for the three agents. The subjects exhale to residual volume and then inhale to total lung capacity.

During this inhalation, they either inhaled from the D-30 mouthpiece or administered themselves one "squirt" of the Medihaler-Iso. At total lung capacity, the subjects held their breath for 10 seconds. After a pause of 30 seconds, the maneuver was repeated for a total of 4 inhalations.

Male subjects, ages 18-30, were recruited through newspaper advertisements that did not mention the use of marihuana. Screening interviews determined that all selected subjects had smoked marihuana previously. Asthmatic subjects were included if they had not used cortico-steroid medication for at least six months and were not taking frequent bronchodilator medications. Cigarette smokers were excluded.

Spirometry, helium dilution, and diffusion capacity (D_LCO) measurements were performed with a standard Stead-Wells type spirometer. Airway resistance (R_{AW}) and the corresponding thoracic gas volume (V_{TG}) were measured in a constant-volume by the plethysmograph (DuBois, Botelho, and Comroe, 1956). The specific airway conductance (SG_{AW}) was calculated (Briscoe and DuBois, 1958) from these measurements. The heart rate was measured with an EKG machine using three chest electrodes; a monitor lead and the integrated rate were inscribed on a multi-channel strip chart recorder.

At each session, the subjects rested for one half-hour before beginning of the testing. Baseline measurements were made in the following order: (1) heart rate, averaging over 90 seconds while the subject was sitting quietly; (2) plethysmographic measurements of R_{AW} and V_{TG}; (3) forced vital capacity (FVC) and its components: forced expiratory volume in the first second ($FEV_{1.0}$) and maximal mid-expiratory flow rate (MMF). The test substance was administered, and these same measurements were repeated in the same order at 5, 20, 50, and 90 minute post-administration.

RESULTS

(1) All subjects had normal chest roentgenograms and 12-lead electrocardiograms. The two "control" subjects had normal histories as well as pulmonary function studies. The three asthmatic subjects had histories of episodic reversable airway obstruction. They showed normal values for total lung capacity (TLC), residual volume (RV), FVC, and D_LCO. Their values for $FEV_1/$FVC% and MMF were reduced. The five subjects are considered together in this preliminary report, as the magnitude of their response to the agents tested was comparable.

(2) The subjects were not able to distinguish the 1.25 percent THC solution from the vehicle alone. No subject experienced more than a transient sense of relaxation following inhalation of either of the substances.

The heart rate (Figure 2) tended to fall throughout the course of each session. The only significant increase in rate occurred 5 minutes after the inhalation of isoproterenol. The mean rate at this time was 17 bpm higher than the mean for the vehicle alone.

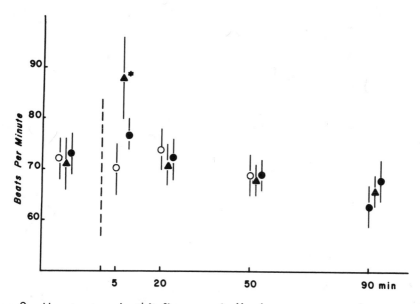

Figure 2. Heart rate. In this figure and all subsequent ones, the open circles
indicate values measured after administration of the vehicle alone;
the filled circle, the values obtained after 0.5 mg of THC and the
triangle, the values after isoproterenol 0.3 mg (see text for dosage
calculations). Each symbol and its vertical line indicates the group
mean value (N=5) and the standard error of the mean. An asterisk
indicates a P value of less than .05; the three treatments were compared by Analysis of Variance and the significantly different points
were ascertained by a paired t-test, as necessary. The vertical
line before the 5-minute mark indicates the drug administration.
In this figure, the heart rate shows an increase only after the administration of isoproterenol.

(3) The vital capacity (Figure 3) was unchanged after the administration of either substance at any time period.

The FEV1% (Figure 4) was increased significantly at 5 and 20 minutes
by both isoproterenol and THC. The MMF (Figure 5) was significantly increased
by THC at all times; the level reached at 20 minutes was maintained at 90
minutes. The MMF peaked sooner after isoproterenol but was no longer significantly elevated by 50 minutes.

The R_{AW} (Figure 6) showed a significant decrease following isoproterenol at all time periods; there was a suggestion that the mean was returning toward baseline at 90 minutes. The THC first achieved a significant reduction
only at 20 minutes but the mean value was apparently not rising yet at 90
minutes. Since the thoracic gas volume (Figure 7) showed no significant
changes, the specific inductance (Figure 8) mirrored the changes in R_{AW}.

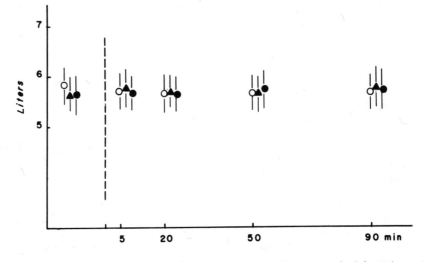

Figure 3. Vital capacity. (See legend of Figure 2 for symbols). There is no change following the administration of either treatment.

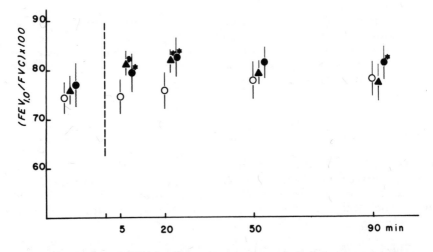

Figure 4. FEV₁%. (See legend of Figure 2 for symbols). Both drugs produce a significant early rise in the FEV₁%; while the values after isoproterenol have returned to baseline by 90 minutes, the effect of THC still appears significant.

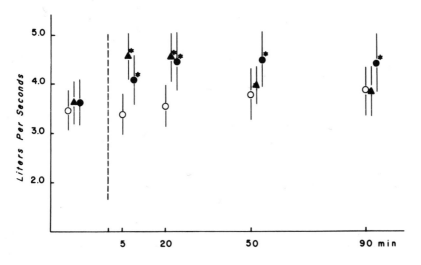

Figure 5. Maximum Mid Expiratory Flow Rate. (See legend of Figure 2 for symbols). The MMF is calculated as the mean flow rate between 25% and 75% of the FVC. Both drugs produce a significant increase; the THC effect seems to start slower but to last longer than that of the isoproterenol.

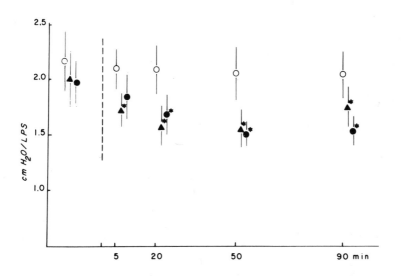

Figure 6. Airway Resistance. (See legend of Figure 2 for symbols). The plethysmographic measurements would also indicate that the action of isoproterenol figures earlier and diminishes earlier than that of THC.

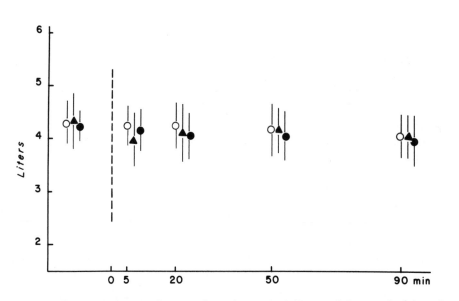

Figure 7. Thoracic Gas Volume. (See legend of Figure 2 for symbols). The measurements of R$_{AW}$ were made at identical lung volume through-out.

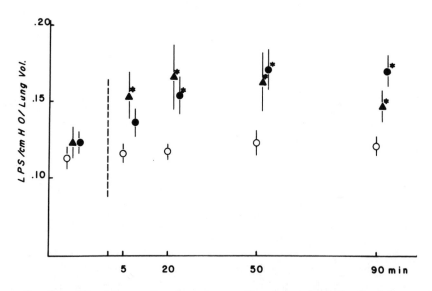

Figure 8. Specific Airway Conductance. (See legend of Figure 2 for symbols). As with R$_{AW}$, there is a strong suggestion that the two aspects have different characteristics regarding the beginning and the duration of their action.

DISCUSSION

The analysis of our preliminary results would suggest that THC, administered as a microaerosol, produces a significant and prolonged bronchodilatation without adverse side effects. Isoproterenol administered from a standard Medihaler-Iso produces more rapid but shorter acting effects on airway function. Both agents appear comparable in the actual magnitude of the airflow changes which they produce.

Previous studies have used dosages of THC comparable to those obtained from marihuana cigarettes, that is, in the range of 5 to 10 mg or more. By refining the delivery system, it would appear possible to produce significant bronchial effects with approximately 0.5 mg. Although this suggests a therapeutic applicability, several questions should be answered first.

The material should be stabilized so that refrigeration is not required for preservation of its activity. Could commercially available nebulizers, producing somewhat larger particles, have the same effect on the airways while also avoiding the cardiovascular and CNS effects? Another question is the potential for abuse of this concentration. Although our subjects did not experience a "high" from the THC, it is perhaps because they received only a limited number of inhalations. Finally, is this concentration range suitable for reversing more severe airway obstruction? This should be studied in spontaneously occurring asthma attacks and in patients with chronic bronchitis.

REFERENCES

Briscoe, W. A. & DuBois, A. B. The relationship between airway resistance airway conductance and lung volume in subjects of different age and body size. J. Clin. Invest., 1958, 37, 1279-1285.

Clark, S. C. Marihuana and the cardiovascular system. Pharm. Biochem. Behav., 1975, 3, 299-306.

Dautrebande, L. Microaerosols. New York: Academic Press, 1962.

DuBois, A. B., Botelho, S. Y., Bedell, G. N., Marshall, R., & Comroe, J. H., Jr. A rapid plethysmographic method for measuring thoracic gas volume: A comparison with a nitrogen washout method for measuring functional residual capacity in normal subjects. J. Clin. Invest., 1956, 35, 322-326.

DuBois, A. B., Botelho, S. Y., & Comroe, J. H., Jr. A new method for measuring airway resistance in man using a body plethysmograph: Values in normal subjects and in patients with respiratory disease. J. Clin. Invest., 1956, 35, 327-335.

Gaoni, Y. & Mechoulam, R. Isolation, structure and partial synthesis of the active constituent of hashish. J. Am. Chem. Soc., 1964, 86, 1646-1647.

Lovejoy, F. W., Jr., Constantin, H., & Dautrebande, L. Importance of Particle Size in Aerosol Therapy. Proc. Soc. Exp. Biol. Med., 1960, 103, 836-838.

Tashkin, D. P., Shapiro, B. J., & Frank, I. M. Acute pulmonary physiological effects of smoked marijuana and oral delta-9-tetrahydrocannabinol in healthy young males. New Engl. J. Med., 1973, 289, 336-341.

Tashkin, D. P., Shapiro, B. J., & Frank, I. M. Acute effects of smoked marijuana and oral delta-9-tetrahydrocannabinol on specific airway conductance in asthmatic subjects. Amer. Rev. Resp. Dis., 1974, 109, 420-428.

Tashkin, D. P., Shapiro, B. J., Lee, Y. E., & Harper, C. E. Effects of smoked marijuana in experimentally induced asthma. Amer. Rev. Resp. Dis., 1975, 112, 337-386.

Vachon, L., Fitzgerald, M. S., Solliday, N. H., Gould, I. A., & Gaensler, E. A. Single-dose effect of marihuana smoke. New Engl. J. Med., 1973, 288, 985-989.

Vachon, L., Mikus, P., Morrisey, W., Fitzgerald, M., & Gaensler, E. A. Bronchial effect of marihuana smoke in asthma. In M. C. Braude and S. Szara (Eds.), The Pharmacology of Marihuana. New York: Raven Press, 1976 (in press).

CHAPTER 9

RESPIRATORY AND CARDIOVASCULAR EFFECTS OF DELTA-9-
TETRAHYDROCANNABINOL ALONE AND IN COMBINATION WITH
OXYMORPHONE, PENTOBARBITAL, AND DIAZEPAM

Theodore C. Smith
Robyn A. Kulp

Department of Anesthesia
University of Pennsylvania
Philadelphia, Pennsylvania

NOTE: The research for this work was supported by U.S.
Public Health Service Grants 5-T01-GM-00215 and 5-P01-
GM-15430. The authors wish to thank Dr. Lee A. Malit
for the initial suggestions and stimulation leading to these
experiments.

Among the clear effects of marihuana and its derivatives are subjective sensations of pleasure, euphoria, dissociation, and mild analgesia.
These are just the sensations an anesthesiologist would wish to induce in his
patients preoperatively. He would like to provide these desirable effects at
little cost to respiratory and circulatory control. Indeed, undesirable side
effects on respiration and circulation constitute the major limitations to the
various classes of premedicants generally in use, that is, opioids, sedatives,
and ataractics. A common approach is to combine two or more types of
drugs so that limited dosage of any one type will limit expression of side
effects. In selecting drugs and dosage the anesthesiologist would like to
have detailed dose response data, especially for respiratory and circulatory
effects, including information on physiological interaction of different
classes. This report considers the cardiovascular and respiratory effects of
delta-9-tetrahydrocannabinol (THC) and its interaction with drugs typical of
the three classes, oxymorphone, pentobarbital, and diazepam. This work is
both preliminary to and more broadly applicable than a clinical trial as a
premedicant. In short, by discriminating and careful physiologic measurements of respiratory control and cardiovascular dynamics, we attempt to
delineate toxic effects and mechanisms of THC alone, and in interaction
with the other depressants. In brief, we found little alarming about large
intravenous doses of THC except for its psychic effects, notably abject fear.
Pentobarbital heightened the effect if anything, but both oxymorphone and

diazepam were therapeutic, the latter at less cost to respiratory and circulatory homeostasis.

METHODOLOGY

The experiments were primarily designed to study the response of
circulatory and respiratory parameters to CO_2 challenge. As will be appre-
ciated from the description below, the set and the setting were conducive
to a study of neither ataractic nor premedication benefits.

Subjects of legal age were recruited from the graduate populations of
three major universities by signs in student aid offices. After a tour of the
laboratory and two informative interviews 24 hours apart, the subjects
appeared in the laboratory in a post-absorptive state. They lay on a standard
operating room table while an internal jugular catheter was placed through
the sternocleidomastoid muscle into the superior vena cava. A second catheter
was placed in a radial or brachial artery. This permitted recording of both
venous and arterial blood pressures by strain gauge and the measurement of
cardiac output by dilution using cardiogreen. The subjects then breathed
through a rubber mouthpiece with the nose occluded by a sponge rubber clip,
inhaling mixtures of dry gas enriched with oxygen with variable carbon dioxide
content. They exhaled into a recycling wedge spirometer. Continuous records
were made of end tidal carbon dioxide tension, inspired carbon dioxide
tension, ventilation (rate and tidal volume), EKG, and venous and arterial
blood pressure. Intermittent measurements were made of cardiac output and
of the inspired oxygen concentration.

The protocol utilized the isohypercapnic alveolar control system of
C. J. Lambertson (Lambertson and Wendel, 1960). Breath by breath the
inspired carbon dioxide concentration is altered to keep end tidal carbon
dioxide tension (P_{ETCO_2}) constant at a preselected elevated value. With

the stimulus of CO_2 thus held level, changes in expired ventilation and
cardiac output are directly relatable to drug effects. Drugs are given intravenously and incremented at intervals to give a cumulative logarithmic
scale. Prior to and following final drug administration, inspired carbon
dioxide tension was altered to provide three or four point steady state
ventilatory responses to carbon dioxide. Immediately before and during all
drug administrations alveolar concentration was controlled manually at
approximately 50 torr.

The initial study involved giving THC alone, starting with 27 $\mu g/kg$
intravenously and progressing in logarithmically scaled increments to provide
a maximum cumulative dose of either 134 or 201 $\mu g/kg$ in five or six doses.
Ten subjects contributed to this study, which has been previously reported
(Malit, Johnstone, Bourke, Kulp, Klein and Smith, 1975). In the second
and third study, the subjects were pretreated with 1 mg of oxymorphone/70
kg and with 100 mg of oxymorphone/70 kg respectively. This work has also
been reported (Johnstone, Lief, Kulp and Smith, 1975). In the fourth study

for which pulmonary data is available in this report, the protocol was altered slightly. Five mg of THC were infused over several minutes and thereafter at ten-minute intervals increments of diazepam were administered intravenously giving cumulative doses of 5, 10, and 20 mg/70 kg.

In all studies the vehicle was 95% ethanol. The dose was not negligible, but one known to have little effect on the measurements. Continuous verbal and physical contact with the subjects assured that they did not doze off, as that is known to alter the response in itself (Smith, 1971).

RESULTS AND DISCUSSION

The effects of 12 to 15 mg of THC alone give a small dextrad shift of the ventilatory response to carbon dioxide, equivalent to about 5 mg of morphine sulfate. There is no change in the slope of the ventilatory response to carbon dioxide. The THC was given incrementally, resulting in a log dose response curve with a significant negative slope in eight of the ten subjects so studied. Several subjects had periods of hyperventilation after one or more doses. One subject had a positive dose response slope, that is, he had apparent stimulation of breathing. Interpolating an average individual dose response curve for a dose of 70 μg/kg, the dose used in the diazepam interaction described below, an average fall of 0.7 liters/min in the hypercapnic ventilation was calculated. The effects on tidal volume were similar to the effects on ventilation, and there was no remarkable change in pattern of breathing.

After establishing the effects of THC alone in this fashion we explored the interaction of THC with the prototypes of commonly used depressant drugs. There were two remarkable differences attributed to the pretreatment with 100 mg of pentobarbital prior to THC. The first was a complete lack of detectable effects on ventilation: it was clearly not seen in the ventilatory response to carbon dioxide which overlay the control response, nor in the tidal volume or frequency of breathing. Pentobarbital given alone in this dose has been previously shown to be a very mild ventilatory stimulant. There was a small increase in dead space, most easily noted in the subjects who received the larger doses, so that one would calculate a small decrease in the alveolar ventilation. However, the resting end tidal carbon dioxide tension did not reflect this. The second remarkable difference was the intolerance of volunteers for the effects of THC following pentobarbital. After THC alone only one of the ten subjects discontinued the study at a low dose, 27 μg/kg, and one stopped at 100 μg/kg. Three more stopped at 134 μg/kg and five tolerated 200 μg/kg. After pretreatment with pentobarbital, one subject of seven stopped at the first dose, 27 μg/kg, three at the second dose, 40 μg/kg, and only three of the seven tolerated 134 μg/kg. None wanted more. The subjects were akisthetic, restless, hyperkinetic, and anxious. Ventilation rose and fell erratically.

Oxymorphone pretreatment provided a different experience. Eight subjects began the study, with 1 mg/70 kg intravenously, and eight received all five planned THC doses totaling 134 $\mu g/kg$. All showed typical opioid depression of ventilation initially, and seven of the eight had significant negative dose response slopes of depressed ventilation on log THC dose. Respiratory rate tended to remain constant and the depth of breathing decreased concomitant with the decrease in ventilation. The final ventilatory response to carbon dioxide was depressed, as measured by both the slope and displacement parameters. The slope change is equivalent to the depression of light surgical anesthesia. Accordingly, our subjects were very hard put to keep awake and responsive, and tended to doze off with only brief pauses in our verbal arousal efforts.

The diazepam study was conducted differently for two reasons. First, we wanted to assure that a single large I.V. dose gave the same effects as a cumulative dose of similar size. Second, we wished to study the situation where THC-induced effects are treated by diazepam, inasmuch as this is an increasingly common therapy for "bad trips." Therefore, we began with a single injection of THC, 5 mg, and followed with 3 doses of diazepam at ten-minute intervals. In Figure 1 you see the control ventilatory response to CO_2 from this study. Following this, the end tidal CO_2 was controlled by breath-by-breath adjustments in inspired CO_2 to provide an end tidal tension of about 50 torr. It is common to find this point, when plotted on ventilation CO_2 diagrams, slightly above the straight line (labeled C in Figure 1). This is attributed to combinations of hysteresis-like response to decreasing CO_2 from the 7% inspired level, and to the cumulative arousal effects of immobility, dry mouth, and augmented CO_2.

The single dose of THC, 5 mg, caused a very slight and statistically insignificant fall in ventilation of 0.3 L/min (a dotted X in Figure 1). The three subsequent doses of diazepam each caused additional depression, totaling 3.3 liters/min after 20 mg of diazepam. This is a statistically significant dose response slope. Again, frequency varied insignificantly and a decrease in tidal volume accounted for the fall in stimulated VE. The post-drug slope of the ventilatory response to carbon dioxide was 63% of the control slope, a value associated in other studies with light sleep. The subjects were responsive for the most part, some actually active, and only one was appreciably difficult to keep awake, although three others would dose quickly and briefly if left alone. The effect of this dose of diazepam has been independently studied and found to have little effect on CO_2 stimulated ventilation at a tension of 50 torr. Further, it gave no noticeable potentiation of subsequent injections of meperidine.

To summarize the ventilatory effects, THC alone and THC with pentobarbital gave little or no effect on CO_2 mediated breathing and did not change the slope of the ventilatory response in any measurable fashion. However, THC with either diazepam or oxymorphone caused obvious depression of the type associated with altered level of consciousness, that is, a slope change.

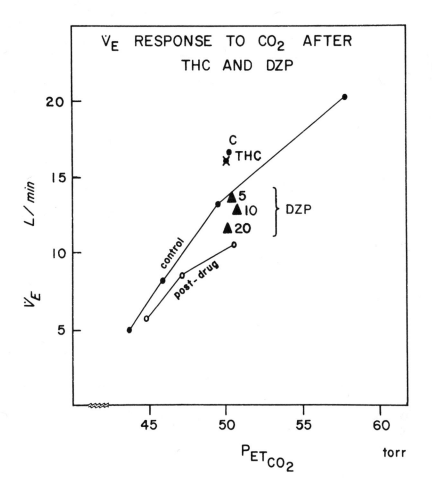

Figure 1. Ventilatory Effect of Delta-9-tetrahydrocannabinol and Diazepam in Six Healthy Volunteers.

After the control steady state response (solid circles connected by lines) the end total CO_2 was controlled at 50 torr $\pm$ 1 (C symbol) and first 5 mg THC and then 3 doses of diazepam (DZP) given intravenously at ten-minute intervals. A final steady state CO_2 response was then obtained (open circles). The post-drug depression of slope by 37% is significant.

The most responsive cardiovascular effect of the variables we studied was the pulse rate change. Figure 2 shows the effect of THC and subsequent diazepam. We have chosen the format of a CO_2 response plot to permit comparison with ventilatory data. We saw a small but real response of heart rate to increased carbon dioxide. During isohypercapnia, THC caused a marked cardioaccelerator response which was subsequently moderated by increments of diazepam and the passage of time, thirty minutes in this case. All subjects had an increase in rate which varied from 24 to 64 beats per minute. Neither the increase nor the final rate was correlated with resting or with the isohypercapnic control rate. Following the diazepam there was a retention of CO_2 responsiveness, albeit at a higher level of pulse rate.

When THC had been given alone, the average result was a dose-related tachycardia with considerable inter- as well as intra-subject variability. There was even more variability of heart rate when oxymorphone or pentobarbital was given as pretreatment. Again, there was a generally progressive rise in pulse, but several subjects were erratic. Serious tachyarrhythmia was seen in two of the subjects after pentobarbital, which was clearly unrelated to the THC dose as it moderated significantly despite additional THC. After pentobarbital, CO_2 responsiveness was retained but it was reversed after oxymorphone.

To return to the effects of THC with diazepam on circulation, we might remark in general that the cardiac output and the blood pressure response parallel the chronotropic effect. The cardiac output increased from 8 to 10 L/min with CO_2 stimulation, demonstrating the usual response to 7% inspired CO_2 of 0.15 L/min/torr. THC during isohypercapnia produced a rise of 3.6 L/min/5 mg THC. Diazepam then caused a dose-related decrease in output of about 1 L/min per doubling of the diazepam dose. These changes in output were almost entirely accounted for by rate changes. The stroke volume was initially 92 ml/beat before THC, 90 ml/beat after THC, and 86, 84, and 80 ml/beat after the last diazepam dose. The cardiac index during isohypercapnia arose 2 L/min with THC and fell to control with diazepam. In comparison, the cardiac index increase after THC alone was 1.9 L/min in the previous study at the level of 70 $\mu g/kg$, 2.0 $L/min/m^2$ after THC with pentobarbital pretreatment, and 1.6 $L/min/m^2$ after THC with oxymorphone pretreatment. In other words, THC increased cardiac output regularly, mostly through chronotropic effect. This luxurious perfusion was not moderated by pentobarbital, was only slightly reduced by oxymorphone, and was returned to normal after diazepam.

Mean arterial blood pressure rose about 4% with CO_2 stimulation. THC caused another 8% rise, progressively reduced after each diazepam dose to the control level. CO_2 response terminally was similar to the control, slightly higher in fact. Mean venous pressure fell 25% with THC and was not altered significantly by the first diazepam dose, but did rise to control level by the last diazepam dose. No CO_2 response in venous pressure was noted before or after the study.

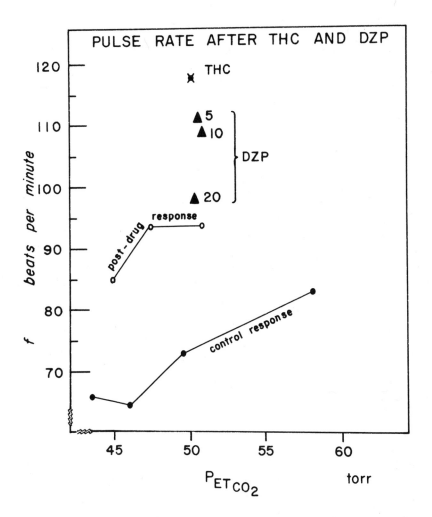

Figure 2.   Chronotropic Effect of Delta-9-tetrahydrocannabinol and Diazepam
in the Same Volunteers.

Ｔhe symbols are the same as in Figure 1. The rate
changes due to each drug injection are significant, but not
the slope of the CO_2 response before or after drugs. Cardiac
output measurements showed similar increase with THC and
return toward normal with diazepam.

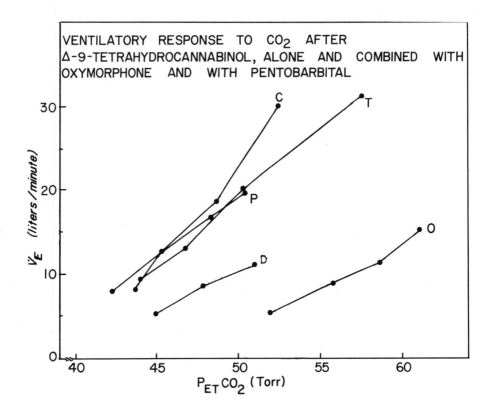

Figure 3. Combined Data From the Several Experiments.

The control response, C, is an amalgam of the before-drug data from all of the studies. The response to THC alone, curve T, is taken from Malit et al. (1975) in which 134 to 201 μg/kg THC were given to nine volunteers. The curves labeled O and P refer to data from Johnstone et al. (1975) wherein 24 to 134 μg/kg THC followed 1 mg oxymorphone (eight subjects) or 100 mg pentobarbital (seven subjects). The curve labeled D refers to the combination of 70 μg/kg THC and 290 μg/kg diazepam in six subjects.

Thus, THC is seen to increase arterial blood pressure, increase cardiac rates and output, the latter largely by stroke rate and not stroke volume, and lower venous pressure. These are the hallmarks of an increase in sympathomimetic stimulation with both beta I and beta II effects, which cannot be CO_2 mediated because the study was entirely isohypercapnic. CNS activation is suggested inasmuch as all variables returned to normal with diazepam.

Anesthetists are expected to look at the eye signs and we did. We regularly saw conjunctival injection. In addition, in the diazepam study the pupils got progressively larger with each dose of each drug. Pupil size in one subject measured photographically began at about 2.3 mm, increased to about 3 mm with THC and a 4.2 mm at the end of the diazepam dosage.

Much more marked were the subjective responses to the study as described in the subjects' words: "At first very pleasant -- geometric drawings were nice to look at as was music -- then strange and foreboding atmosphere -- time dilation -- tripped out -- you're all just torturing me -- nightmarish -- horrible -- caught in cyclic repetition -- never end -- vision of hell -- in a shell with partially anesthetized senses -- depersonalized -- injection of valium -- almost immediate relief -- began to enjoy things -- little recollection -- relaxed -- mental blankness -- had fried eggs and toast and went to bed after the study."

Another subject described the results this way: "Helpless blown-up balloon -- my will taken away -- voice from a distance -- disembodied -- X-ray vision -- sense of laser beams in the air -- wanted to move -- afraid to -- started calling to be let down -- singing to give the doctor's graphs some human interest -- abundance of energy, yellow, orange, and brown -- fear of loss of control -- diamond thinking was deep blue -- what did you mean by breaking into my fantasies."

In summary, healthy young men tolerate large to excessive doses of delta-9-THC with little important change in breathing and circulation, and of CNS control of these vital systems (see Figure 3). They do get scared, "out of their gourd." Pentobarbital makes things worse -- unequivocally! Oxymorphone and, we would guess, any other opioid, are effective in treating the toxic psychosis, but at a cost to ventilation that we judge excessive and hazardous, despite the maintenance of cardiac output. Diazepam, and we would guess other benzodiazepines and perhaps other ataractics as well, similarly soothe the psyche with less deleterious effects on respiration and no worrisome cardiac depression.

REFERENCES

Johnstone, R.E., Lief, P.L., Kulp, R.A., & Smith, T.C. Combination of delta-9-Tetrahydrocannabinol with oxymorphone or pentobarbital. Anesthesiol., 1975, 42, 674-683.

Lambertson, C.J., & Wendel, H. An alveolar P_{CO_2} control system. J. Appl. Physiol., 1960, 15, 43-48.

Malit, L.A., Johnstone, R.E., Bourke, D.I., Kulp, R.A., Klein, V., & Smith, T.C. Intravenous delta-9-Tetrahydrocannabinol. Anesthesiol., 1975, 42, 666-673.

Smith, T.C. Pharmacology of respiratory depression. Internal. Anesthesiol. Clinics, 1971, 9, 125-143.

DISCUSSION

Mechoulam: I want to ask you whether there are any available animal models so that one can study a larger variety of compounds.

Tashkin: Yes, in fact there are animal models of asthma. We are gearing up to do such studies.

Smith: I would like to defend the use of humans, at least in some regard. I think there is some therapeutic information that is necessary because people do come into emergency rooms with bad trips and have to have something done to them. A dog is ten times as tolerant to morphine as a human being is, and a cat gets rather berserk when given morphine. I'm not sure how I would interpret an animal's actions, so that some sort of comparison is absolutely necessary in human beings to indicate just which animal models are appropriate.

Mechoulam: But what I am shooting at is we won't have a new anti-asthmatic drug until we have screened a variety of compounds, and obviously you can't screen them on humans.

Sallan: I have a question for Dr. Tashkin. You mentioned that you were doing radioimmunoassays on your subjects, and I think I missed your data.

Tashkin: They are being done by Drs. Gross and Soares, and they have only analyzed samples on two subjects.

Smith: I would like to ask Dr. Tashkin -- he undoubtedly appreciates the value of the aerosol particle size. Can you tell us something about the device you use?

Tashkin: We used a device that produces a polydispersed aerosol; that is, the particles are from 1 - 10 microns. Extrapolation from other data suggests that no more than 10 percent of the particles are deposited in the tracheobronchial tree. The rest are deposited in the oropharynx and are probably swallowed.

Hepler: I would like to ask Dr. Smith what he thinks of dilated pupils in his subjects.

Smith: I haven't the foggiest idea; I was concerned that the pupil dilatation increased during this study. It was quite common to see rather large pupils at the end of the study, particularly when people were dozing off and having whatever dreams they were having. I have the feeling that if you are going to have a dream, it might be frightening or it might be pleasant, and you would have autonomic reactions to the fright or the pleasantness, which would change pupilary size, but I could not correlate their subsequent reports of their post-experimental feelings with what I observed.

Sallan: I would like to ask any of the pharmacologists in the audience -- Dr. Robins mentioned the temperature lability of the drug and the fact that we are told the delta-9-THC has to be kept refrigerated. Yet it is shipped from wherever it is shipped from, and I don't know how long it is in the mail. I was really wondering what the realities are about the temperature.

Braude: It is shipped in an alcohol solution in which it is fairly stable at ordinary temperatures.

Vachon: Our material is shipped in bulk form -- it's 99 and some fraction percent pure. We take it back to Arthur D. Little Co. who manufactures it in the first place, and they say now on paper we have 10 grams to draw on from the bank. When I go and pick it up, I take it refrigerated in an insulated package and I keep it in my air-conditioned car for about 15 minutes, then I put it in my refrigerator in the hospital, and we are very careful to bring it to room temperature only at the time we are going to use it. This is why I had ADL do a study on what happens to it when I bring it up to room temperature.

Harris: The stuff that's in the sesame oil solution is relatively stable, but everything is relative. If it is kept refrigerated, it stays around longer. If it stays at room temperature, if you keep it a week at room temperature, you are not going to have any significant loss. If you keep it two months at room temperature, it's going to be a greater loss than if you keep it two months in the refrigerator. So everything is relative. The stuff that's being used by aerosol is a horse of a different color. You are putting a high percentage of oxygen into a thin layer of material, and the rate of oxidation is undoubtedly going to be much higher in that formulation.

Cohen: One of the speakers mentioned that only a few tenths of a milligram was the actual delivered dose in the lungs, and I would like him to explain why.

Robins: I don't know about effective delivered dose. I think this is the amount that comes out of the top of the aerosol generator.

Cohen: On that amount, they do or do not have psychological symptoms?

Robins: They did not. At most, they felt a slight relaxation. They did not feel high.

Burstein: It might be interesting to collect some of the aerosol, condense it, and determine how much THC is present.

Vachon: It's very difficult to do because you are dealing with an extremely small amount. This is the total dose offered, not what gets into the lungs. We had our material repeatedly tested after a week, and over 90 percent of the original THC activity was still present. That is, preparing the solution, put it in a vial, stopper it, keep it at $4°C$, then in the afternoon take it out, leave it on the shelf for one hour, then put it back in the refrigerator. You do that five times, then on Friday afternoon, put it in the gas chromatograph and 90 percent of the THC activity is there.

Mental Functioning

CHAPTER 10

STIMULANT EFFECTS OF MARIHUANA ON THREE NEUROPSYCHOLOGICAL

SYSTEMS

Shirley Y. Hill
Donald W. Goodwin

Department of Psychiatry
Washington University School of Medicine
St. Louis, Missouri

NOTE: This work was supported in part by U. S. Public
Health Service Grants DA-00282, DA4RG008, and
AA-00209.

The present report deals with three separate studies examining the effects of marihuana on three neuropsychological systems: memory, pain perception, and vision. The results suggest there may be a commonality in the way marihuana affects these systems.

The studies all involved inhalation of marihuana smoke. Combustion and administration of the smoke utilized a procedure described by Renault (1971). A 9-liter spirometer with attached crucible was used. One gram of marihuana placebo or marihuana containing 1.5% (-)-delta-9-transtetrahydro-cannabinol (THC) was burned in the crucible by pulling air through the material as the inner cannister of the spirometer was raised, trapping the smoke with minimal loss. Pulling air through the material in this manner resulted in almost total combustion of the 1 g dose. The crucible was then replaced with a rubber mouthpiece for inhalation. Subjects inhaled the smoke for 5 seconds, held their breath for 15 seconds, and resumed breathing for 35 seconds. This was done until three cannisters of smoke were inhaled, requiring about 15 minutes. Assuming minimal loss of smoke by this method, the dose delivered was calculated to be approximately 12 mg of THC.

The present paper reports results of three separate experiments performed in our laboratories. Male subjects between the ages of 21-30 were used. All were experienced marihuana smokers who had smoked marihuana at least twice weekly for a year prior to testing. More than half had smoked for four or more

years at least once a week. They were required to abstain from smoking marihuana or using other drugs for 48 hours before the test session. All subjects
were screened for inclusion in the study using a structured medical and psychiatric interview; none showed evidence of medical or psychiatric illness.
The studies were run single blind; that is, the subjects were not told that a
placebo would be given.

STATE-DEPENDENT LEARNING

The abuse potential of marihuana has been widely debated as the use
of the drug has increased in Western countries. Overton (1972) has suggested
that the abuse potential of various drugs may parallel their capacity for producing "state-dependent" effects in animals and man. State-dependent or
"dissociated" learning refers to a phenomenon observed in animal and human
studies wherein certain behavior learned in particular drug states transfers more
readily when the same drug state is reintroduced than if subsequent testing
occurs under the influence of another drug or in a non-drug state. This phenomenon has been demonstrated primarily with sedative and hypnotic drugs,
such as barbiturates and alcohol, which are relatively susceptible to abuse.
In general, drugs with little abuse potential (for example, phenothiazines)
dissociate weakly or not at all.

Barry and Kubena (1972) have shown that delta-9-transtetrahydrocan-
nabinol produces state-dependent effects in rats. In the study reported here,
we examined the effects of smoking marihuana on various tasks, to see whether
the drug produces state-dependency in man. If Overton's hypothesis is correct,
detection of state-dependent effects from marihuana would be associated with
its possible abuse potential.

Subjects were randomly assigned to one of four treatment groups. One
(MM) received marihuana on both days. A second group (PP) received marihuana placebo on both days. A third group (MP) received marihuana on Day 1
and placebo on Day 2. The fourth group (PM) received placebo on Day 1 and
marihuana on Day 2. Use of this factorial design permits analysis of drug,
day, and change-state effects.

Tests were chosen in order to include verbal, non-verbal, and visual
motor abilities. In addition, some of the tests required ordering of responses
while others did not.

Tests included a visual avoidance task; a word association recall task;
a verbal learning task measuring memory for "word strings" of varying degrees
of meaningfulness; and a test measuring recall of ordered objects. Upon completion of smoking, tests were given in a counter-balanced order during a
period of one hour. All tests except the visual avoidance task were designed
to measure positive transfer of learning from Day 1 to Day 2. The avoidance
task measured interference or negative transfer. Where positive transfer is
measured, dissociative learning is suggested when mean error scores in the
same-state groups are lower than in the change-state groups. In the avoidance

task, designed to measure negative transfer, dissociation would be reflected by fewer errors in the change-state groups than in the same-state groups.

In the avoidance task, four patterns of lights were randomly presented. Each pattern could be extinguished by a specific switch controlled by right and left hands and feet. An incorrect response or failure to respond within 3 seconds resulted in presentation of a noxious tone. The criterion was 20 correct responses, with number of errors to reach criterion taken as the measure of performance. The task was identical on both days, except that on Day 2 the pattern-switch relation was altered. Thus, performance on Day 2 was assumed to reflect interference; that is, the greater the number of errors on Day 2, the greater the degree of interference.

This test requires visual-motor coordination in that responses must be made within 3 seconds, or they are counted as an error. In addition, the subject must simultaneously respond to a given pattern with the correct switch while holding information concerning other alternate patterns. In this respect, the test requires discrimination learning.

The rote learning task involved memorizing 4 five-word "word strings" of varying meaningfulness (normal sentence, anomalous sentence, anagram, and word list) (Marks and Miller, 1964). On Day 2 subjects were asked to recall the word strings memorized on Day 1 after which a relearning session was conducted. The following word strings were used: (a) the normal sentence was: "Soapy detergents dissolve greasy stains"; (b) the anomalous sentence was: "Pink accidents cause gallant storms"; (c) the anagram was: "Neighbors sleeping noisy wake parties"; (d) the nonsense word list was: "give odors snows fatal violent." Performance was measured in terms of errors of sequence and omission. Only the (d) type word string requires memorization of the proper word sequence unaided by language cues.

For the word association test, 20 words of low association value (Palermo and Jenkins, 1964) were presented. Subjects were instructed to respond to the stimulus words with the first word that came to mind. On Day 2 the stimulus words were repeated and subjects were asked to recall their responses on Day 1. Performance was measured in terms of errors made on Day 2 recall.

In the object recall test, subjects were shown seven plastic objects from the Kahn test of symbol arrangement (Kahn, 1953). They were asked to name each so that subsequent deficits in recall presumably would reflect memory loss rather than inattention. The subjects were then asked to order the objects from left to right. On Day 2 subjects were asked to recall the seven objects and then arrange them in the same order as on Day 1.

All measures of performance were subjected to 2 by 2 factorial analyses of variance. Table 1 presents the interaction F values for the four tasks and the mean errors for each group. The interaction effect tests the marihuana state change effect. Thus, any significant interaction may be taken as evidence of dissociation.

Table 1. Mean Errors and F Values for Change of State

Task	Day 2 -- Mean Errors				F Value
	PP	PM	MP	MM	
Ordered Object Recall	0.25	3.13	2.88	1.13	12.46[a]
Avoidance	14.25	13.88	15.38	10.88	0.64
Word Association	0.50	2.50	1.25	3.13	0.01
Word Strings					
Type a	0.69	1.75	1.32	0.94	1.00
Type b	2.19	3.07	2.19	2.37	0.15
Type c	1.94	2.75	2.62	2.00	0.63
Type d	3.06	4.82	6.19	3.94	5.78[b]
Types (a-d) (combined)	20.50	17.56	20.06	20.00	1.00

Data are based on analysis of four groups of eight subjects each. The first letter refers to the condition on Day 1 and the second letter refers to the condition on Day 2.

[a] $P < 0.01$

[b] $P < 0.05$

As Table 1 shows, the recall of ordered objects revealed a significant interaction effect ($P < 0.01$). The dissociative effect arose from the MP and the PM groups making more errors than either the PP or MM groups. Analysis of simple principal effects indicated that both the PM and MP groups differed significantly from the PP group ($F = 9.63$, $P < 0.01$; and $F = 8.03$, $P < 0.01$, respectively). Also, the PM group differed significantly from the MM group ($F = 4.66$, $P < 0.05$).

Neither the avoidance task nor the word association task revealed a significant interaction effect. In the word string task, with errors analyzed by type of string, there was evidence of dissociation for the type (d) string (Table 1) in which both syntax and meaningfulness are missing. The other three types of word strings provided these cues. The normal sentence provided both syntax and meaningfulness, while the anomalous sentence provided syntax, and the anagram provided meaningfulness.

Although an interaction effect was not found in the word association task, a significant drug effect was evident ($F = 8.73$, $P < 0.01$). Thus, marihuana disrupts memory for self-generated word associations, though this effect is no more pronounced in the change-state groups than in the same-state groups.

The significant results found in the ordered object recall and the type (d) word string (Table 1) suggest that tasks involving sequential memory may be most sensitive to dissociation. The lack of dissociation found for the (a), (b), and (c) type word strings may be explained by the fact that recall of the sequence is aided by long-term memory for sentence structure or meaningfulness of words. In contrast, the type (d) string must be recalled sequentially without the aid of either. This task seems to have much in common with sequential recall of the plastic Kahn objects, where meaningfulness also plays an insignificant role.

The results of the present study suggest that marihuana produces statedependent learning when tasks sensitive to dissociation are used. In other studies of state-dependent learning, using other drugs, similar differential effects were found, depending on the task and the drug administered. Stillman, Weingartner, Wyatt, Gillin, and Eich (1974) have also found that tasks requiring ordering of stimuli are much more sensitive to the disruptive effects of marihuana in a state-dependent design. They found especially clear statedependent effects on a test of picture arrangement in which sequential arrangement rather than the content of the pictures had to be remembered.

CRITICAL FLICKER FUSION

In reviewing marihuana literature, one is impressed by the rather small attention sensory processes have received. Further, clinical studies have often noted a phenomenon called "perceptual sharpening." This refers to the fact that visual and auditory sensations seem, to the marihuana user, to be heightened (Tart, 1970).

Critical flicker fusion (CFF) has been used for decades in studies on the psysiology of vision. CFF refers to the minimal number of successive flashes of light per second that produces a sensation of steady light. The effects of a variety of drugs on the fusion threshold have been studied (Simonson and Brozek, 1952) suggesting that CFF is a sensitive measure of drug effects on central nervous system (CNS) excitability. Amphetamines raise the CFF threshold (Simonson, Enzer and Blankenstein, 1941), while CNS depressants, such as barbiturates (Rohack, Krasno and Ivy, 1952) and alcohol (Hill, Powell and Goodwin, 1973), usually lower the threshold.

Thirty-one male subjects were studied in this experiment. Testing was conducted in a quiet, dark, windowless room. The subject sat facing the flash lamps of a photostimulator (Lafayette Instrument Co., Model 1202A). The subject's forehead was aligned against the head rest of a telebinocular ophthalmic lens device (Keystone View Co., Model 46C), with the subject viewing two lamps. The photostimulator was placed behind the lens at a distance approximately equal to the focal length of the lens (25 cm). Two NE 34 lamps, each having a diameter of 2 cm, provided 1.1 log foot lamberts of constant intensity throughout the frequency determinations. An exposure photometer (Salford Electrical Instruments) was used to determine light intensity at the surface of the telebinocular lens. The flicker frequency was varied manually by rotation of dials on the photostimulator, frequency varying at a rate of approximately 0.5 cycles per second. Each day before testing began the photostimulator was calibrated against two reference frequencies (24 and 40 cps).

Using the method of limits, stimuli were presented in alternating ascending and descending series. Ten pairs of ascending and descending measures were obtained. Four practice trials were run before testing to insure subjects understood the directions and were responding consistently. The light was varied from 20 to 60 cycles per second. Subjects were asked to report "stop" as soon as the light stopped flickering on ascending trials and report "start" on descending trials. A pre-post design was employed. Subjects in both the marihuana and placebo groups were tested 15 minutes before smoking and within one hour following smoking.

Results

A comparison of the pre-post differences in the marihuana and placebo groups was made. A t-test (random groups) was performed on the difference scores for each subject. This analysis revealed a significant drug effect ($t=1.80$, $df=29$, $p<.05$, one tail). The drug effect was in the direction of enhancement of the CFF; that is, an increase in the flash frequency was necessary to produce fusion.

The mean increase in flicker frequency was 1.33 cycles per second. Statistically significant changes have been found following the administration of numerous drugs (Hill, 1973; Simonson and Brozek, 1952). Because of the small standard error of the mean (0.35 cps) associated with this method, it is possible to detect significant drug-induced changes.

Discussion

The increase in CFF threshold suggests that smoking of marihuana is associated with increased excitability of the visual system. This inference is based on the fact that benzedrine, a known CNS excitant, similarly raises the CFF threshold (Simonson, Enzer and Blankenstein, 1941). This increased ability to discriminate successive exposures of light is consistent with previous clinical reports of "perceptual sharpening" from marihuana (Hollister, 1971). In another study, Sharma and Moskowitz (1972) found that marihuana increased visual autokinetic motion. Benzedrine produces a similar increase in apparent motion (Sharma and Moskowitz, 1972), further suggesting that marihuana acts as a visual excitant. Marihuana apparently fails to affect visual acuity (Moscowitz, Sharma and Schapero, 1972) in contrast to its effect on CFF and autokinesis. This indicates that marihuana may have its greatest effect on time-related processing of information.

In an earlier report by Clark and Nakashima (1968), results of a CFF study indicated that marihuana failed to effect the fusion threshold. However, this finding is difficult to interpret because no statistical data were presented nor was the THC content of the marihuana known.

MARIHUANA AND ANALGESIA

In our third study, the effects of marihuana smoking on perception of both painful and non-painful stimulation in a laboratory setting were investigated. Marihuana, hashish, and other preparations of <u>Cannabis sativa</u> have been used for centuries to relieve pain (Mikuriya, 1969). Whether cannabis actually has analgesic properties has not previously been studied systematically in man. However, case history reports (Noyes and Baram, 1974) indicate the possibility that cannabis may produce analgesic effects in some individuals.

In the present study, 26 healthy male subjects were assigned to a marihuana group (N=20) and a placebo group (N=6). Subject selection, delivery of the marihuana, and the THC content of the marihuana were the same as that described in previous experiments.

Because of the reported influence of psychological factors in the determination of pain thresholds (Wolff and Horland, 1967), subjects were given a structured set of instructions regarding the reporting of sensations.

Stimulation was produced electrically with a Gross Model S4 stimulator. The output was wired in series with a 10,000 ohm resistor so that current received by the subject could be determined. The output signal was fed into a Tektronix oscilloscope (561A) with a dual trace amplifier (3A1), so voltage and amperage could be read and photographed (oscilloscope camera C-12); parallel output was applied to the subject. Electrode paste (Sanborn Redoux Creme) was applied to the subjects' second and fourth fingers, and electrodes were attached.

With the use of the method of limits, ascending and descending thresholds were determined for non-painful and painful stimulation. Pain tolerance was determined by gradually increasing the current above the ascending pain threshold until the subject could no longer tolerate it.

The following instructions, after Wolff and Horland (1967), were given:

> This test uses electrical stimulation to your fingers. You need not worry about any danger associated with the electricity because everything is controlled and safe. I am going to take several measurements with this test. I would like you to give me five verbal responses, which I shall explain to you now. When I first turn on the current you will not feel anything. I will slowly increase the current and I want you to say "now" as soon as you begin to feel the slightest amount of any kind of sensation, such as faint touch or tickling. As the current continues to increase I want you to say "pain" as soon as the first

sensation changes to pain. I repeat: whenever the sensation changes into any kind of pain, ache, or hurting
sensation, I want you to say "pain." As the current continues to increase I want you to say "stop" when you do
not want to take any more of this painful sensation. As
soon as you say "stop" I will turn down the current. As
the current decreases I want you to say "pain gone" as soon
as all the pain has disappeared. Likewise say "sensation
gone" when you no longer feel it. The five responses I
want you to make are listed on this card. We will repeat
this procedure three times.

Use of the oscilloscope camera made it possible to record pain tolerance
(the point at which the subject said "stop") with minimum discomfort. When
the subject said "stop," the camera was immediately triggered and the current
was turned off.

The ascending and descending detection thresholds were based on the
"now" and "all gone" responses, respectively. The ascending and descending
pain threshold was based on the "pain" and "pain gone" categories, respectively, and the subject's pain tolerance was inferred from the point at which
he said "stop." Sensation and pain thresholds as well as tolerance for pain
were measured before smoking began and starting 15 minutes after smoking
ended.

Results

Mean values for sensation and pain thresholds and for pain tolerance
may be seen in Table 2. The placebo and marihuana groups did not differ significantly with respect to baseline presmoking means. Also, no pre-post differences were significant in the placebo group, indicating that repetition of
the procedure did not alter the determination of the thresholds obtained. In
the marihuana group, three significant pre-post differences were found: two
thresholds were decreased (descending sensations and ascending pain), as was
pain tolerance.

Animal studies suggest that marihuana analgesia may occur (Dewey,
Harris, Howes, Kennedy, Granchelli, Pars and Razdan, 1970; Gill, Patton
and Pertwee, 1970; Bauxbaum, Sanders-Bush, and Efron,1969). This may be
due to the fact that near hypnotic doses are often used in these studies. Injection of delta-8-THC and delta-9-THC in mice, in doses sufficient to produce
analgesia, also produces significant decrements in spontaneous motor activity
(Dewey et al. (1970).

Determination of pain thresholds in animal experimentation usually
relies on a motor response such as jumping or tail flicking. In these studies,
failure to make the motor response in a given amount of time is interpreted as
evidence of analgesia. This may or may not be truly indicative of threshold

Table 2. Mean Current Level Before and After Smoking Marihuana or Placebo (In μA)

Response Parameter	Placebo (N=6)				Marihuana (N=20)			
	Pre	Post	Differ-ence	t Value	Pre	Post	Differ-ence	t Value
Ascending Sensation	415.50	433.39	17.89	0.06	425.31	388.23	-37.08	-0.79
Descending Sensation	514.50	563.33	48.83	0.61	622.73	539.60	-83.13[a]	-2.37
Ascending Pain	783.61	887.28	103.67	1.35	1231.52	1006.12	-225.40[a]	-2.25
Descending Pain	952.44	1303.33	350.89	2.39	1188.96	1075.61	-113.35	-1.82
Pain Tolerance	1345.00	1544.88	199.88	0.60	1959.07	1803.15	-155.92[a]	-2.09

[a] $P \leqslant 0.05$ (two-tailed t-test)

changes of experienced pain if the animal's capacity for making a response is retarded.

The present study was designed to evaluate the analgesic effects of a moderate dose (12 mg) of THC in humans. The results indicate that the dose administered failed to decrease sensitivity to painful stimulation and produced, in some cases, a heightened sensitivity to the electrically produced painful stimulation.

There are definite limitations involved in the study of pain in a laboratory setting. One has to do with the fact that there are many types of "experimental" pain available, including aching pain produced by tourniquet (Smith, Egbert, Markowitz, Mosteller and Beecher, 1966), ice-water immersion (Wolff, Kantor, Jarvik and Laska, 1966a, 1966b), and cutaneous stimulation produced thermally (Clark, 1969) or electrically (Wolff et al., 1966a, 1966b). Our results are based on only one type of pain, namely, culaneous electrical stimulation. However, this method has been found to be a reliable and sensitive method of evaluating analgesic agents by other investigators (Wolff et al., 1966a, 1966b).

Among the obvious advantages of electrical stimulation is the quantification and control of the noxious stimulation. Also, each of the 20 subjects given marihuana was used as his own control. Pain and sensation thresholds, as well as pain tolerance, were measured before and after smoking the marihuana. A placebo group was used to evaluate the effects of repeated testing on pain thresholds and tolerance. The placebo group tended to show a decrease in sensitivity on repeated testing, possibly due to habituation to the noxious stimulation. It is of interest, therefore, that the marihuana group showed an increased sensitivity to the painful stimulation following the smoking period.

The relative loading of physiological and psychological factors in the determination of pain thresholds and tolerance is an important question.

Gelfand (1964) has discussed this problem and has assumed that measures of pain tolerance have proportionally higher loading of psychological factors whereas pain threshold measures are loaded more heavily with physiological factors. If this assumption is correct, the significant decrease in ascending pain threshold and pain tolerance indicates that THC affects both physiological and psychological aspects of pain.

However, Clark (1969) has criticized the use of traditional psychophysical methods in the study of pain for their inability to separate sensory and non-sensory variables. He has studied pain in the laboratory setting using a method based on signal detection theory (Green and Swets, 1966) which makes it possible to divide the threshold into two components of observer performance, physiological (sensory) and psychological (non-sensory).

The present study was based on traditional psychophysical methods. Therefore, we are unable to state the relative degree of psychological and physiological loading. Further work, using a signal-detection paradigm (Green and Swets, 1966) is needed to determine how much of the marihuana-induced change in thresholds and tolerance are a result of altered sensory sensitivity and how much is due to changes in response bias, the general tendency of subjects to inhibit or emit the response "pain." Nevertheless, the joint effect of these factors revealed heightened sensitivity to painful stimulation, casting doubt on the usefulness of marihuana as an analgesic drug.

GENERAL DISCUSSION

Results of these experiments allow the following conclusions: marihuana in moderate doses (12 mg THC) (1) produces state-dependent disruption of recall, (2) elevates the critical flicker fusion threshold, and (3) fails to produce analgesia in a laboratory setting.

Certain aspects of marihuana usage on the central nervous system (CNS) may explain these effects. Marihuana has generally been thought of as having sedative effects (Hollister, 1971). This is largely based on subjective reports of marihuana users, indicating relaxation and sleepiness. These "depressant" effects are also suggested by laboratory studies showing decremental effects on motor and memory function (Manno, Kiplinger, Scholz and colleagues, 1971; Melges, Tinklenberg, Hollister and colleagues, 1970). However, on the basis of our findings that marihuana increases sensitivity to intermittent light and to painful and non-painful stimulation, we would conclude that marihuana has, as one of its prominent actions, a stimulating effect on the CNS.

Subjectively, marihuana users often report a heightened "perceptual awareness" (Hollister, 1971; Tart, 1970), suggesting that the drug may have stimulant as well as depressant properties. Also, Kopell, Tinklenberg, and Hollister (1972) have found that contingent negative variation (CNV) amplitudes are enhanced following the use of marihuana. CNV amplitudes are thought to be a measure of complex changes in attention-arousal functions. An enhancement of CNV amplitude is indicative of increased attention and arousal. In another study of CNV amplitudes, Roth, Galanter, Weingartner, and co-workers (1973) found that subjects receiving marihuana had much smaller CNV amplitudes (hence less arousal) for irrelevant stimuli than subjects receiving a placebo.

It is possible, in fact, that the stimulant properties of marihuana apply mainly to experiences that are relevant to the subject, relevant being defined as that which is meaningful because of familiarity or because of the demand characteristics of the experiment.

For example, this may explain the task specificity of state-dependent effects produced with marihuana. In our study, subjects had the most difficulty with tasks having the fewest salient cues, namely, ordered recall of objects or words. When word strings were presented which were meaningful, state-dependent decrements were not evident.

Interpretation of our results concerning the analgesic properties of marihuana may also be seen in light of the "stimulus relevancy" hypothesis. In the present study, subjects were doing their utmost to concentrate on the painful stimulus and respond accordingly as the experimenter demanded. Thus, the painful stimulation may be thought of as highly "relevant" for the subjects. For this reason, it might be expected that they showed a greater sensitivity to pain. To what extent these findings are limited to the laboratory setting is unknown.

A biphasic effect of marihuana has been suggested by Tinklenberg (1975) in which marihuana may be thought of as having stimulant effects soon after smoking, followed by a later depressant effect. This phenomenon might explain our enhancement effect. However, measures in the present study were taken as much as one hour following the smoking period so that if a depressant effect did occur, it would have to have occurred at least one hour following smoking. It seems more likely that marihuana simultaneously produces both depressant and stimulant effects that are, at least in part, determined by the setting in which it is used.

REFERENCES

Barry, H. & Kubena, R. K. Drug addiction: Experimental pharmacology, 1, 3. Mt. Kisco, N.Y.: Futura, 1972.

Bauxbaum, D., Sanders-Bush, E., & Efron, D. H. Analgesic activity of tetrahydrocannabinol (THC) in the rat and mouse. Fed. Proc., 1969, 28, 735.

Clark, W. C. Sensory-decision theory analysis of the placebo effect on the criterion for pain and thermal sensitivity (d'). J. Abnorm. Psychol., 1969, 74, 363.

Clark, L. & Nakashima, E. Experimental studies of marihuana. Am. J. Psychiatry, 1968, 125, 379-384.

Dewey, W. L., Harris, L. S., Howes, J. F., Kennedy, J. S., Granchelli, F. E., Pars, H. G., and Razdan, R. K. Pharmacology of some marijuana constituents and two heterocyclic analogues. Nature, 1970, 226, 1265-1267.

Gelfand, S. The relationship of experimental pain tolerance to pain threshold. Can. J. Psychol., 1964, 18, 36-42.

Gill, E. W., Patton, W. D., & Pertwee, R. G. Preliminary experiments on the chemistry and pharmacology of cannabis. Nature, 1970, 228, 134-136.

Green, D. M., & Swets, J. A. Signal detection theory and psychophysics. New York: Wiley, 1966.

Hill, S. Y., Powell, B. J., & Goodwin, D. W. Critical flicker fusion: Objective measure of tolerance? J. Nerv. Ment. Dis., 1973, 157, 46-50.

Hollister, L. E. Marihuana in man: Three years later. Science, 1971, 171, 21-29.

Kahn, T. C. Manual for the Kahn test of symbol arrangements, Beverly Hills: Western Psychological Services, 1953.

Kopell, B. S., Tinklenberg, J. R., & Hollister, L. E. Contingent negative variation amplitudes. Arch. Gen. Psychiatry, 1972, 27, 809-811.

Manno, J. E., Kiplinger, G. F., Scholz, N., & Forney, R. B. The influence of alcohol and marihuana on motor and mental performance. Clin. Pharmacol. Ther., 1971, 12, 202-211.

Marks, L. E. & Miller, G. A. J. Verb. Learn. Verb. Behav., 1964, 3, 1.

Melges, F., Tinklenberg, J., Hollister, L. E., & Gillespie, H. A. Mari-
    huana and temporal disintegration. Science, 1970, 168, 1118-1120.

Mikuriya, T. H. Marihuana in medicine: Past, present and future. Calif.
    Med., 1969, 110, 34-40.

Moskowitz, H., Sharma, S., & Schapero, M. A comparison of the effects of
    marihuana and alcohol on visual functions. In M. F. Lewis (Ed.),
    Current Research in Marihuana, New York: Academic Press, 1972,
    129-150.

Noyes, R. & Baram, D. A. Cannabis analgesia. Comprehensive Psychiatry,
    1974, 15, 531-535.

Overton, D. A. In B. Kissin and H. Begleiter (Eds.) The biology of alcoholism,
    2, Physiology and behaviour. New York-London: Plenum, 1972.

Palermo, D. S. & Jenkins, J. J. Word association norms: Grade school through
    college. Minneapolis: University of Minnesota Press, 1964.

Renault, P. F., Schuster, C. R., Heinrich, R., & Freedman, D. X. Mari-
    huana: Standardized smoke administration and dose effect curves on
    heart rate in humans. Science, 1971, 174, 589-591.

Rohack, G. S., Krasno, L. R., & Ivy, A. C. Drug effects of flicker fusion
    threshold. J. Appl. Physiol., 1952, 4, 566-574.

Roth, W. T., Galanter, M., Weingartner, H., Vaughan, T. B., & Wyatt,
    R. J. The effect of marihuana and the synthetic-THC on the auditory
    evoked response and background EEG in humans. Biol. Psychiatry,
    1973, 6, 221-233.

Sharma, S., & Moskowitz, H. Effect of marihuana on the visual autokinetic
    phenomenon. Percept. Mot. Skills, 1972, 35, 891-894.

Simonson, E. and Brozek, J. Flicker fusion frequency background and appli-
    cations. Physiol. Rev., 1952, 32, 349-379.

Simonson, E., Enzer, N., & Blankenstein, S. Effect of amphetamine (benze-
    drine) on fatigue of the central nervous system. War Med., 1941, 1,
    690-695.

Smith, G., Egbert, L., Markowitz, R., Mosteller, F., & Beecher, H. An
    experimental pain method sensitive to morphine in man: The sub-maxi-
    mum effort tourniquet technique. J. Pharmacol. Exp. Ther., 1966,
    154, 324-332.

Stillman, R. C., Weingartner, H., Wyatt, R. J., Gillin, C., & Eich, J.
    State-dependent (dissociative) effects of marihuana on human memory.
    Arch. Gen. Psychiatry, 1974, 31, 81-85.

Tart, C. T. Marihuana intoxication: Common experiences. Nature, 1970,
    226, 701-704.

Tinklenberg, J. R. Laboratory and field investigation: Interactions and
    differential advantages. In R. Blum, D. Bovet, and J. Moore (Eds.),
    International Handbook for Drug Classification. Rome: United Nations
    Social Defense Research Institute, 1975.

Wolff, B., & Horland, A. Effect of suggestion upon experimental pain: A
    validation study. J. Abnorm. Psychol., 1967, 72, 402-407.

Wolff, B., Kantor, T. G., Jarvik, M. E., & Laska, E. Response of ex-
    perimental pain to analgesic drugs. I. Morphine, aspirin and placebo.
    Clin. Pharmacol. Ther., 1966a, 7, 224-238.

Wolff, B., Kantor, T. G., Jarvik, M. E., & Laska, E. Response of experi-
    mental pain to analgesic drugs. II. Codeine and placebo. Clin.
    Pharmacol. Ther., 1966b, 7, 323-333.

CHAPTER 11

HYPNOTIC PROPERTIES OF THC: EXPERIMENTAL COMPARISON OF THC,

CHLORAL HYDRATE, AND PLACEBO

Carlos Neu

Assistant Clinical Professor of Psychiatry
Tufts University School of Medicine
Boston, Massachusetts

Alberto DiMascio

Director of Psychopharmacology Research
Commonwealth of Massachusetts
and
Professor of Psychiatry
Tufts University School of Medicine
Boston, Massachusetts

George Zwilling

Research Associate

INTRODUCTION

Tetrahydrocannabinol (THC) was found by Mechoulam in 1964 to be the active ingredient of marihuana (Mechoulam, 1965) which reproduces in man all the mind-altering effects found in marihuana users. Besides the well-known psychological effects of this psychoactive ingredient of particular importance for this study are the reports of its sedative and calming properties which were initially reported by O'Shaughnessy in the middle of the nineteenth century. He found cannabis (generic for marihuana) to have muscle-relaxant anticonvulsant and analgesic properties. Perhaps the most important finding, which still holds, was that even with the large doses of cannabis that had been given to different animals, no one died. O'Shaughnessy's findings awakened great interest in Europe where numerous reports sprouted, indicating a wide gamut of actions: soporific and sleep-inducing, for the treatment of menstrual cramps, coughs, insomnia, and as a mild somnificant (Wood, 1886; Hare and Chrystie, 1892).

Turning to the more recent literature, Grinspoon (1971) reports of the safety of cannabis. Increase in pulse rate and occasional transitory hypotension are the only noteworthy physiological changes caused by cannabis (Grinspoon, 1971; Hollister, 1971; Gorodetzky and Jasinski, 1967). Depersonalization and transitory psychotic-like breaks have only been reported at high doses (Melges, Tinklenberg, and Hollister, 1970). As stated by Cousens and DiMascio (1973), because of THC's low lethality and absence of serious toxic effects, the advantages of this drug over the standard hypnotic sedative drugs are obvious.

Preliminary studies on sleep EEG using smoked marihuana reported by Kales, Hanley, and Rickles (1971) showed that the "initial smoking produces a decrease in REM sleep, but very quickly there is a return to REM sleep baseline levels and above baseline levels as the smoking is continued over a short period."

OBJECTIVES

The study had two separate phases, both with similar experimental designs. In the first phase, the aims of the study were to examine the hypnotic properties for (-) delta-9-THC -- its efficacy in both inducing and maintaining sleep in insomniacs -- and to examine the benefit/side effect ratio at various dosage levels. The second phase, which was based on the results of the first, aimed to further examine the hypnotic properties of the drug at doses not expected to induce the hangover effect reported at the higher doses of the first phase. A further objective was to compare THC with a known sedative-hypnotic agent.

EXPERIMENTAL PROCEDURE

General Design

In both phases of the study, a similar general design was followed. In the first study, 9 healthy male subjects were tested once a week for a 6-week period to determine the effects of (-) delta-9-THC. The first two sessions were adjustment trials to the laboratory. The results to be reported correspond to the last four sessions during which the subjects were given 10 mg, 20 mg, and 30 mg of the experimental drug and a placebo. During the second phase, 10 male subjects were tested weekly for 6 weeks to determine the effects of three doses of THC (5 mg, 10 mg, 15 mg), chloral hydrate (500 mg), and placebo in altering their usual sleep pattern. The first session was used for familiarizing the subjects to the environment and each other.

In both phases, the subjects were given, in accordance with a replicated latin square design, the THC, placebo and, in the second phase, the chloral hydrate as well. The study was double blind (to the subjects and the sleep observer-recorder) while the researchers (Cousens in the first; Neu in the second) knew the code in order to prepare and administer the preparation at each session. One-half hour after administering the liquid, the researchers left the laboratory, remaining on call for the duration of each session.

Subject Selection

Advertising through a local newspaper for healthy males, 21 to 40 years of age with sleep difficulties, to participate in a sleep study with a new (FDA-approved) potential medication, were asked to call the laboratory. No mention of marihuana was made.

On the initial phone contact, callers were asked about their sleep habits; if they were currently using hypnotics or other psychoactive medications; as well as whether they had experience with marihuana. Questions regarding their physical and mental health were also asked. Only after these questions were answered, the callers were told that the investigational drug was synthetic marihuana. Those who were in good physical and mental health, not currently on sedative or psychoactive medication, with experience in the use of marihuana -- but not currently heavy users (1-2 week maximum), and reporting that they usually required at least one hour to fall asleep, were asked to answer three questionnaires to be mailed out. The forms mailed included: (1) a questionnaire about their sleep habits, (2) the Langner Psychiatric Impairment Scale (Shader, Ebert, and Harmatz, 1971), and (3) the Taylor Manifest Anxiety Scale (Taylor, 1953).

Eligible candidates were required to have a rating of less than 5 in the Langner Scale and less than 23 in the Taylor Anxiety Scale ($\bar{x} = 15$ in Phase I; $\bar{x} = 11.7$ in Phase II). These subjects were further screened by a personal interview with the project psychiatrist in order to further rule out those with any psychotic or marked neurotic symptoms, as well as those with physical contraindications. Subjects were instructed not to ingest any psychoactive drugs for a week prior to the onset of the study, as well as throughout its duration.

Setting

In the first phase of the study, all 9 subjects slept in one large room with dividers between the beds. In the second phase, two dormitory rooms housed six and four beds (no dividers were used this time). In both phases, two additional rooms were available for studying and TV watching.

Drugs and Dosage

THC was (-)-trans-delta-9-tetrahydrocannabinol 95% in dehydrated alcohol prepared and obtained from the National Institute of Mental Health. In the second phase, liquid chloral hydrate (Noctec®) was used. To mask the flavors of these drugs, they were placed in a drink composed of Fresca®, Bitter Lemon®, cherry juice, and drops of almond extract. The placebo was the drink without the drugs.

The three dose levels of THC used were 10, 20, and 30 mg. These dosages spanned a range that has been noted to induce sleep and have some psychoactive effects, yet not cause the subjects to lose contact with reality.

The THC dose levels used during the second phase reflected the findings of the first in which the two highest were accompanied by a hangover effect sufficiently severe to render the use of these unadvisable. Chloral hydrate was used at a 500 mg level.

Once the preparation was given to the subjects, they were allowed to socialize in moderation for one hour. After that, all interaction was stopped, although reading or watching TV was permitted until each individual felt like going to sleep.

Data Collection

An experienced sleep observer-rater was present from the time of drug ingestion until the next morning. He recorded the subjects' activities prior to retiring, and at 15-minutes intervals he made a bed-sleep check for all subjects throughout the night. The rater recorded time at which a subject went to bed, when he fell asleep, and whether he was awake or asleep during each subsequent bed-sleep check.

In the morning, subjects filled out a questionnaire pertaining to the quality of their sleep and changes noticed from their usual sleep pattern.

Data on side effects were collected on three occasions: (a) pre-medication, (b) on awakening the next morning, and (c) the following evening to record persistence of side effects ("hangover effects"). The side effects checklist was based on a form used by Linton and Langs (1962) to capture effects of psychotomimetic drugs and one developed by DiMascio and co-workers for the general drug side effects.

RESULTS

Data were examined with regard to: sleep induction, sleep interruption, quality of sleep, and side effects.

Sleep Induction

Two measures of sleep induction were recorded: the time it took to go to bed after ingesting the medication, and the time it took to fall asleep. In addition, a total sleep induction measure was obtained by summing these two measures. To test the significance of difference among the various treatment cells, analysis of variance (repeated measurements) were carried out.

In the first study, while analyses of variance of the "time to bed" measure and the "time to fall asleep" measure failed to show statistically significant differences, the "total time to fall asleep" was significant at $P < 0.05$. While all three doses of THC shortened the "total time to fall asleep" as compared to placebo, the 20 mg dose shortened the time the most; its mean difference from the placebo was 62 minutes ($P < 0.01$) (Table 1).

In the second study, the data tended to indicate that it took patients longer to decide to get into bed if they had taken THC, in comparison to placebo or chloral hydrate. However, once in bed with the two lower doses of THC, the subjects tended to go to sleep more rapidly. As stated above, none of these drug condition times were statistically significant from the placebo times.

Table 1

Total Time to Fall Asleep

Phase 1

Dosage	Time	Mean Difference from Placebo	P Value from Placebo
Placebo	3.00*	---	
10 mg. THC	2.28	0.72	< 0.05
20 mg. THC	1.96	1.04	< 0.01
30 mg. THC	2.10	0.90	< 0.05

Phase II

Placebo	2.80*	---	Ⓐ
CLH [+]	2.77	0.03	
5 mg. THC	3.05	-0.25	
10 mg. THC	3.00	-0.20	
15 mg. THC	3.40	-0.60	

* Hours after medication ingested
+ Chloral hydrate (500 mg.)
Ⓐ No statistical significance

Sleep Interruption Data

Throughout the night, the subjects' sleep was checked. Once the sleep observer had found them to be asleep, the number of awakenings were recorded during the night. Each subject was observed at 15-minute intervals. Each "awakening unit" was measured as 15 minutes. The total number of 15-minute units was then counted as the frequency of awakenings.

Whereas during the Phase I study, fewer awakenings and less time awake were noticed during the first half of the night, with the trend becoming greater as the dose of THC was increased, during Phase II, the number of awakenings did not differ statistically under any drug condition (chloral hydrate included). There was a tendency for the highest dose of THC given during Phase II (15 mg) toward fewer awakenings during the first half of the night. This finding is in line with those described above for Phase I.

Side Effect Data

In order to establish a baseline for the emergence of side effects and to determine the psychotomimetic properties of THC, a side effect checklist was administered to the participants before each session and repeated upon awakening in the morning and the following evening. The striking finding of the analysis of side effects data is that none were severe. In the study where the higher doses of THC were used, a number of subjects talked about being "spaced out," "stoned," or "hung over" during the next day for a range from several hours to 24 hours. As the dosage increased (10 mg to 20 mg and 30 mg), so did the degree and duration of these feelings, as well as the number of subjects reporting such experiences (after 10 mg, 1 subject; after 20 mg, 5 subjects; after 30 mg, 5 subjects). There seemed to be a pronounced subjective distinction between the middle and highest doses, with the latter producing a "stoned" sensation of a longer time span.

The other side effects reported included dry mouth, particularly in the second study in all treatment modalities (this may have been caused by very dry atmospheric conditions in the laboratory). "Objects look different," "feelings of unreality," and "hard to concentrate" were effects reported by subjects in both studies with a tendency to get worse at the higher doses.

Cousens (Phase I) reported that THC given at night time had a beneficial sleep-inducing effect. When 20 mg or 30 mg were given, the hypnotic effect was accompanied by an unpleasant "hangover effect." In that first study, it was found that the subjects fell asleep on the low dose of THC (10 mg) an average of 43 minutes earlier than with placebo and without the hangover effect found with the higher doses. In the Phase II study, it was decided to span Cousens' optimum dose (10 mg) 5 mg in either direction so that a greater resolution of the dose-response curve could be obtained.

The results of the second phase indicate that at the doses of THC used, contrary to findings in the first phase, the hypnotic properties of THC were limited. However, the data on chloral hydrate (500 mg), surprisingly, also failed to produce hypnotic activity. In comparison to the placebo, none of the active treatment cells facilitated sleep induction nor did they extend the actual duration of sleep.

In contrast to objective data, subjective reports indicated that it took less time to go to bed after the THC ingestion (especially the high dose) than after the placebo. The subjects also reported that on the next day they were "tired, hungover, and groggy" after the high dose of THC as compared to the other four treatment situations.

It was found that those side effects noted in the first phase to be most commonly reported were also reported more frequently by the subjects of the second experiment.

While the negative findings on the objective measurements of sleep induction and duration (which contrast with those found by Cousens at 10 mg) deserve explanation, we have been unable to come up with solid reasons. The possibility of the decomposition of the THC was discounted after laboratory testing by the National Institute of Mental Health on this possibility. Like-wise, the chloral hydrate was potent. The laboratory and experimental condi-tions of the present study were basically similar to Cousens', but one major difference may have contributed to the disparity of the findings. While Cousens ran his study during the spring, this project took place during the winter. During this season, unfortunately, the control of room temperature was diffi-cult, causing either very warm or very cold conditions in the laboratory. Some of the participants complained about these temperature changes, and it is pos-sible that it caused serious enough discomfort, thus reducing greatly the drug effect.

In conclusion, the second project failed to show significant hypnotic properties for THC as well as for chloral hydrate. Perhaps because of unfortu-nately great variability in the laboratory conditions, this second study failed to confirm Cousens' findings. Neither study finding should be considered con-clusive. The very important advantages of THC (that is, safety and low inci-dence of side effects) over many other currently used hypnotics warrant more extensive research.

References

Cousens, K. and DiMascio, A. (-) Delta-9-THC as an hypnotic. Psycho-
     pharmacologia (Berlin), 1973, 33, 355-364.

Gorodetzky, C. W. & Jasinski, I. H. Effect of (-) delta-9-trans. tetrahydro-
     cannabinol. Psychopharmacologia (Berlin), 1967, 11, 184-188.

Grinspoon, L. Marihuana reconsidered. Cambridge: Harvard University
     Press, 1971, 227-228.

Hare, H. A. & Chrystie, W. A system of practical therapeutics. Vol. 3.
     Philadelphia: Lee Brothers, 1892.

Hollister, L. E. Marihuana in man: Three years later. Science, 1971, 172,
     21-28.

Kales, A., Hanley, J., & Rickles, W. Effects on marihuana administration
     and withdrawal in chronic users and naive subjects. Presented at First
     International Congress of the Association of the Psychophysiological
     Study of Sleep, June, 1971.

Linton, H. B. & Langs, R. J. Subjective reactions to lysergic acid diethyla-
     mide. Arch. Gen. Psychiat., 1962, 6, 352-368.

Mechoulam, R. J. & Gaoni, Y. A total synthesis on dl-tetra -detrahydrocan-
     nabinol, the active constituent of hashish. J. Amer. Chem. Soc.,
     1965, 87, 3273-3275.

Melges, F. T., Tinklenberg, J. R., & Hollister, L. E. Temporal disintegra-
     tion and depersonalization during marihuana intoxication. Arch. Gen.
     Psychiat., 1970, 23, 204-210.

O'Shaughnessy, W. B. On the preparation of Indian hemp or gunjah (Cannabis
     indica). Trans. Med. Phys. Soc. Bombay, 1842.

Shader, R. I., Ebert, M. H., & Harmatz, J. S. Langner's psychiatric impair-
     ment scale: A short screening device. Amer. J. Psychiat., 1971,
     128, 5, 596-601.

Taylor, J. A. A personality scale of manifest anxiety. J. Abn. Soc. Psychol.,
     1953, 48, 285-290.

Wood, H. C. J. Treatise on Therapeutics, 6th Ed. Philadelphia: Lippincott,
     1886.

CHAPTER 12

THE EFFECT OF BETA-ADRENERGIC BLOCKADE ON ACUTE MARIHUANA INTOXICATION

L. Vachon
A. Sulkowski

Boston University School of Medicine
Boston, Massachusetts

NOTE: This study was supported by National Institute
on Drug Abuse research grant DA00067.

There is at present a considerable body of experimental data documenting both the peripheral and the CNS effects of acute marihuana intoxication. So far, however, there is little information concerning the neuropharmacologic mechanisms involved. Sympathomimetic and anticholinergic hypotheses have been proposed (Beaconsfield, Ginsberg and Rainsbury, 1972; Drew and Miller, 1974); the amino acid neurotransmitters and prostaglandins have been also considered as possible biochemical mediators of the "high" and its behavioral correlates (Sklenovsky, Navratil and Hrbek, 1974; Burstein and Raz, 1975). The sympathomimetic hypothesis has been supported in respect of the cardiovascular changes of which tachycardia remains the most reliable sign of intoxication. The beta adrenergic blockade has been consistently reported to be effective in preventing this striking effect (Clark, 1975). The results of analogous experiments with the drugs affecting the cholinergic neurotransmission have been largely inconclusive, at least in human volunteers (Beaconsfield, 1972; Freemon, Rosenblatt and El-Yousef, 1975).

In the report where the beta-adrenergic receptor blockade has been shown to counteract effectively the marihuana-induced rise in heart rate and blood flow (Beaconsfield et al., 1972), there was no report of the subjective psychological experience nor of any objective tests of psychomotor performance. In the study (Drew and Miller, 1974) where an effort was made to study the effects of propranolol on marihuana induced cognitive dysfunctioning, there was no evidence of propranolol activity by itself nor of modification of the marihuana effect. The dose of delta-9-THC delivered in the smoke was less than 1.0 mg, which is a small dose by most standards.

We felt that the question should be reinvestigated with careful simultaneous and more sophisticated monitoring of subjective, behavioral, and physiological variables. The propranolol and the marihuana should be administered in effective dosages, separately and in combination. It has been shown rather convincingly that propranolol does cross the blood-brain barrier and is distributed throughout the CNS in rabbits, monkeys, and man (Hayes and Cooper, 1971; Myers, Lewis, Reid and Dollery, 1975).

SUBJECTS, MATERIALS, AND METHODS

Six male subjects were recruited through a newspaper advertisement asking for volunteers in a physiological experiment. No mention was made of marihuana. The subjects were interviewed by a psychiatrist and given a battery of psychological tests and a physical exam. Only subjects with good health, a good adaptation to their life situation, and who had prior marihuana experience were admitted to the study. They were given a complete description of the procedure and purpose of the project as well as the name of the medication and the possible side effects. They signed a statement of informed consent.

Propranolol, 120 mg., was given by mouth one hour before smoking. The placebo for this medication was a similar looking tablet which contained 100 mg of Vitamin C. The marihuana cigarettes, 1 gram containing 2% delta-9-THC, were supplied by NIDA. Reanalysis at the end of the experiment showed that their content was 1% delta-9-THC. The placebo cigarettes were made with marihuana from which the THC had been extracted.

There were three test days: On one the subject received propranolol and the placebo marihuana. On another he received the placebo for propranolol and the active marihuana, and on the third he received both active medications. The order of administration was balanced between the subjects.

Each session consisted of a pre-treatment session before the medications were administered and a post-treatment session where the same tests were repeated in the same order. The sequence was (1) reaction time, (2) CPT, (3) matching tests, (4) ADSST and tests of memory. The heart rate and blood pressure were measured and conjunctival reddening rated (0-4 points scale) during rest intervals between the tests.

The reaction time was measured as the time to press a hand-held micro-switch button with the thumb in response to a signal. First the stimulus was the letter "X" flashed on a random interval (1.0 to 3.0 seconds) for 3 minutes. This was followed by the auditory stimuli: This time a tone (1000 Hz) was administered as the visual stimulus had been. Finally, both the tone and the flash were presented simultaneously. The response to the visual stimulation is in the order of 200 milliseconds while the response to the auditory stimulus is faster by about 15 milliseconds. The response to the bisensory stimulation is again faster than either by 10 to 15 milliseconds. Optimally, when both are presented simultaneously, the two stimuli should not be exactly simultaneous but offset by the difference in response time characteristic of each individual. In the present pilot exploration in the use of this test we have not built such a difference into our apparatus.

For the Continuous Performance Test (CPT), the "A-X" task was used. The subject was asked to press a button within 0.75 seconds after the appearance of the letter X if it was just preceded by an "A." The trial lasted 5 minutes with the presentation of approximately 200 stimuli, 25% of which were critical. To increase the difficulty of the CPT, we have reduced the duration of the stimulus to 50 milliseconds (1/2 of the usual duration) and the presentation of the stimuli is randomized between 0.75 to 1.5 seconds.

The Automated Digit Symbol Substitution Test (ADSST) is an electronic version of the well-known paper and pencil test. The subject was presented with letters flashing in a random sequence and was asked to press the corresponding number button on a touch tone keyboard according to a code placed next to the stimulus display. A new stimulus followed one second after each response. The code was presented to the subject only during a trial. Each trial lasted 3 minutes; there were 5 trials, interrupted by two-minute rest periods. The scoring system was designed to reflect the learning process.

A response was classified as "correct" (C) when it was according to the code and within two seconds after the appearance of the stimulus. It was "late correct" (L) when it occurred more than two seconds after the stimulus (S) but still according to the code; it was "incorrect" if it did not correspond to the code or occurred more than 4 seconds after the stimulus. If a subject pressed twice in response to a stimulus, the second response was considered an "over-push" (Op). The result of each trial is calculated as the General Index (GI). The general index (GI) is weighted for both speed and accuracy of performance:

$$GI = (2C + 2S + L) - Op$$

The Matching Task was administered essentially the same way as the ADSST except that the stimulus was a number and the subject was to press the corresponding identical number on the touch-tone. The scoring was exactly as for the ADSST.

The Test of Memory (TOM) was presented at the end of each ADSST trial. The subject was presented each letter once and asked to press the corresponding code number he remembered. The trial took only 30 seconds.

The heart rate was measured from the monitor leads of an EKG recording. The blood pressure was measured by the usual sphygmomanometric method.

Finally, at the end of each experimental session the subjects rated the intensity of the subjective "high" on a 0-100 point scale where 0 corresponds to "not high at all" and 100 to "the most intense high I have ever experienced after marihuana."

RESULTS

The marihuana preceded by the placebo-propranolol resulted in the well-known pattern of physiologic changes: clear tachycardia, rise in systolic blood pressure, and conjunctival injection. The propranolol followed by the placebo marihuana caused a moderate but significant drop in heart rate (by 10 bpm) and in systolic blood pressure (by 18 mm) without eye reddening. The interaction of both treatments (propranolol and marihuana) resulted in a slight but clear increase in the heart rate immediately after smoking, and a gradual decrease afterwards. This reduction in the tachy-cardia is highly significant when compared either with the baseline ($p < .025$) or the post-marihuana values ($p < .005$). The conjunctival injection ratings after combined propranolol and marihuana fell midway between the ratings performed after each of these drugs administered with the other placebo ($p < .05$).

The analysis of the Continuous Performance Test (CPT) and matching test (MT) showed that there is no significant treatment nor trial effects.

The ADSST learning curve was, however, markedly depressed following the administration of the placebo-propranolol with the active marihuana. The propranolol with the placebo marihuana was without effect but beta blockade prevented the marihuana-induced decrease in performance when both active medications were combined.

The retention of the code was tested after each ADSST trial: Marihuana with the placebo-propranolol reduced the number of correct recalls and again the propranolol appeared to prevent this effect; propranolol with the placebo marihuana did not interfere with the correct responding.

The visual reaction time was not significantly affected by the different treatments in this small sample ($N = 5$ for this test). The administration of marihuana, with or without propranolol, prolonged the auditory reaction time by about 15%, which is in contrast with the small change after the propranolol without the active marihuana ($p < .05$). The bisensory reaction time is also unchanged by the administration of propranolol without active marihuana. But after the active marihuana (and the placebo-propranolol) it is prolonged by 18%; this prolongation is significantly reduced by the interaction of both active medications ($F = 9.876$, $p < .01$).

The self-rated intensity of subjective "high" varied between treatments ($F = 29.24$, $p < .01$). It followed the pattern of physiological and behavioral variables with the highest values for placebo propranolol plus marihuana treatment. Propranolol reduced significantly the intensity of the marihuana high ($p < .005$) but did not bring it down to the propranolol and placebo-marihuana treatment level ($p < .001$).

DISCUSSION

The physiological effects of marihuana which we observed here are similar to those reported by others and ourselves before. As expected, the propranolol prevented the tachycardia and the rise in systolic blood pressure.

Similarly, the psychomotor performance and subjective rating of "high" after marihuana are replications of those of our previous reports (Vachon, Sulkowski and Rich, 1974; Vachon and Sulkowski, 1976). The addition of the Matching Task and Test of Memory made the analysis of ADSST performance more precise. The matching allows us to estimate the changes in simple psychomotor responding, which does not involve learning and information processing. The memory test permits us to assess the contribution of impaired retention (short-term memory). The matching task is not affected by marihuana; the recall of the code is. The memory test needs further improvement; the variance is very high because the subjects are presented with each letter only once per trial for a total of only 10 stimuli.

A neuropsychological prototype of central (cortical) information processing and integration is the difference between reaction times to unisensory and bisensory stimuli (Hershenson, 1962; Anreassi and Greco, 1975). We introduced this experimental technique to test our hypothesis that marihuana-induced changes in ADSST performance reflect an impairment of these central processes and cannot be explained by psychomotor slowdown and/or memory deficit. The present results lend some support to our hypothesis: Marihuana prolonged reaction time to bisensory stimulation and this effect was significantly reduced by pretreatment with propranolol.

The reduction by propranolol of the marihuana "high" may be due to propranolol peripheral action with or without simultaneous effect at the level of the CNS. It would seem, however, that the prevention of the slight memory impairment, the reduction of the clear impairment of learning on the ADSST, and of the attenuation of the bisensory disintegration, should be assigned to the interaction of the beta-blocker and marihuana in the CNS itself. This would suggest that the brain adrenergic pathways are involved in the production of some of the marihuana effects.

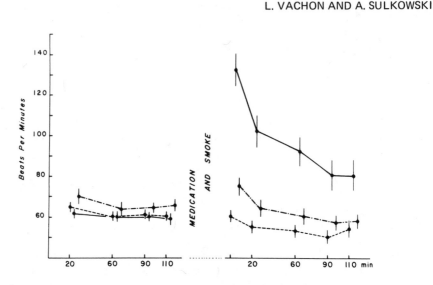

Figure 1. Heart rate ($\bar{x} \pm$ SEM) before and after (1) propranolol (dotted line), (2) propranolol followed by marihuana (dot and dash line), and (3) marihuana (solid line) treatments. See text for details.

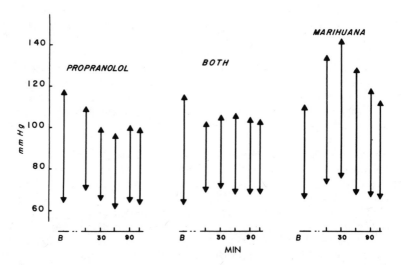

Figure 2. Blood pressure ($\bar{x}$) during baseline (B) and following the administration of the three treatments. Only the changes in systolic BP are significant: (1) Propranolol was followed by a reduction ($p < .01$) from 30 minutes after the treatment on; (2) the combined treatment resulted in a slight drop ($p < .05$) only immediately after the smoking; (3) marihuana caused marked elevation immediately ($p < .01$) and 30 minutes ($p < .05$) after the smoking.

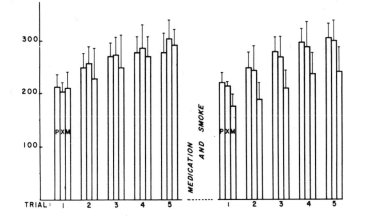

Figure 3. ADSST performance (General Index: $\bar{x} \pm$ SD of each trial) before and after propranolol (P), marihuana (M), and the combined treatment (X). The pre-treatment trials show a clear learning effect but no difference between the three conditions. The post-treatment trials show a definite differential effect between the treatments (F = 11.2, p < .005). After active marihuana (M) the scores of each trial are significantly lower than those obtained after either of the other two treatments (p values are less than .025 for the first 3 trials and less than .01 for the last 2). There is clearly no difference between the trials after propranolol followed by either the placebo marihuana or the active marihuana.

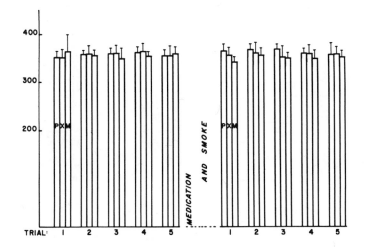

Figure 4. Matching Task performance (General Index, $\bar{x} \pm$ SD) before and after propranolol (P), marihuana (M), and the combined treatment (X). There is no learning effect nor any difference between the treatments.

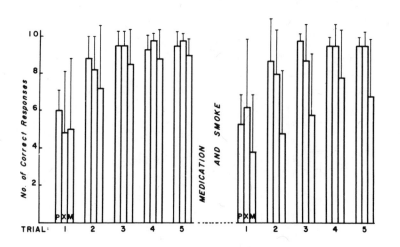

Figure 5. Test of Memory. This shows the number of letters recalled correctly ($\bar{x} \pm$ SD) during a single sequential presentation of the 10 letters after each ADSST trial. There is a significant treatment effect (post treatment: F = 4.2, p < .05) despite the large intersubject variability.

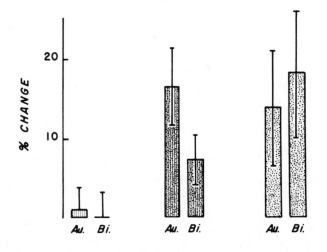

Figure 6. Reaction time. The reaction time is presented in milliseconds ($\bar{x} \pm$ SEM) after propranolol (vertical lines), marihuana (dots), and the combined treatment (vertical lines and dots) for the auditory (Au) and bisensory (Bi) stimuli.

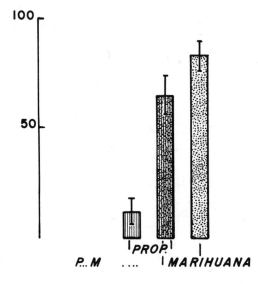

Figure 7. "High" Rating. The subjective rating ($\bar{x}$ + SD) of the "high" on a scale of 0 ("not high at all") to 100 ("highest ever") are shown for propranolol (vertical lines), marihuana (dots), and the combined treatment (vertical lines and dots).

REFERENCES

Andreassi, J.L., & Greco, J.R. Effects of bisensory stimulation on reaction time and the evoked cortical potential. Physiol. Psychol., 1975, 3, 183-194.

Beaconsfield, P., Ginsburg, J., & Rainsbury, R. Marihuana smoking: cardiovascular effects on man and possible mechanisms. New England J. Med., 1972, 287, 210.

Burstein, S. & Raz, A. Inhibition of prostaglandin E_2 biosynthesis by delta-1-tetrahydrocannabinol. Prostaglandins, 1972, 2, 369-374.

Clark, S.C. Marihuana and the cardiovascular system. Pharm. Biochem. Behav., 1975, 3, 299-306.

Drew, W.G., Kiplinger, G.F., Miller, L.L, et al. Effects of propranolol on marihuana-induced cognitive dysfunctioning. Clin. Pharmacol. Therap., 1972, 13, 526-533.

Drew, W.G. & Miller, L.L. Cannabis: Neural mechanisms and behavior -- a theoretical review. Pharmacol., 1974, 11, 12-32.

Freemon, F.R., Rosenblatt, J.E., & El-Yousef, M.K. Interaction of physostigmine and delta-9-tetrahydrocannabinol in man. Clin. Pharmacol. Ther., 1975, 17, 121-126.

Hayes, A. & Cooper, R.G. Studies on the absorption, distribution and excretion of propranolol in rat, dog, and monkey. J. Pharmacol. Exp. Ther., 1971, 176, 302-311.

Hershenson, M. Reaction time as a measure of intersensory facilitation. J. Exp. Psychol., 1962, 63, 289-293.

Myers, M.G., Lewis, P.J., Reid, J.L., & Dollery, C.T. Brain concentration of propranolol in relation to hypotensive effect in the rabbit with observations on brain propranolol levels in man. J. Pharm. Exp. Ther., 1975, 192, 327-335.

Sklenovsky, A., Navratil, J., & Hrbek, J. Effect of delta-9-tetrahydrocannabinol on free amino acids in the brain. Activ. Nerv. Sup., 1974, 16, 216-217.

Vachon, L., Sulkowski, A., & Rich, E.S., Jr. Marihuana effects on learning, attention and time estimation. Psychopharmacologia (Berl.), 1974, 39, 1-11.

Vachon, L., & Sulkowski, A. Attention, learning and speed in psychomotor
    performance after marihuana smoking. In M.C. Braude & S. Szara
    (Eds.), The Pharmacology of Marihuana. New York: Raven Press, 1976,
    in press.

CHAPTER 13

THE USE OF MARIHUANA IN THE TREATMENT OF ALCOHOLISM

Chaim M. Rosenberg

Boston University School of Medicine

Boston, Massachusetts

The past decade has seen an increasing awareness of the impact on
man of alcohol abuse. The skid-row stereotype of alcoholism has slowly
given way to the realization that this illness ranges from mild and reversible
to severe and chronic and that all strata of the population are affected. Not
only does alcoholism impair the physical and mental health of the individual
but it also diminishes his social and economic well-being and that of his
family.

In spite of a very considerable effort to provide effective treatment
for alcoholic persons, success has largely eluded us. All too often people
who develop clear signs of alcoholism deny their addiction and avoid seeking
treatment until their condition has entered a destructive stage. Those who
enter treatment frequently continue to drink episodically and most soon drop
out and are lost to follow-up. It would seem that the power of alcohol on the
person is so strong that a tremendous resolve is required before the drug is
given up completely.

Several models have been developed in an effort to treat the alcoholic.
Most of these models insist upon continuous sobriety as a basic requirement
before psychological and social rehabilitation can occur. Unfortunately, the
use of psychotherapy alone or combined with tranquilizers or antidepressant
medication has not proved very effective in reducing drinking or improving
clinic attendance (Ditman, 1966; Kissin, Platz and Su, 1971; Gerrein,
Rosenberg and Manohar, 1973; Rosenberg, 1974). The drug disulfiram
(Antabuse) blocks a stage in the metabolism of alcohol and if taken at the
same time as alcohol it causes a severe reaction. Many alcoholics take this
drug as added protection against the impulse to drink. When disulfiram was
introduced in 1948 it was hailed as a considerable advance in the treatment
of alcoholism. With the passage of time, however, the enthusiasm for it has
dwindled. The disulfiram-alcohol reaction is feared and many patients

refuse to take the drug. The majority of those who do agree to take disulfiram soon discontinue its use and return to the use of alcohol. Several explanations are given why patients stop taking the drug. Firstly, failure to comply with treatment is not unique to alcoholism but occurs in all illnesses, especially those which are of long duration (Davis, 1968; Blackwell, 1973; Marston, 1970). Secondly, disulfiram blocks the effects of alcohol but provides nothing in its place. Alcohol is more than a beverage to the alcoholic. It is a way of life -- involving barroom atmosphere, friendships, and a way to fill time. The patient is faced with a choice and usually choses to give up disulfiram and return to his old haunts. Since there are no withdrawal symptoms from stopping disulfiram, the return to alcohol is possible after a few days.

Methadone maintenance in the treatment of heroin addiction provides us with another model for the treatment of addictions. Not only does methadone "block" the euphoric effects of heroin but it also prevents heroin withdrawal symptoms. The addict soon becomes dependent on methadone and needs to attend the clinic very regularly to receive the drug. While he attends, progress can be made towards his integration into society and moving him away from crime. Complete abstinence is a difficult goal to reach. The methadone model suggests that if one drug is to be given up, then something should be substituted in its place. We speculate that an alcoholic would be willing to give up alcohol and take disulfiram on a regular basis only if an acceptable alternative to alcohol is provided. At the present time, however, there is no substance available in the treatment of alcoholism that is equivalent to methadone use in heroin addiction. Perhaps marihuana -- or some similar preparation -- could serve as a reinforcer for disulfiram and as a substitute for alcohol?

We first became interested in this idea some four years ago. At that time it was commonly believed that while each drug could provide a "high" the use of one precluded the use of the other. Marihuana was the part of the youth counterculture, while alcohol was the drug of the establishment. Thus, Zinberg and Weil (1970) stated that where the use of marihuana became more regular, so "the use of alcohol, especially distilled spirits, declined proportionately or even more steeply." Becker (1963) suggested that when people begin to use larger amounts of alcohol, barbituates, or opiates they reduce their use of marihuana. The passage of time, alas, has shown that the assumed antagonism between alcohol and marihuana was more the result of societal forces than a pharmacological incompatibility. Nowadays both drugs are used by young people -- often at the same time.

A look into the literature shows that the therapeutic use of marihuana in alcoholism is not a new idea. Kane in 1881 described a patient who took hashish in an effort to control her addiction to alcohol. Thompson and Proctor (1953) used a marihuana derivative -- pyrahexyl -- in the treatment of alcohol withdrawal states.

At the present time marihuana does not seem to be widely used by alcoholic persons. We surveyed 240 new patients seen at the alcoholism clinic at Boston City Hospital. Each patient was questioned about his drug and alcohol use during the month before coming to the clinic. Nearly one-third admitted to using tranquilizers on at least four days during each week. Five percent had used barbiturates but less than 2% had used either ampheta-mines or opiates. Nearly 7% of the 240 patients admitted to using marihuana up to four times a week but less than 1% had used the drug more than four times a week. Younger patients were more likely to have been using mari-huana than older patients. Thus, nearly 20% of those under 36 years of age had used the drug during the previous month as compared to only 3% among those age 36 or older.

During 1972 we invited subjects who had completed treatment for alcohol intoxication to participate in an experiment involving the use of marihuana. Out of 25 patients we approached only 5 agreed to try the drug (one of whom developed an acute paranoid reaction). Most placed marihuana in the same category as heroin and considered it more dangerous even than alcohol. It is possible, however, that this extreme view has softened with time and that nowadays a greater proportion of alcoholics, especially those who are younger, will be willing to participate in an experiment with this drug.

Before testing the potential therapeutic uses of marihuana in alco-holism it was necessary to proceed through a number of steps and to seek answers to the following questions: (1) What are the acute effects of mari-huana on alcoholics as compared to normals? (2) What are the acute effects of marihuana as compared to the effects of alcohol when these drugs are administered to normals and alcoholics? (3) What are the effects of disulfiram and marihuana when given at the same time? (4) Will alcoholics agree to take marihuana over a fairly lengthy period and at the same time agree to take disulfiram?

Advertisements were placed in local daily newspapers and student magazines calling for male subjects to participate in our drug studies. Ninety-one men responded and were asked to come in to complete a question-naire dealing with their psychological and physical health and their patterns of drug use. In this part of the study we recruited healthy subjects who were only light users of alcohol, marihuana, and other drugs and had no history of serious physical or mental disorder. Thirty normal subjects completed the experiment (two others experienced a transient paranoid reaction after smoking marihuana and did not complete the procedure). The normal subjects varied in age from 21 to 32 years. Nearly all had attended college with an average of 15 years of education each. At the time of the study most of them were attending one or another of the universities in metropolitan Boston. They participated in the study out of curiosity as well as for the opportunity to smoke "good" marihuana. No doubt, the chance to earn some money also played a part.

We separately advertised in the same newspaper for persons who were experiencing difficulties with their use of alcohol. A total of 52 persons responded to this advertisement. We did not consider persons who had a

history of serious physical or mental disorder or had never smoked marihuana.
We used the Michigan Alcoholism Screening Test (MAST) to determine the
stage of alcoholism each of them had reached. To match our normal sample,
we selected younger persons whose alcohol addiction was of intermediate
severity and who did not show gross economic and social decompensation.
The final group of 30 alcoholics were closely matched with the normals in
age (mean 27 years, range 21 to 36 years). They had an average of 13 years
of education but fewer of them were attending universities at the time of the
study.

An immediate difference between the groups was that while only one
normal subject failed to show up for the experiment, as many as 10 alcoholics
did not come. Those who failed to attend were replaced by the next candidate. Since we offered each subject $3 an hour -- and a chance to earn up
to $15 -- the poor attendance of the alcoholic group indicates that even the
inducement of money is not always a strong reinforcer of behavior.

Our comparisons between normals and alcoholics included measures
of physiological response (heart rate and forearm blood flow), mood changes,
and mental acuity. All subjects were measured at rest and during mental
stress. Heart rate and forearm blood flow were recorded on a polygraph using
an EKG lead for heart rate and a plethysmograph with strain gauge to record
blood flow. The subject lay comfortably on his back on the bed. The strain
gauge was placed around the left forearm and the EKG lead was attached and
linked to the polygraph. Blood flow to the left hand was stopped by means of
a blood pressure cuff inflated to 180 mm Hg. The left upper-arm blood
pressure cuff was inflated to a pressure of around 50 mm Hg. whereby the
venous return was intermittently occluded while the arterial inflow continued
without interference. In this way, changes in forearm blood flow altered the
girth of the forearm. The resulting changes of tension in the strain gauge
were recorded on the polygraph.

Two types of emotional stress were used. Firstly, each subject was
asked to speak for three minutes into a videotape camera on a topic which
he had previously disclosed as one that caused him much personal anxiety.
While making the speech he could see himself on the monitor and was told
that the videotape would later be played back to a panel of experts who
would rate the speech for content of thought. Secondly, each subject was
asked to solve mental arithmetic problems under pressure of time. The mental
arithmetic consisted of groups of 20 problems of varying degrees of complexity.
The subject was told that he would be paid according to the number of correct
answers. Thus, in addition to acting as a stressor, this test also served as a
measure of mental acuity. Both public speaking and mental arithmetic have
been established as laboratory models of clinical anxiety and are associated
with physiological arousal as shown by increases in heart rate, forearm blood
flow, and finger sweating (Droppleman and McNair, 1971).

Changes in mood during each rest and stress period were measured by
means of subject self-evaluation using items selected from the Psychiatric
Outpatient Mood Scale (POMS). This scale measures feeling states such as

friendliness, anxiety, anger, depression, and drowsiness. Finally, the subjects who were given alcohol or marihuana were asked to rank the drug "high" on a scale where 0 = no "high" at all, and 4 = extremely "high".

Ten normals and ten alcoholics were tested under control conditions and were not given any drug throughout the procedure. Ten others from each group smoked marihuana and a further ten from each group drank alcohol. The marihuana was obtained from the Center for Studies of Narcotics and Drug Abuse. The dosage we used was approximately 0.4 Gr. of cigarette/ 50 lb. of body weight (the equivalent of 7.5 mgm Delta THC/50 lb. body-weight). Alcohol was consumed in the form of 100-proof vodka mixed with orange juice; the dosage was 2 ml. vodka/kgm bodyweight. Breathalyzer readings were taken before any subject participated to ensure that none had been drinking prior to the study. For those who received alcohol a further breathalyzer reading was made one half-hour after ingestion. The mean blood alcohol level was 0.06% (range 0.05 - 0.08%).

Each subject was tested for a period of 140-160 minutes. Resting levels of heart rate and blood flow were obtained. The subject was then told to speak for three minutes while looking into the videotape camera. Following the speech the subject was asked to relax and resting levels were recorded for 15 minutes. He was then subjected to additional stress by being asked to solve mental arithmetic problems within a limited time period. After this procedure the subject was asked to relax and further resting readings were taken. At this stage alcohol or marihuana was administered while the third group acted as controls. One half-hour after taking the drugs the procedure was repeated in the same sequence -- viz. resting, public speaking, rest, mental arithmetic, and rest.

Following each rest and stress procedure the subject was given the questionnaire to complete to measure changes in anxiety, confusion, depression, anger, drowsiness, and friendliness. Lastly, we recorded the number of correct answers obtained by each subject during the mental arithmetic tests.

These data provided us many comparisons of marihuana and alcohol effects as well as comparisons between normals and alcoholics.

Before taking marihuana or alcohol, the 30 normal subjects had a mean heart rate of 64 beats/minute at rest. The rate increased by some 20-30% during periods of stress but returned rapidly to baseline levels once the stress was over. The 30 alcoholics as a group had a mean resting level somewhat higher than the normals but their response during stress was less, with the rate of increase only half that of the normals. The normal and alcoholic subjects who were given alcohol showed no appreciable change in their initial baseline rate nor in their response to stress. However, following each stress the heart rate for both normals and alcoholics failed to return to baseline but remained raised by some 5-10%. Both the normals and the alcoholics who smoked marihuana showed a dramatic rise in resting heart rate of about one-fourth above pre-marihuana levels. The responses to stress

were proportionately similar to those in the pre-marihuana conditions. Again
the normals showed an increase above baseline of some 20% during stress
while the stress response of the alcoholics was only half as great.

The results with forearm blood flow at rest and during stress were in a
similar direction to those of the heart rate. We concluded that alcoholic
subjects had resting heart rate and blood flow levels somewhat higher than
normals. However, the response of alcoholics to stress was lower. When
given alcohol or marihuana the alcoholics responded similarly to normals but
throughout their response to stress was attenuated. In both normals and
alcoholics, marihuana markedly increased heart rate and blood flow but did
not impair the relaxation response at the end of each stress. Alcohol, by
contrast, impaired this relaxation response.

Changes in mood states were more difficult to evaluate than measures
of physiological response. In general, the normal subjects showed a greater
responsiveness to stress than the alcoholics by becoming less friendly but more
alert and anxious. When alcohol was given to alcoholics they experienced
increases in anger and depression. Marihuana, by contrast, did not intensify
these mood states. For both normals and alcoholics, the marihuana "high"
was substantially greater than the alcohol-induced "high". In both normals
and alcoholics the ability to solve mental arithmetic problems was reduced
after smoking marihuana by 10%. Alcohol, in the doses we gave, did not
impair mental acuity in either group.

We have interpreted the data as follows: Alcoholics are less responsive
to stress than normal subjects, and they are more likely to "give up" and
withdraw from the stress situation. Among alcoholics and normals alike, the
drug alcohol interferes with the defense reaction of "flight or fight" by
preventing complete relaxation after stress. Among alcoholics, this drug has
the added effect of increasing anger and depression (see also, McNamee,
Mello and Mendelson, 1968; Warren and Raynes, 1972). Marihuana, by
contrast, produced more positive mood states and did not interfere with the
arousal reaction. Marihuana, however, is not without negative effects.
It greatly increases heart rate and sometimes produces an acute psychiatric
syndrome of which we saw 3 among 27 subjects tested. These findings confirmed our belief that marihuana could have a place in the treatment of
alcoholism. Careful screening of subjects is necessary to avoid giving the
drug to persons who are prone to psychiatric disturbances. Also a smaller
dose should be used to reduce the effect of the drug on the cardiovascular
system.

We have studied the interaction of disulfiram and marihuana on 15
male subjects who were in good health and had a history of some prior marihuana usage. The subjects were asked to fill out a medical screening
questionnaire before being admitted to the research ward.

Baseline measures of heart rate, blood pressure, and temperature were
recorded 3 times at 15-minute intervals before administration of the two
drugs. Each subject was asked about his alcohol consumption in the preceding

24-hour period to ensure that his system was free from alcohol before the administration of 250 milligrams of disulfiram crushed and dissolved in orange juice. The subject was then given a marihuana cigarette to smoke.

The subject was monitored immediately after ingestion, then at 15-minute intervals for the first hour, 30-minute intervals for the second hour, and 60-minute intervals for the third and fourth hours. Approximately 15 minutes after smoking the marihuana cigarette the subject was asked to rate his high on a scale of 0-4; 0 representing no subjective effects and 4 representing extreme effects. Finally, each subject was reminded that he would not be able to drink any kind of alcoholic beverage for at least five days.

The results indicate that there is no subjectively discernible interaction between marihuana and disulfiram. One subject developed a headache one hour after administration of the two drugs but reported later that it had disappeared.

We are now entering the fourth phase of our study. This involves testing the value of marihuana as a reinforcement for the use of disulfiram (Antabuse) by persons with alcohol problems. Our previous research has shown that giving alcoholics disulfiram twice weekly under staff supervision improves clinic attendance and leads to reduced drinking over our research period of two months. However, less than half of all alcoholics will accept disulfiram. Many who start discontinue its use. Our purpose is to see if marihuana can be used as a positive reinforcer or inducement for alcoholics to accept and continue taking disulfiram under our twice-weekly supervision.

Sixty subjects will be tested. Persons with a history of excessive alcohol use will be invited to come to our office to complete a questionnaire dealing with alcohol and drug use as well as physical and mental status. Persons who are judged to be early- or intermediate-stage alcoholics will be invited to participate in the study. Each of these 60 subjects who agrees to participate will be paid $1.00 per visit to meet travel expenses. Since we plan to measure return rates we do not wish to offer a large sum of money because it is likely that some of the subjects may be coming principally for the money and this will seriously impair the study as a whole.

Our purpose is to determine whether the smoking of marihuana will reinforce the use of disulfiram in patients with alcohol problems. We, therefore, plan to see whether the smoking of marihuana will (1) increase the attendance patterns of alcoholic subjects, (2) increase their willingness to take disulfiram, and (3) alter the drinking patterns of alcoholic subjects.

Subjects will be allocated at random to one of four groups each with 15 subjects: (1) Control Group -- This group will not receive drugs of any kind. (2) Disulfiram only -- Each time they attend the subjects in this group will be invited to ingest 250 mgm of disulfiram crushed in orange juice. On each occasion they will be informed about the alcohol-disulfiram reaction and strongly urged to avoid all forms of alcohol. Only persons sober for 24

hours will be given disulfiram. All persons will be given a card to carry
stating they are taking disulfiram in case of an alcohol-disulfiram reaction.
(3) Marihuana only -- Each time they attend the subjects in this group will
be permitted to smoke up to one marihuana cigarette. (4) Disulfiram-
Marihuana together -- The subjects in this group will be permitted to smoke
up to one marihuana cigarette after they have ingested 250 mgm disulfiram
crushed and mixed with orange juice. They will be warned about the alcohol
reaction and strongly urged to avoid any form of alcohol. If subjects in this
group refuse to take disulfiram, they will not be given marihuana.

For each group, subjects will be told to come twice weekly on
Monday and Thursday or Tuesday and Friday at a fixed time. Each time a
subject comes he will see an alcoholism counselor for 30-45 minutes of
individual therapy. He will then be interviewed by a research worker who
will inquire about his job status, drinking behavior, and living arrangements.
In addition, the research assistant will record the number of visits made by
each subject as well as conducting a breathalyzer test to determine present
blood-alcohol levels. The maximum time each patient can remain in the
study will be 28 days involving 8 visits. After this period he will be invited
to continue treatment in the Outpatient Alcoholism Clinic at Boston City
Hospital.

A study of this kind is bound to meet a considerable degree of resistance and we have encountered more than our fair share. We have now
obtained all necessary authority to proceed with the study. We have contacted the various alcoholism programs in Boston and have placed advertisements in local papers. These advertisements invite persons with alcohol
problems to contact us with regard to participating in a study involving
alcohol education, counseling and drug management with disulfiram and/or
marihuana.

From November, 1975 to January 31, 1976, 101 persons responded by
telephone to over 20 separate advertisements. The purpose and nature of the
study was explained to them but only 62 agreed to come in for an appointment.
The most frequent reason for not coming was the refusal to take disulfiram
(13 out of 39; 33%). Only 2 people refused to smoke marihuana. Most of
the remaining 24 who refused to come in were looking for a job or money
rather than treatment. Only 27 of the 62 who agreed to come for an appointment actually did so. A further 7 dropped out before starting the study
leaving only 20 persons who actually received disulfiram; marihuana; disulfiram and marihuana or served as controls. The five subjects who served as
controls attended 40 percent of the possible visits. While they remained in
the study, the controls admitted to drinking alcohol on 17 percent and smoking
marihuana outside of the study on 20 percent of the days. Two of the controls
completed the 28 day study but neither of them later continued in the outpatient clinic. The 5 patients who received disulfiram alone attended 45
percent of the possible visits. None of them was drinking but as a group they
smoked marihuana on 16 percent of the days they were in the study. Two of
them completed the study and one continued in the outpatient clinic. The
5 subjects who received marihuana alone attended on 64 percent of the

possible visits. Compared with the controls, they drank alcohol (49 percent of days) and smoked marihuana on their own (32 percent of days) more often. Three of them completed the study, but none continued in the outpatient clinic. Finally, the 5 subjects who received both <u>disulfiram and marihuana</u> attended on 63 percent of possible visits. While they remained in the study, they were unable to drink alcohol, but they did smoke marihuana outside of the study on 48 percent of the study days. Three of the five subjects on disulfiram and marihuana completed the study, and all continued in the outpatient clinic.

The results of the study must remain tentative until we have tested more subjects. The reluctance of many alcoholics to disulfiram is known (Gerrein, Rosenberg, and Manohar, 1973; Rosenberg, 1974) but it would also seem that neither is marihuana particularly attractive to them. The smoking of marihuana by itself in a research setting seems to increase outside use of both marihuana and alcohol. However, when marihuana is given with disulfiram, this combination blocks alcohol use but boosts the outside use of marihuana. Overall, the combination of disulfiram and marihuana appears to be the most effective both in terms of continued attendance and reduced alcohol intake. Adverse reactions were limited to one subject who became anxious while smoking marihuana. No untoward effects were reported with the combination of disulfiram and marihuana.

We plan to continue this prospective study for several more months to determine the possible value of marihuana in the treatment of chronic alcoholism. Our preliminary findings indicate that marihuana by itself is neither sought after nor particularly useful in alcoholism treatment. However, as a reinforcer to disulfiram, it may well be of value.

REFERENCES

Becker, H.S. Outsiders: Studies in the sociology of deviance. New York: Macmillan, 1963.

Blackwell, B. Drug therapy - patient compliance. New England Journal of Medicine, 1973, 289, 249-252.

Davis, M. Variations in patients' compliance with doctors' advice: An empirical analysis of patterns of communication. American Journal of Public Health, 1968, 58, 274-286.

Ditman, K.S. Review and evaluation of current drug therapies in alcoholism. Psychosomatic Medicine, 1966, 28, 667-677.

Droppleman, L.F., & McNair, D.M. An experimental analog of public speaking. J. Consult. Clinical Psychology, 1971, 36, 91-96.

Gerrein, J.R., Rosenberg, C.M., & Manohar, V. Disulfiram maintenance in the outpatient treatment of alcoholism. Archives of General Psychiatry, 1973, 28, 798-802.

Kane, H.H. Drugs that enslave. Philadelphia, 1881.

Kissin, B., Platz, A., & Su, W.H. Selective factors in treatment choice and outcome in alcoholics. In N.K. Mello & J.H. Mendelson (Eds.), Recent Advances in Studies of Alcoholism. Washington, D.C.: Government Printing Office, Public Health Service Publication No. (HSM) 71-9045, 1971, 781-802.

Marston, M. Compliance with medical regimens: A review of the literatures. Nursing Research, 1970, 19, 312-323.

McNamee, H.B., Mello, N.K., & Mendelson, J.H. Experimental analysis of drinking patterns of alcoholics: Concurrent psychiatric observations. American Journal of Psychiatry, 1968, 124, 1063-1069.

Rosenberg, C.M. Drug maintenance in the outpatient treatment of chronic alcoholism. Archives of General Psychiatry, 1974, 30, 373-377.

Thompson, L.J., & Proctor, R.C. Pyrahexyl in the treatment of alcoholic and drug withdrawal conditions. N. Carolina Med. Journal, 1953, 14, 520-523.

Warren, G.H. & Raynes, A.G., Mood changes during three conditions of alcohol intake. Quarterly Journal of Studies of Alcohol, 1972, 33, 979-989.

Zinberg, N.E. & Weil, A.T. A comparison of marihuana users and non-users. Nature, 1970, 226, 119-123.

DISCUSSION

Rubin: I would like to make two comments based on the Jamaican study: one on alcoholism and one on mental function. Jamaica, as you must know, is a rum-producing country, as is the rest of the Caribbean, and there are not many teetotalers there. For the most part, people there are very relaxed about drinking. However, there are some very interesting differences in statistics of admissions to mental hospitals. In the Bahamas, where ganja is not used very much, the rate of annual admissions to mental hospitals for alcoholism is 55 percent, whereas in Jamaica, where ganja is endemic, the rate of annual admissions for alcoholism is less than one percent. I think this is a very interesting idea for Dr. Rosenberg to know about. On the question of mental function, I have been somewhat concerned all day long that a great many studies that are being presented on the acute effects of cannabis are presented without regard to any long-term study, and it seems to me they have to be placed in perspective. In the Jamaica study, there were 30 smokers and 30 nonsmokers. The 30 smokers had a history of smoking from 7 to 37 years with a mean of 17.5 years; they also smoked more heavily and with a higher THC content than is the case in this country, as you probably know. We gave a panel of 19 psychological tests, including neuropsychological, psychomotor, and personality tests. No significant differences were found between smokers and nonsmokers on any of the tests. But the important thing is that there was no indication whatsoever of disturbance of mental function or brain damage or anything that matches some of the findings that appear in acute studies. My reason for bringing this up is that I believe that acute reactions have to be seen in relation to the perspective of the effects of long-term chronic use.

Lemberger: I want to ask Dr. Vachon a question. You were talking about propranalol blocking some of the effects of marihuana. I am sure you realize that propanalol is not only a beta-blocking agent but it also affects many other functions. One of the major things it does affect is blood flow, and thereby would be affecting the metabolism of the marihuana and many other subsequent effects.

Harris: It would be nice if some kind of a dose-response relationship could have been shown. I always get concerned with one fixed dose of one drug vs. one fixed dose of another drug. It would have been nice if you had fixed the dose of one and then had done a dose-response curve with the other. That would have given you a much better idea of whether you have a true interaction.

Miller: Did you use a 25 mg THC dose?

Vachon: No, it was a one-gram cigarette containing either 1 percent or 2 percent of THC.

Stillman: I want to ask you, is it possible that the tranquilizing or sedative effect of propranalol would reduce the depth of pulmonary inspiration, thus resulting in a lower dose of marihuana? Your reduction in marihuana effects would then result not from a direct effect of propranalol but simply from a lower delivered dose of marihuana.

Vachon: The smoking of the joint is timed. We ask the subject to inhale and we time his inhalation, and so on.

Hanley: I have a question for Dr. Neu. How did you determine this stage of sleep after the subjects retired?

Neu: There was an observer who walked into the room every 15 minutes with a small flashlight. When the subjects were obviously awake, there was no problem. A couple of subjects were faking that they were asleep, but when he put the flashlight close to their eyes, they would blink or make some sign that they were awake.

Cohen: I would like to ask Dr. Hill about her placebo. It seemed from her slides that it has an enormous effect on thresholds and on sensitivity, and in fact more so than the active drug but in the opposite direction.

Hill: We did find changes when we repeated the test. I think it should be pointed out that when you repeat the procedure there is a tendency to get a decrease in thresholds. The fact that we got opposing findings with the marihuana even further dramatizes the effect of marihuana.

Phillipson: I would like to go back to the point Vera Rubin made about findings in the Jamaica study. I believe it was not really the custom in Jamaica to inhale deeply and to retain that inhaled smoke for a long period of time. I got the idea that they didn't smoke it the way we do up here.

Rubin: I can't give you an exact measure of that, but there is some measure of it from the substudy that was done with videotaping to try to assess work performance.

Phillipson: I definitely remember being told about videotapes where the Jamaicans who might be chronic users might sort of puff the joints like a young American girl smoking her first cigarette.

Petersen: Someone did try to get them to inhale deeply and apparently deep inhalation was not the custom, but they certainly inhale some of it. But in Jamaica they don't inhale as deeply as they do here where material is scarce.

Harris: Isn't it a question of a dose-response thing? When you've got good stuff and plenty of it, you don't have to spend a lot of time trying to extract everything out of it. It's the same thing with nicotine. You give people good heavy-nicotine cigarettes, and they smoke it quite differently than they smoke low-nicotine filter cigarettes. My experience is that people who smoke marihuana smoke just enough to get the feeling that they want to get.

Rubin: We have chain smokers in Jamaica, you know, who smoke the way I smoke cigarettes.

Hill: I would just like to say that recently I had the opportunity to hear Dr. Dornbush talking about the Greek study, and although it is often said that there is no long-term effect of marihuana on brain functioning, and so on, actually there was very little done in the way of psychological testing in that study, and those that were given did not make it possible to conclude an absence of brain damage from chronic marihuana smoking. But I would like to say that we are trying to look at heavy users of marihuana in St. Louis -- which requires interviewing over 50 people to get 10 daily users. But our results show that using the computerized brain scan -- none of the people tested so far give any indication of abnormality.

Neu: I want to ask Dr. Rubin, regarding the statistics you mention of 55 percent on one island and one percent on another island: Is the pattern for hospitalization for other illnesses throughout the year parallel? Were different criteria used for admission on the two islands?

Rubin: I don't have the figures for that. We were primarily interested in the figures for alcoholism.

CHAPTER 14

THE THERAPEUTIC ASPECTS OF MARIHUANA:

COMPUTER ANALYSES OF ELECTROENCEPHALOGRAPHIC DATA FROM
HUMAN USERS OF CANNABIS SATIVA

John Hanley
Eleanore D. Tyrrell
Pierre M. Hahn

Departments of Psychiatry and Computer Science
and Laboratory of Environmental Neurobiology
Center for the Health Sciences
University of California
Los Angeles, California

NOTE: This research was supported by contract #HSM 42-71-89
and computing assistance from Health Sciences Computing
Facility, UCLA, supported by National Institute of Health
Special Research Resources Grant RR-3.

INTRODUCTION

This report summarizes computer analyses of brain wave (EEG) data
derived from 18 subjects who participated in a 94-day study conducted at
the Neuropsychiatric Institute, UCLA. These subjects were smokers of
Cannabis sativa by their own accounts. They continued to inhale this
compound during their hospital stay. Comparisons were made between this
experimental group and a comparison group, age- and sex-matched (male).
The comparison group attested to non-use of the compound or, in a few
instances, of use not more recent than two years previously. Comparisons
were also obtained within the experimental group. The between group study
was performed before the hospitalized subjects began their use of cannabis
provided by the investigators. The within group studies were done during the
hospital stay. These within studies were undertaken during a no-intoxication
period and also before and after using one marihuana cigarette. The cigarettes
consisted of a 2.2% concentration of delta-9-THC in 900 mgm of cannabis.
During the course of the 94-day study, the 18 subjects smoked each an average
of 4.79 ± 2.43 cigarettes a day. The range extended from a minimum of
1.7 to 10.0 per day.

187

SUMMARY COMMENTS ON THE EEG

The electroencephalogram of man was discovered and recorded by Hans Berger (1929). It consists essentially of continuous trains of waves that are aperiodic in nature, occupy the frequency spectrum between 1 and 100 H_z (cycles per second), are in the microvolt range, and require amplification to be visible. The wave train can then be seen to consist of complex waves; that is, they are not pure sine or cosine waves.

With conventional amplification and quantitative analytic approaches to the wave train the energy spectrum appears to be principally distributed over a frequency from 1-32 H_z. During life, the activity is virtually ceaseless and dynamic, ever fluctuating throughout the day and changing dramatically throughout the nocturnal sleep cycle (Loomis, Harvey and Hobart, 1937; Aserinsky, 1953; Oswald, Taylor and Treisman, 1960; Rechtschaffen and Kales, 1968). The electromagnetic wave process appears to be generated in dendritic substances as a seemingly unique phenomenon in cerebral neurons (Adey, Walter and Hendrix, 1961; Adey, 1969; Pasik, Pasik, Hamori and Szentagothai, 1973; Creutzfeld, Fuster and Lux, 1964; Elul, 1972; Fujita and Sato, 1964).

Because the waveform is complex, there are severe limitations on the ability of the unaided human eye to accomplish their resolution. Despite such difficulties, and despite the early disappointment that the EEG did not fulfill the perhaps unthinking optimism of the expectations of some early workers, clinical electroencephalographers have become sufficiently skilled to recognize normal and abnormal EEGs and classify the abnormalities (Hill and Parr, 1950; Gibbs, 1950). In normal states, it has become possible to visually observe patterns related to alertness and concentration, relaxed inattention, and the stages of sleep. We will discuss the use of the computer to assist in the resolution of the wave form later in the chapter. We turn our attention now to the method of data acquisition.

ELECTRODES AND THEIR PLACEMENT

Because the acquisition of EEG data was primarily to be obtained from subjects in relaxed, relatively immobile states, conventional scalp disk gold electrodes were employed (Grass ESG.) and a suitable conducting paste. No attempt was made to obtain recordings during the actual smoking of the cigarette; hence, special electrode approaches required because of inherent difficulties caused by movement were not needed (Hanley, Adey, Zweizy and Kado, 1971; Hanley, Hahn and Adey, 1974).

The scalp disk electrodes were placed at locations prescribed by the International 10-20 system advocated by Jasper (1958). The system permits convenient monitoring of different anatomic locations and has the advantage of being standardized among widespread laboratories, facilitating ease of communication among investigators. Eight electrodes were used in a bipolar montage and were positioned as follows (Figure 1):

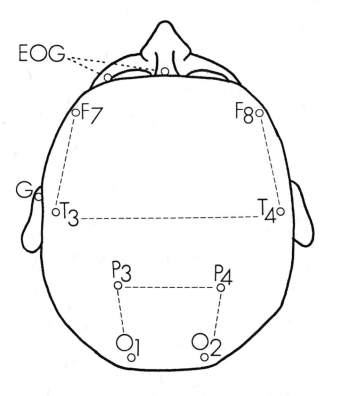

ELECTRODE PLACEMENT

Figure 1.

F7-T3   F8-T4   P3-O1   P4-O2   T3-T4   P3-P4

The alpha-numeric designations denote anatomic locations on the head with odd numbers referring to left and even numbers referring to right symmetrical locations. Two more electrodes were placed at the nasion and the left outer canthus of the eye to permit monitoring of the electrooculogram (EOG) in order to identify eye movement artifact in the EEG. An ear clip electrode served as a ground lead.

RECORDING METHODS

Signals acquired by the above sensors were amplified by a Beckman type R dynograph and written out as a conventional paper trace. They were simultaneously stored on FM analog magnetic tape with the use of an Ampex FR 1300 recorder. In addition, a binary coded decimal marker, designed and built in house by coauthor P. M. Hahn, was recorded on paper and tape for coordination of these traces and for provision of a signal recognizable by computers for EEG epoch identification.

COMPUTER ANALYSES OF THE EEG DATA

Selected sections of the analog tape were digitized at a sampling rate of 256/sec (Nyquist, 1924) using a Digital Equipment Corporation PDP-81 computer in the preparation of a 7-track digital tape reel. This data was then submitted to an IBM 360-91 general purpose digital computer for spectral and discriminant analyses. For efficient computation, Fast Fourier Transform (FFT) algorithms are utilized in the spectral analysis program (BMD 03T) available at the UCLA Health Science Computing Facility (Cooley and Tukey, 1965; Dixon, 1973).

Spectral analysis provides:

(1)   Estimates of autospectral "intensity" -- sum of spectral densities at each frequency of interest: this is proportional to the mean square of the EED amplitude and is a measure of the power in the particular frequency pass-band.

(2)   Mean frequency within the bands of interest -- division of the frequency band is under the control of the investigator: for the purpose of communication with clinically oriented electro-encephalographers, we selected arbitrary divisions which correspond closely to the so-called delta, theta, alpha, and beta bands, that is, 1-3 Hz, 4-7 Hz, 8-13 Hz, 14-19 Hz, and 20-25 Hz. This is near the dominant frequency if one is present.

(3)   <u>Band width with the band</u> -- this expresses
        the invariability of the dominant frequency

        (Rhodes, Reite, Brown and Adey, 1965).
        Two measures are derived from comparison
        of any two wave trains from two different
        anatomical locations. These cross spectral
        terms are:

(4)   <u>Coherence</u> -- this is analogous to the correla-
        tion coefficient of classical statistics
        (Koopmans, 1965). It was introduced to the
        EEG literature by D. O. Walter. It can be
        determined at each frequency, or band of
        frequencies, across the spectrum.

(5)   <u>Phase relations</u> -- this quantitatively
        describes the degrees of lead and lag
        between two wave processes when they are
        not in phase. This measure will be perhaps
        made clear by consulting Figure 2, which
        illustrates one of the results of the analysis.

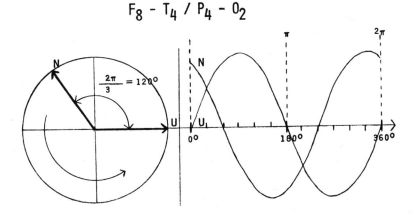

SCHEMATIC SUMMARY OF PHASE DIFFERENCES BETWEEN USERS (U) AND NON-USERS (N) OF MARIJUANA

$$F_8 - T_4 / P_4 - O_2$$

Figure 2.

The resulting generation of spectral estimators from multichannel recordings across a band of frequencies from 1-25 H_z numbers into the hundreds and provides an immense amount of data which is even more bewildering to the human eye than the original raw data, despite precise quantification. This increasing complexity provided motivation for the development and use of discriminant analysis programs (Dixon, 1973). We now briefly discuss them because of their value in selection of significant EEG features in patterns of huge dimensionality. Because of space limitations, the discussion will be succinct and unfortunately will lack mathematical rigor. This may be remedied by consulting the references.

DISCRIMINANT ANALYSIS

This program is a hybrid of pattern recognition and classical statistics (Dixon, 1973; Anderson, 1950). It is a linear, stepwise process in which the above spectral estimators are divided into two disjoint sets. One set is for variables not yet entered into the discriminant function. From this set the program chooses that variable for which the ratio of the between-group variance to within-group variance (F value) is greatest. The value of this "F" indicates by its magnitude the desirability of entering the variable into the discriminating function. The second set is used to evaluate which variable already entered would be best removed. The separate measures are thus competed against each other until the most effective features have been selected. The program also scores its own performance and prints out the actual classification and percent success. It is important to note here that if, for example, a variable has 80% success in discriminating between two groups, this does not mean that each selected epoch has an 80% chance of being correct; it means that 80% of the data were correctly discriminated and 20% were wrongly discriminated.

Finally, on the basis of the best two selections, the program prints a "scattergram" of the distribution within calculated cartesian coordinates as illustrated in Figure 3. Further details of the program and its applications may be sought in references (Walter, Rhodes and Adey, 1967; Hanley, Walter, Rhodes and Adey, 1968; Sklar, Hanley and Simmons, 1973). The most lucid description of the multivariate classifier has been provided, in our opinion, by Nilsson (1965).

CAUTIONARY REMARKS

We are fully aware of considerations that limit the utility of these approaches to the data that are somewhat inherent in the data itself. For instance, the times series approach to the EEG relies on stochastic, stationary assumptions (Weiner, 1963). That is, the data is presumed to be a random process whose statistical properties are not perturbed by a translation in the origin for time. Anyone familiar with the EEG knows that these assumptions are violated by this time-varying signal. We do not choose,

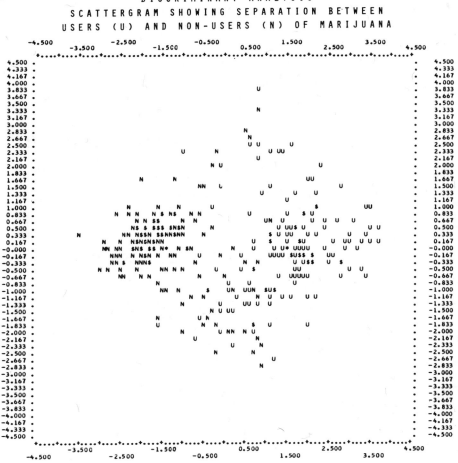

Figure 3.

however, EEG epochs that vary so obviously; also, the methods are adequate for even weakly stationary processes (Blackman and Tukey, 1959).

It is also certainly true that the mathematics for demonstrating significance have not yet been developed for stepwise discriminant analysis (Dixon and Sklar, n.d.). It is possible, however, to use the strategies of training and testing sets and to scramble data into pseudogroups. Because of insufficient computing funds we were not able to pursue these tactics here; we did so in a similar experiment with the EEGs of dyslexic children with satisfying results (Sklar, Hanley and Simmons, 1973). We have also examined the F statistics extensively and list them in the section on results. We now tabulate the overall results.

Between Group Studies[a]

DISCRIMINANT ANALYSIS RESULTS

Lead Pairs	Parameter	Band (Hz)	Success (%)
1. Users (U) vs. Non Users (N)			
F8-T4/P4-02	PHASE	14-19	85
F7-T3/P3-P4	PHASE	14-19	86
P4-02	SUMSPEC[b]	1- 3	90
2. Moderate Users (M) vs. Heavy Users (H)[c]			
P3-P4	FBAR	20-25	74
P3-01/P4-02	COH	1- 3	69
P3-01/P4-02	COH	8-13	75
3. Heavy Users (H) vs. Non Users (N)			
P4-02	SUMSP	1- 3	83
F7-T3/P3-P4	PHASE	14-19	87
F8-T4/P4-02	PHASE	14-19	91
4. Moderate Users (M) vs. Non Users (N)			
F8-T4/P4-02	PHASE	14-19	89
F8-T4/P3-P4	PHASE	14-19	89
F8-T4/P4-02	PHASE	8-13	91

---

[a] Based on history of drug habits prior to entering the study.

[b] Computer abbreviation for autospectral intensity.

[c] Users were divided into Moderate Users (3-6 joints/week) and Heavy Users (more than 6 joints/week).

Within Group Studies[a]

DISCRIMINANT ANALYSIS RESULTS

Lead Pairs	Parameter	Band (Hz)	Success %		

1. Pre-Intox (B) vs. Post-Intox (A) (days 46 and 72)

Lead Pairs	Parameter	Band (Hz)	Success %	B	A
T3-T4/P3-P4	COH	20-25	65	.26	.16
P3-P4	FBAR	8-13	71	10.1	9.86
T3-T4	SUMSPEC	4- 7	72	.19	.16

2. Post-Intox (day 46) vs. Post-Intox (day 72)

Lead Pairs	Parameter	Band (Hz)	Success %	day 46	72
P3-01/P4-02	PHASE	14-19	54	0	6
T3-T4/P3-P4	COH	1- 3	63	.12	.16
F8-T4	SUMSPEC	1- 3	63	.60	.53

3. Baseline (day 5) vs. Detox (day 78)

Lead Pairs	Parameter	Band (Hz)	Success %	day 5	78
F7-T3/P4-02	PHASE	8-13	61	62	31
P4-02/T3-T4	COH	20-25	59	.06	.04
F7-T3	FBAR	14-19	62	16.3	16.4

4. Baseline (day 5) vs. Post-Intox (day 72)

Lead Pairs	Parameter	Band (Hz)	Success %	day 5	72
P4-02	SUMSPEC	1- 3	61	.34	.24

---

[a] Smokers only from data obtained during the study.

Between Group Studies

TABLE OF F VALUES

(Using all variables for lead pairs where P is less than 1×10^{-7})

Non Users (N)   Users (U)

200 Variables, 177 Cases (N), 158 Cases (U)

Lead Pairs	Variable	Band (Hz)	F	Average (N)	(U)
F7-T3	SUMSP	1- 3	32	.49	.56
F8-T4	SUMSP	1- 3	153	.44	.64
P3-01	SUMSP	1- 3	37	.20	.28
P4-02	SUMSP	1- 3	109	.17	.34
T3-T4	SUMSP	1- 3	53	.33	.45
P3-P4	SUMSP	1- 3	85	.21	.35
F7-T3/P3-01	PHASE	1- 3	39	128	64
P3-01/P4-02	COH	1- 3	32	.20	.33
F8-T4	FBAR	4- 7	36	5.4	5.2
P4-02	SUMSP	4- 7	51	.097	.14
P4-02	FBAR	4- 7	77	5.6	5.3
T3-T4	SUMSP	4- 7	35	.15	.18
T3-T4	FBAR	4- 7	34	5.4	5.3
F7-T3/P3-01	PHASE	4- 7	75	141	55
F7-T3/P4-02	PHASE	4- 7	40	147	82
F7-T3/P3-P4	PHASE	4- 7	141	36	145
F8-T4/P3-P4	PHASE	4- 7	62	145	67
F8-T4/P4-02	PHASE	4- 7	90	166	73
F8-T4/P3-P4	PHASE	4- 7	99	133	33
P3-01/P4-02	COH	4- 7	35	.32	.43
F7-T3	SUMSP	8-13	77	.30	.18
F7-T3	FBAR	8-13	45	9.8	10.1
F7-T3	BW	8-13	45	2.7	3.3
F8-T4	SUMSP	8-13	147	.32	.15
F8-T4	BW	8-13	33	2.6	3.1
P3-01	SUMSP	8-13	30	.60	.50
P4-02	SUMSP	8-13	93	.64	.45
T3-T4	SUMSP	8-13	101	.39	.25
T3-T4	BW	8-13	35	2.9	3.3
P3-P4	SUMSP	8-13	69	.55	.40
F7-T3/F8-T4	COH	8-13	51	.31	.18
F7-T3/P3-01	COH	8-13	50	.26	.14
F7-T3/P3-01	PHASE	8-13	109	152	56
F7-T3/P4-02	COH	8-13	48	.21	.10
F7-T3/P4-02	PHASE	8-13	88	149	62

Lead Pairs	Variable	Band (Hz)	F	Average (N)	(U)
F7-T3/P3-P4	PHASE	8-13	148	50	150
F8-T4/P3-01	COH	8-13	50	.24	.13
F8-T4/P3-01	PHASE	8-13	172	168	56
F8-T4/P4-02	COH	8-13	79	.33	.16
F8-T4/P4-02	PHASE	8-13	161	162	54
F8-T4/P3-P4	PHASE	8-13	246	143	17
F8-T4	SUMSP	14-19	53	.071	.043
F7-T3/P3-01	PHASE	14-19	157	164	52
F7-T3/P4-02	PHASE	14-19	75	152	73
F7-T3/P3-P4	PHASE	14-19	221	30	152
F8-T4/P3-01	PHASE	14-19	143	165	63
F8-T4/P4-02	PHASE	14-19	283	186	67
F8-T4/P3-P4	PHASE	14-19	172	143	30
F7-T3/P3-01	PHASE	20-25	58	128	49
F7-T3/P4-02	PHASE	20-25	31	129	74
F7-T3/P3-P4	PHASE	20-25	152	31	146
F8-T4/P3-01	PHASE	20-25	38	137	75
F8-T4/P4-02	PHASE	20-25	165	165	54
F8-T4/P3-P4	PHASE	20-25	147	147	35
P3-01/P4-02	COH	20-25	50	.25	.38

Moderate Users (M)   Heavy Users (H)

200 Variables, 98 Cases (M), 60 Cases (H)

Lead Pairs	Variable	Band (Hz)	F	(M)	(H)
P3-P4	SUMSPEC	8-13	34	.45	.31
P4-02	FBAR	20-25	37	21.6	22.0
P3-P4	FBAR	20-25	43	21.7	22.1
P3-P4	BW	20-25	42	3.2	3.8

Heavy Users (H)   Non Users (N)

200 Variables, 60 Cases (H), 177 Cases (N)

Lead Pairs	Variable	Band (Hz)	F	(H)	(N)
F8-T4	SUMSPEC	1- 3	88	.66	.44
P3-01	SUMSPEC	1- 3	68	.35	.20
P4-02	SUMSPEC	1- 3	144	.41	.17
T3-T4	SUMSPEC	1- 3	47	.47	.33

Lead Pairs	Variable	Band (Hz)	F	Average	
				(H)	(N)
P3-P4	SUMSPEC	1- 3	114	.42	.21
F7-T3/P3-O1	PHASE	1- 3	31	55	128
P3-O1/P4-O2	COH	1- 3	66	.44	.20
P3-O1	SUMSPEC	4- 7	41	.16	.11
P4-O2	SUMSPEC	4- 7	67	.16	.10
P4-O2	FBAR	4- 7	67	5.3	5.6
T3-T4	SUMSPEC	4- 7	54	.20	.15
T3-T4	FBAR	4- 7	40	5.2	5.4
P3-P4	FBAR	4- 7	40	5.3	5.5
F7-T3/P3-O1	PHASE	4- 7	44	.05	.07
F7-T3/P3-P4	PHASE	4- 7	75	147	36
F8-T4/P3-O1	PHASE	4- 7	33	68	145
F8-T4/P4-O2	PHASE	4- 7	46	78	166
F8-T4/P3-P4	PHASE	4- 7	37	43	133
P3-O1/P4-O2	COH	4- 7	48	.51	.32
F7-T3	SUMSPEC	8-13	47	.17	.30
F7-T3	BW	8-13	39	3.4	2.7
F8-T4	SUMSPEC	8-13	90	.13	.32
P3-O1	SUMSPEC	8-13	60	.41	.60
P4-O2	SUMSPEC	8-13	116	.36	.64
T3-T4	SUMSPEC	8-13	78	.22	.39
T3-T4	BW	8-13	30	3.5	2.9
P3-P4	SUMSPEC	8-13	96	.31	.55
F7-T3/F8-T4	COH	8-13	30	.16	.31
F7-T3/P3-O1	COH	8-13	112	26	152
F7-T3/P4-O2	PHASE	8-13	93	33	149
F7-T3/P3-P4	PHASE	8-13	87	157	50
F8-T4/P3-O1	PHASE	8-13	143	40	168
F8-T4/P4-O2	COH	8-13	68	.10	.33
F8-T4/P4-O2	PHASE	8-13	86	58	162
F8-T4/P3-P4	PHASE	8-13	92	24	143
F8-T4	SUMSPEC	14-19	32	.04	.07
P4-O2	FBAR	14-19	32	16.2	16.5
F7-T3/P3-O1	PHASE	14-19	116	31	164
F7-T3/P4-O2	PHASE	14-19	61	58	152
F7-T3/P3-P4	PHASE	14-19	139	158	30
F8-T4/P3-O1	PHASE	14-19	79	64	165
F8-T4/P4-O2	PHASE	14-19	131	77	186
F8-T4/P3-P4	PHASE	14-19	45	62	143
P3-P4	FBAR	20-25	43	22.1	21.8
P3-P4	BW	20-25	36	3.8	3.2
F7-T3/P3-P4	PHASE	20-25	88	152	31
F8-T4/P4-O2	PHASE	20-25	99	48	165
F8-T4/P3-P4	PHASE	20-25	50	59	147

Moderate Users (M)   Non Users (N)

200 Variables, 78 Cases (M), 177 Cases (N)

Lead Pairs	Variable	Band (Hz)	F	Average	
				(M)	(N)
F8-T4	SUMSPEC	1- 3	99	.64	.44
P4-02	SUMSPEC	1- 3	59	.30	.17
T3-T4	SUMSPEC	1- 3	31	.43	.33
P3-P4	SUMSPEC	1- 3	36	.31	.21
P4-02	FBAR	4- 7	46	5.4	5.6
F7-T3/P3-01	PHASE	4- 7	57	58	141
F7-T3/P4-02	PHASE	4- 7	30	84	147
F7-T3/P3-P4	PHASE	4- 7	105	144	36
F8-T4/P3-01	PHASE	4- 7	50	67	145
F8-T4/P4-02	PHASE	4- 7	83	70	166
F8-T4/P3-P4	PHASE	4- 7	83	27	133
F7-T3	SUMSPEC	8-13	44	.19	.30
F7-T3	FBAR	8-13	59	10.2	9.8
F8-T4	SUMSPEC	8-13	83	.16	.32
P4-02	SUMSPEC	8-13	47	.51	.64
T3-T4	SUMSPEC	8-13	55	.27	.39
F7-T3/F8-T4	COH	8-13	31	.19	.31
F7-T3/P3-01	COH	8-13	30	.14	.26
F7-T3/P3-01	PHASE	8-13	49	75	152
F7-T3/P4-02	PHASE	8-13	40	79	149
F7-T3/P3-P4	PHASE	8-13	95	144	50
F8-T4/P3-01	PHASE	8-13	102	65	168
F8-T4/P4-02	COH	8-13	33	.19	.33
F8-T4/P4-02	PHASE	8-13	121	53	162
F8-T4/P3-P4	PHASE	8-13	228	13	143
P3-01/P4-02	COH	8-13	37	.69	.57
F8-T4	SUMSPEC	14-19	31	.04	.07
F7-T3/P3-01	PHASE	14-19	92	66	164
F7-T3/P4-02	PHASE	14-19	45	82	152
F7-T3/P3-P4	PHASE	14-19	146	149	30
F8-T4/P3-01	PHASE	14-19	121	62	165
F8-T4/P4-02	PHASE	14-19	289	61	186
F8-T4/P3-P4	PHASE	14-19	222	10	143
F7-T3/P3-01	PHASE	20-25	39	50	128
F7-T3/P3-P4	PHASE	20-25	105	142	31
F8-T4/P4-02	PHASE	20-25	122	58	165
F8-T4/P3-P4	PHASE	20-25	160	21	147
P3-01/P4-02	COH	20-25	52	.39	.25

Within Group Studies

TABLE OF F VALUES

PRE-INTOX (B)   POST-INTOX (A)

200 Variables, 340 Cases (B), 329 Cases (A)

Lead Pairs	Variable	Band (Hz)	F	Average (B)	(A)
T3-T4	SUMSP	4- 7	50	.19	.16
P3-01	FBAR	8-13	40	9.95	9.66
P4-02	FBAR	8-13	45	9.92	9.63
T3-T4	FBAR	8-13	44	10.1	9.86
P3-P4	FBAR	8-13	54	10.2	9.86
T3-T4	SUMSP	14-19	30	.081	.10
T3-T4	FBAR	14-19	37	16.2	16.4
F7-T3/F8-T4	COH	14-19	30	.080	.053
F7-T3	SUMSP	20-25	41	.041	.064
T3-T4	SUMSP	20-25	51	.045	.071
T3-T4/P3-P4	COH	20-25	101	.26	.16

FINDINGS

The most obvious findings from these results are the relative ease of the separation between smokers and non-smokers; the more difficult (but still separable) classification of heavy and moderate smokers; and the poor, scarcely better-than-chance results of the variety of combinations within the group in hospital, before and after cannabis use. In addition to the discriminant analysis results, surveys of the entire data reveal that the inhalation of cannabis decreases the energy in the EEG signal. This is most easily seen in the symmetrical placements across the head as illustrated in Figure 4. Though our experiments have not been aimed at establishing therapeutic uses of marihuana (the title of this symposium), nevertheless, the potential for anticonvulsant properties in this compound are suggested by this energy decrease since electrical concomitants of seizures include sudden increases in the energy of the EEG signal. Further, the phase differences which attend the use of the compound may be of value in petit mal which exhibits phase synchrony and characteristic energy increase.

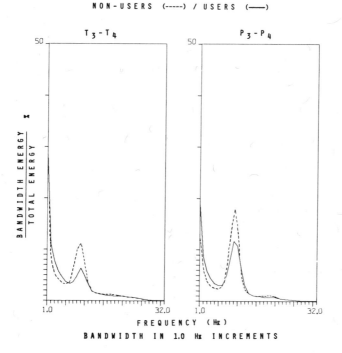

POWER SPECTRAL DENSITY

MARIJUANA STUDY

NON-USERS (-----) / USERS (———)

Figure 4.

REFERENCES

Adey, W.R. Spectral analysis of EEG data from animals and man during sorting, orienting and discriminating responses. In T. Mullholland, C. Evans (Eds.), Attention in Neurophysiology. London: Butterworth, 1969.

Adey, W.R., Walter, D.O., & Hendrix, C.E. Computer techniques in correlation and spectral analyses of cerebral slow waves during discriminative behavior. Expte. Neurol., 1961, 3, 501-524.

Anderson, T.W. Introduction to Multivariate Statistics. New York: Wiley, 1950.

Aserinsky, E. Ocular motility during sleep and its application to the study of the rest activity cycles and dreaming. Ph.D. Dissertation, University of Chicago, 1953.

Berger, H. Uber das Elektroenkephalogram des Menschen. Arch. Psychiat. Nervenkr., 1929, 87, 525-570.

Blackman, R.B. & Tukey, J.W. The Measurement of Power Spectra. New York: Dover, 1959.

Cooley, J.W. & Tukey, J.W. An algorithm for the machine calculation of complex Fourier series. Math. of Comput., April, 1965, 19, 297-301.

Creutzfeld, O.D., Fuster, J.M., Lux, J.D., & Nacimento, A.C. Experimenteller Nachweis von Beziehungen zwischen EEG-wellen and Activitat corticaler Nervenzeller. Naturwissen schaften, 1964, 51, 61-77.

Dixon, W.J. BMD 07M: Stepwise discriminant analysis. Biomed. Computer Programs. Berkeley: University of California Press, 1973.

Dixon, W.J. BMD 03T Time Series Spectral Estimation. BMD Biomedical Computer Programs. Berkeley: University of California Press, 1973.

Dixon, W.J. & Sklar, B. Personal communication.

Elul, R. The genesis of the EEG. Internat. Rev. Neurobiol., 1972, 15, 228-272.

Fujita, Y. & Sato, T. Intracellular records from hippocampal pyramidal cells in rabbit during theta rhythm activity. J. Neurophysiol., 1964, 27, 1012-1025.

Gibbs, F.A. Atlas of electroencephalography (3 vols.). Cambridge, Mass.: Addison-Wesley, 1950.

Hanley, J., Adey, W.R., Zweizy, J.R., & Kado, R.T. EEG electrode amplifier harness. Electroencephalog. & Clin. Neurophysiol., 1971, 30, 147-150.

Hanley, J., Hahn, P.M., & Adey, W.R. Electrode systems for recording the EEG in active subjects. In Biomedical Electrode Technology, 283-313. New York: Academic Press, 1974.

Hanley, J., Walter, D.O., Rhodes, J.M., & Adey, W.R. Chimpanzee Performance: Computer analysis of electroencephalograms. Nature, 1968, 220, 879-881.

Hill, D., & Parr, G. (Eds.), Electroencephalography: A Symposium of its Various Aspects. London: McDonald & Co., 1950, 184-191.

Jasper, H.H. The ten-twenty system of the International Federation. Electroencephalog. & Clin. Neurophysiol., 1958, 10, 371-375.

Koopmans, L.H. Ann. Math. Stat., 1965, 35, 352.

Loomis, A.L., Harvey, E.N., & Hobart, G.A. Cerebral states during sleep as studied by brain potentials. J. Exp. Psychol., 1937, 21, 127.

Nyquist, H. Certain factors affecting telegraph speed. Bell System Tech. J., 1924, 3, 324-346.

Nilsson, N.J. Learning machines. New York: McGraw-Hill, 1965.

Oswald, I., Taylor, A.M., & Treisman, M. Discriminative responses to stimulation during human sleep. Brain, 1960, 83, 440.

Pasik, P., Pasik, T., Hamori, J., & Szentagothai, J. Interneurons in monkey lateral geniculate nucleus: Participation in "Triadic" and "NonTriadic" Synapses. Proc. 3rd Ann. Meet. Soc. NeuroScience. San Diego: 1973, 28.

Rechtschaffen, A., & Kales, A. A manual of standardized terminology, techniques and scoring systems for sleep stages of human subjects. National Institutes of Health, Publication #204, 1968.

Rhodes, J.M., Reite, M.R., Brown, D., & Adey, W.R. Aspects anatomo-fonctionnels de la physiologie du sommeil. Proc. CNRS Symp. (Lyons, France), 1965, 451.

Sklar, B., Hanley, J., & Simmons, W.W. A computer analysis of EEG spectral signatures from normal and dyslexic children. IEEE Trans. Biomed. Engrg. BME, 1973, 20, 20-26.

Sklar, B., Hanley, J., & Simmons, W.W. An EEG experiment aimed at identifying dyslexic children. Nature, 1973, 240, 414-416.

Walter, D.O., Rhodes, J.M., & Adey, W.R. Discriminating among states of consciousness by EEG measurements: A study of four subjects. Electroencephalog. & Clin. Neurophysiol., 1967, 22, 22-29.

Weiner, N. The Extrapolation, Interpolation, and Smoothing of Stationary Time Series. New York: Wiley, 1963.

CHAPTER 15

MARIHUANA, COGNITIVE STYLE, AND LATERALIZED HEMISPHERIC
FUNCTIONS

Richard A. Harshman

Department of Psychology
University of Western Ontario
London, Ontario, Canada
(affiliation at time of research: UCLA)

Helen Joan Crawford

Hypnosis Laboratory, Department of Psychology
Stanford University
Stanford, California

Elizabeth Hecht

Department of Psychology
University of California
Los Angeles, California

NOTE: This study was conducted as part of a research
program on the Pharmacological Effects of Cannabinoids
in Man, supported by U. S. Public Health Service Contract HSM 42-71-89, whose principal investigator was
Dr. Sidney Cohen, co-principal investigator Dr. Ira Frank.

ABSTRACT

Two hypotheses concerning the psychological effects of marihuana are
proposed: (a) that the process of becoming "high" on marihuana consists, in
part, of shifting into a new cognitive style or mode which involves less reliance
on analytical, sequential, verbal processing, and more reliance on synthetic,
holistic, imagistic processing; (b) that one of the ways that marihuana produces
this shift is by decreasing left, and increasing right hemisphere participation
in cognitive activities. To test these hypotheses, 25 male subjects were administered a battery of psychological tests which tap either analytic or synthetic

(or "mixed") cognitive processes by means of tasks lateralized either to the left or to the right hemisphere (or both hemispheres). Each subject was tested in both nonintoxicated and intoxicated states, according to a counterbalanced design. A differential pattern of marihuana effects was observed: verbal analytic tasks were impaired, holistic-nonverbal closure tasks were facilitated, and "visualization" tasks showed mixed results. Performance on "low level" perceptual tasks was not affected. To further test the relationship between marihuana effects and brain lateralization, the subject sample was split into a "high lateralized" and a "low lateralized" group, based on nonintoxicated performance on dichotic listening tasks. Separate analyses indicated that "low lateralized" subjects showed no enhancement of closure ability when intoxicated, whereas "high lateralized" subjects showed a strong enhancement of this ability. Further differences in drug effects were also noted, consistent with the hypothesis that an individual's reaction to marihuana depends, in part, upon his particular pattern of brain lateralization.

INTRODUCTION

Source of the Experimental Hypotheses

If one compares "normal" cognition with that which is reportedly experienced during marihuana intoxication, one finds a pattern of differences which seem to parallel recently established differences between the cognitive functioning of the left and right cerebral hemispheres. Those cognitive activities reportedly experienced as impaired or less prominent during marihuana intoxication often resemble those cognitive functions which have been found to be more characteristic of the left hemisphere. Similarly, those reportedly experienced as enhanced or more prominent during marihuana intoxication often resemble cognitive functions found more characteristic of the right hemisphere. A short summary of the relevant neuropsychological and psychopharmacological data will serve to bring out this parallelism.

Hemisphere specialization data. There is an increasing body of evidence which indicates that the left and right cerebral hemispheres in man are specialized to perform higher-level processing in different ways (for reviews, see Blakemore, Iverson, and Zangwill, 1972; Bogen, 1969; Dimond and Beaumont, 1974; Milner, 1971). While the specialization of the left hemisphere for language and the right for certain visuo-spatial functions is well established (see reviews just cited), the discovery of additional hemispheric specializations has led some authors (for example, Bogen, 1969; Levy, 1969, 1973; Ornstein, 1972; TenHouten and Kaplan, 1973) to suggest a broader interpretation of each hemisphere's role. They propose that the information processing methods of the left and right hemispheres may represent two different cognitive "modes" which play fundamental and complementary roles in human thought: the left hemisphere is characterized as using verbal, analytical, linear-sequential processing, while the right hemisphere is characterized as nonverbal, nonanalytical, nonlinear, and as using instead synthetic, gestalt-holistic, parallel processing.

Marihuana intoxication data. Experiential reports of the marihuana intoxication state (for example, Anonymous, 1969; Solomon, 1966, section two) and in particular the results of a questionnaire study of 150 marihuana users (Tart, 1971) suggest that being "high" may involve a coordinated shift in perceptual and cognitive activities which might be appropriately described as a change in cognitive "mode." There is a reported impairment or decrease in verbal and linear-sequential cognitive activity and a reported enhancement and increase in nonverbal processing, particularly for musical, visual, and kinesthetic stimuli.

Specific parallels. The evidence for the parallelism between these two types of data can be developed in terms of specific examples.

(a) Reported impairments: At higher levels of marihuana intoxication, experiential reports commonly mention verbal difficulties such as "I find it difficult to read while stoned" (Tart, 1971: 172), "memory span for conversations is somewhat shortened," and "I may forget what the start of a sentence was about even before the sentence is finished" (Tart, 1971: 154). Such reported effects can be interpreted as indicating an impairment of left hemisphere verbal functions, since there is evidence supporting left hemisphere mediation of reading comprehension (Weisenburg and McBride, 1935) and verbal short- and intermediate-term memory (Black, 1973; Cohen, Noblin, and Silverman, 1968; Milner, 1962, 1967, 1971). These experiential reports have been verified in several laboratory experiments with intoxicated subjects (for example, Clark, Hughes, and Nakashima, 1970; Weil and Zinberg, 1969). Laboratory studies have also indicated interference (at high doses) with complex, sequential thought processes (for example, Melges, Tinklenberg, Hollister, and Gillespie, 1970) which is also consistent with left hemisphere impairment.

(b) Reported enhancements: On the other hand, at both moderate and strong dose levels, marihuana users frequently report enhancement of musical perception, enhanced visual depth sensation, and the enhanced perception of "patterns, forms, figures, meaningful designs" in material that might normally seem "just a meaningless series of shapes or lines" (Tart, 1971: 59). Each of these enhancement effects relates to a cognitive or perceptual process which is predominantly a function of the right hemisphere. (For experimental evidence on the right hemisphere lateralization of these functions, see the following: re aspects of music, see Bogen, 1969; Gordon and Bogen, 1974; Kimura, 1964; Milner, 1967; re depth perception, see Kimura, 1973; Kimura and Durnford, 1974; re closure for visual patterns, see Bogen, DeZure, Ten-Houten and Marsh, 1972; DeRenzi and Spinnler, 1966; Lansdell, 1970; Newcombe, 1969; Warrington and James, 1967.) In addition, marihuana users report a general enhancement of various kinds of nonverbal awareness and cognition, including bodily sensations not usually in awareness, imagery, and "intuitive insights" (Anonymous, 1969; Solomon, 1966; Tart, 1971). While there is little specific data on the lateralization of such functions, their experiential enhancement seems consistent with a shift toward the cognitive mode postulated for the right hemisphere. Evidence that marihuana enhances waking suggestibility (Crawford, 1974) is also relevant, in light of recent evidence

(Gur and Gur, 1974) that hypnotic suggestability is associated with right hemispheric functioning.

Statement of the Hypotheses

The parallels described above lead naturally[1] to the following hypotheses:

(1) The process of becoming "high" on marihuana consists, in part, of shifting into a new cognitive style or "mode" which involves less reliance on analytical, sequential, verbal processing, and more reliance on synthetic, holistic, imagistic processing.

(2) One of the ways that marihuana produces this shift is by decreasing left, and increasing right hemisphere participation in cognitive activities.

These two hypotheses are to some extent independent. It is possible, for example, that (1) could be true and (2) disconfirmed by subsequent experimental test. In order to clarify how this could happen, we must explain the notion of a "cognitive style shift" independently of any reference to hemisphere functions. We must also explain what sort of cognitive changes would not constitute a shift in "cognitive style" or "cognitive mode," so that hypothesis (1) does not seem to be trivially true.

The idea of "cognitive style" antedates the idea that there are different cognitive processing "modes" for the two cerebral hemispheres. For over thirty years, psychologists have been comparing the ways that different individuals organize and use their cognitive-perceptual processes (for example, see Tyler, 1965, Ch. 9 for a review). We are merely extending that notion to include possible differences in "cognitive style" within the same individual across different states of consciousness.

While the term "cognitive style" suggests an easily modified choice of cognitive approach to a problem, many of the "styles" studied by psychologists consist of firmly rooted patterns of behavior that contribute to (or are caused by) differences in ability to use particular cognitive approaches. For example, highly "field dependent" subjects (see below for definition) are generally unable to change to a more analytic style, even when the task demands it, whereas highly "field independent" subjects are unable to adopt a more global approach when this would be beneficial. It is this stronger interpretation of "cognitive style" that is used in this paper.

Not all changes in consciousness would constitute a change in cognitive style. For example, the various effects of marihuana apparently include impairment of attention and memory (see, for example, Darley, Tinklenberg, Roth, Hollister, and Atkinson, 1973; DeLong and Levy, 1973). But such changes in abilities do not in themselves provide evidence of a change in cognitive style; they might merely indicate less efficient performance in the same cognitive style. However, we have noted above that experiential reports of marihuana intoxication often include impressions of a reduction in verbal-sequential processing and simultaneous impressions of enhancement of several forms of nonverbal-holistic processing. Such reports suggest a selective pattern of shifts in several related cognitive abilities. If such a systematic pattern of changes in abilities could be objectively verified, it would indicate a shift in cognitive style.

We are not the first to suggest an interpretation of marihuana's effects in terms of "cognitive style." Dinnerstein (1968) has speculated that marihuana intoxication might move subjects toward a more "field dependent" mode (where the perception of an element is more strongly influenced by the surrounding perceptual field, see Witkin, Lewis, Hertzman, Machover, Meissner, and Wapner, 1954; Witkin, Dyk, Faterson, Goodenough, and Kays, 1962). Dinnerstein's suggestion is not incompatible with our hypotheses. In fact, the interpretation he suggests might be a special case of the more general cognitive shift which we hypothesize (see Cohen, Berent, and Silverman, 1973). However, the relationship between "field dependence" and hemisphere functions is not yet well established. For example, the Embedded Figures Test, which is often used to measure "field dependence," probably taps functions of both hemispheres (see discussion below). To date, marihuana studies incorporating tests of "field dependence" have obtained mixed results (Carlin, Bakker, Halpern, and Post, 1972; Hollister and Gillespie, 1970; Jones and Stone, 1970; Meyer, Pillard, Shapiro, and Mirin, 1971; Pearl, Domino, and Rennick, 1973). One advantage of the broader cognitive and neuropsychological hypotheses proposed here is that they are subject to a wider variety of experimental tests.

METHOD

The hypothesized shifts in cognitive style and hemispheric participation were tested by administering a battery of cognitive, perceptual, and preference tests (Table 1) to 25 subjects, and comparing their performance in the intoxicated vs. nonintoxicated state, counterbalanced for treatment order. The tests are so selected that lowered scores on one subset of tests and unchanged or raised scores on another subset would indicate a shift in cognitive style.[2] A more or less uniform change across all cognitive tests would indicate a general sedative or stimulant effect with no specific effect on cognitive style.

In addition to their role in the measurement of cognitive abilities, many of the psychological tests selected for this study were chosen because they tap lateralized functions (i.e., functions which tend to be localized in a single cerebral hemisphere). For example, the Street and Gollin tests of closure ability, as well as very similar closure tests, have previously been used to study the effects of unilateral brain damage and are known to be much more impaired by right hemisphere damage than by left hemisphere damage (Bogen, DeZure, TenHouten, and Marsh, 1972; DeRenzi and Spinnler, 1966; Lansdell, 1970; Newcombe, 1969; Warrington and James, 1967). More information on lateralization of tests is provided in Appendix 4. For those tests which are known to tap lateralized functions, systematic patterns of change

Table 1

Classification of Major Psychological Tests and Variables

I.   Cognitive Ability Tests and Variables

    A.   "Verbal" (analytical-verbal propositional ($\underline{P}$) function)

        1.   Nonsense Syllogisms
        2.   Inference Test
        3.   Composite "Verbal" Score (sum of A1 + A2 raw scores)

    B.   "Closure" (holistic-nonverbal appositional ($\underline{A}$) function)

        1.   Street Test
        2.   Gestalt Completion Test
        3.   Harshman Figures
        4.   Gollin Figures (error score)
        5.   "Closure" Composite Score (sum of B1 + B2 + B3 – B4 raw scores)

    C.   "Cognitive Style" indices

        1.   A/P Ratio (closure composite divided by verbal composite)
        2.   A-P Balance (closure composite minus verbal composite)

    D.   "Disembedding" (mixed analytic-holistic-nonverbal)

        1.   Hidden Figures Test

    E.   "Visualization" (originally hypothesized to be mostly $\underline{A}$ function, however more recently discovered to be mixed analytic-holistic-nonverbal)

        1.   Form Board
        2.   Surface Development
        3.   Paper Folding
        4.   "Visualization" Composite Score (sum of E1 + E2 + E3 raw scores)

II.   Perceptual Ability Tests and Variables

    A.   Nonverbal (right hemisphere, low level appositional ($\underline{A}$) functions)

        1.   Timbre Test
        2.   Arc-Circle Test

    B.   Verbal (left hemisphere, low level propositional ($\underline{P}$) functions)

        1.   Matched Syllables Dichotic Test
        2.   Matched Words Dichotic Test

III. Preference Tests

    A.   Preference for type of stimulus (aesthetic preference)

        1.   Design Judgment Test

    B.   Preference for type of cognitive task (verbal vs. spatial)

        1.   Grouping Test

    C.   Unconscious preference for processing mode

in test performance can provide indirect evidence of shifts in cerebral participation in perceptual-cognitive activities.

Testing Procedure

Experimental design. To insure that testing was accomplished during the period of 1 to 1.5 hours after intoxication, the battery of tests was divided into two parts (A and B), which were administered in separate intoxication periods on two successive mornings. Tests were given according to the schedule in Table 2. In this schedule, tests of right and left hemisphere functions were distributed throughout each testing period to balance the effects of any changes in intoxication level during the testing session. Order of conditions (intox vs. nonintox) and of parallel test forms were counterbalanced across subjects. Each subject was assigned to one of four test conditions: nonintox, form A (six subjects); intox, form A (six subjects); nonintox, form B (seven subjects); intox, form B (six subjects). Subjects were administered the opposite treatment and form conditions on retest.

Subjects. Twenty-five male subjects between the ages of 21 and 35 were obtained from a larger study of the effects of chronic marihuana intoxication.[3] All subjects were heavy users of marihuana before joining the research project and were carefully screened for physical and psychological problems before being admitted to the chronic study. Once admitted, each subject lived in special quarters at UCLA for 94 days where he participated in various testing programs (including this study) according to a standardized schedule. Subjects were paid $800 for their 94 days of participation, plus additional fees earned by performing specific tasks. Every subject admitted to the 94-day chronic study after September, 1973 participated in this cognitive style/hemisphere dominance study; 27 subjects began testing; however, one subject dropped out before retest and one had invalid data due to experimenter error.

Drug administration and testing conditions. Subjects were individually tested in a private office adjacent to their living area at UCLA. When tested in the nonintoxicated condition, subjects had not smoked for at least two days prior to testing. When tested in the intoxicated condition, subjects had been smoking marihuana on previous days. On the morning of testing, each subject refrained from smoking until just before the beginning of the testing session. At that time, he completely smoked one marihuana cigarette containing approximately .9 grams of marihuana assayed at 2.2 percent natural THC (19.8 mg THC). He was then tested for 1 to 1.5 hours after which he resumed other activities connected with the 94-day project.

Approximately two weeks elapsed between test and retest. However, because of scheduling conflicts or other problems, a few subjects were retested as few as 8 or as many as 21 days after initial test.

Table 2
Testing Schedule

Test Name (Source)	Length	Cognitive Function Tested	Lateralization
Part A (first morning)			
1. Street Test (Street)	1.5 min	gestalt closure	Right
2. Gestalt Completion (ETS)	3 min.	gestalt closure	Right
3. Nonsense Syllogisms (ETS)	4 min.	verbal analytic syllogistic	Left
4. Form Board Test (ETS)	8 min.	visualization	Right (?) ***
5. Inference Test (ETS)	6 min.	verbal analytic syllogistic	Left
6. Surface Development (ETS)	6 min.	visualization	Right (?) ***
7. Grouping Test (Galin)	1-4 min.*	verbal-spatial preference	L-R preference (?)
8. Harshman Figures (Harshman)	20 sec. x 11	gestalt closure	Right
9. Gollin Figures (Gollin)	5 sec. x 50	gestalt closure	Right
10. Paper Folding Test (ETS)	3 min.	visualization	Right (?) ***
11. Hidden Figures Test (ETS)	10 min.	non-verbal analytic	Left bilateral
Part B (second morning)			
1. Timbre Test (Seashore)	4.2 min.	auditory tone quality perception	Right
2. Matched Syllables (Berlin)	5 min.	(dichotic monosyllables)**	L-R use
3. Matched Words (Benson)	5 min.	(dichotic words)**	L-R use
4. Matched Words, Part II	5 min.	(dichotic words)**	L-R use
5. Matched Syllables, Part II	4.2 min.	(dichotic monosyllables)**	L-R use
6. Timbre Test, Part II	10-30 min.*	auditory tone quality perception	Right
7. Arc-Circle Test (Nebes)	2-5 min.*	part-to-whole judgment	Right
8. Design Judgment Test (Graves)	5-10 min.*	aesthetic judgment (?)	Right (?)
9. Reflective Eye Movements (Bakan, Day, Kinsbourne, etc.)		---	L-R use

* No time limit.

** Dichotic listening tasks are not used as tests of a cognitive function proper, but rather as a means of getting left and right ear scores which can be compared to measure hemispheric use asymmetry during a controlled task of a precise kind (in this case, syllable and word perception/discrimination/identification under conditions of dichotic competition).

*** Subsequently reevaluated and determined to be mixed left and right. See Appendix 5.

The Test Battery

Table 1 presents a list of the major tests (and related composite variables), classified into three basic groups: cognitive ability tests, perceptual ability tests, and tests of preference for particular stimuli or modes of cognitive processing ("preference tests"). Of these three groups, the largest and most important for our hypothesis testing is the group of cognitive ability tests. Most of these tests were selected from the Educational Testing Service's "Kit of Reference Tests for Cognitive Factors" (French, Ekstrom, and Price, 1963), and were thus believed to represent relatively factorially pure measures of the ability in question. Test descriptions and references are given in Appendix 3 and 4.

Composite variables. In order to obtain more reliable estimates of each cognitive ability under examination, several different tests of each ability[4] were included in the test battery. Because of the relatively small number of subjects tested in this study, interesting trends exhibited by a single test might fall short of statistical significance (see Appendix 1, "Problems of sample size"). However, with composite variables spanning several related tests, we have a better chance of detecting a real difference as statistically significant, since these composites are more stable and reliable. Further, since composite scores are less affected by peculiarities of any single test's format, they provide the most appropriate means of representing the general ability common to several closely related tests. In this study, composites were computed by simply summing raw scores of the constituent tests.

Two special composite variables were constructed to contrast different cognitive abilities. These are the Cognitive Style Indices listed under Section I-C of Table 1. They provide a means of directly measuring the predicted shifts in cognitive style. To explain these indices, however, we must first provide some additional background and terminology.

Definition of "Appositional," "Propositional," and the "Cognitive Style Indices." We will adopt the terminology suggested by Bogen (1969) for describing the distinctive cognitive modes of the left and right hemispheres. He proposed that the term "propositional" (first suggested by Hughlings Jackson) be adopted to represent the analytical-verbal-sequential functioning mode of the left hemisphere, and that the term "appositional" be used to refer to the holistic-nonverbal (and not yet well understood) functioning mode of the right hemisphere.

Subsequently, Bogen, DeZure, TenHouten, and Marsh (1972) have suggested that the overall relative emphasis or relative development of these two modes in one individual be measured by comparing his performance on appositional vs. propositional tasks. Specifically, they suggested a simple "A/P Ratio" as a measure of cognitive style. In their article they had only one appositional and one propositional task, and they simply took the ratio of the raw scores on these two tasks (Street Closure Test and WAIS Verbal Similarities) to compute their ratio. Since we have several tasks representing each of these cognitive abilities, we used the closure composite score as the appositional numerator and the verbal composite score as the propositional denominator for our A/P Ratio.

In addition to the (nonlinear) ratio measure suggested by Bogen et al. (1972), we also compared the relative magnitude of the A and P scores by computing an A-minus-P "balance" score. This provides a slightly different (linear) supplementary measure of cognitive style.

Experimental Predictions

With the terminology and variables defined above, we can now state more precisely the predicted changes implied by the experimental hypotheses. The first (cognitive style shift) hypothesis implies the following results:

1. **Relative Cognitive Shift Predictions.** During marihuana intoxication, the relative performance of a subject should shift in the direction of appositional functions:

   (a) the A/P Ratio should become larger;
   (b) the A-P Balance should shift in the positive direction.

These predictions would be fulfilled if marihuana changed cognitive performance in any one of five ways: (a) it could depress both A and P functions, but have a greater depressant effect on P functions; (b) it could selectively depress only P functions; (c) it could selectively stimulate A functions; (d) it could stimulate both A and P functions, but have a significantly greater facility effect on A functions; or (e) it could stimulate A functions and depress P functions. Considered by themselves, these alternative modes of action might seem to be decreasingly likely as one proceeds from (a) to (e). However, consideration of the second experimental hypothesis (of a "hemispheric shift") leads us to predict what otherwise might seem the least likely of these modes of action:

2. **Absolute Cognitive Shift Predictions.** During marihuana intoxication, the absolute performance levels of a subject should be altered as follows:

   (a) A functions should be enhanced;
   (b) P functions should be depressed;
   (c) Mixed A-and-P tests should show mixed results, depending on the relative importance of A vs. P functions for performance on each test.[5]

RESULTS AND DISCUSSION I:
COGNITIVE AND HEMISPHERIC SHIFTS

First, we will consider cognitive task data since they provide the most direct test of the "cognitive shift" hypothesis, as well as an indirect test of the "hemispheric shift" hypothesis. Subsequently, we will consider data for the perceptual tasks, which allow experimental testing of additional predictions implied by the "hemispheric shift" hypothesis.

Cognitive Ability Tests

Relative-shift results. An A/P Ratio and A-P Balance score were computed separately for each subject in both nonintox and intox conditions. Adjusted means for each condition were then computed across subjects (see Appendix 1 for details). The results are shown in Table 3. Both cognitive style indices show a statistically significant shift toward greater "appositionality," consistent with predictions 1-a and 1-b.

Absolute-shift results. Adjusted means for each cognitive ability composite are presented in Table 4 and Figure 1. In the intoxicated condition, the "appositional" closure composite score is significantly higher, consistent with prediction 2-a, while the "propositional" verbal composite score is significantly lower, consistent with prediction 2-b. At the same time, the A-P "mixed" disembedding score shows only a small shift. While a small shift on this test is consistent with prediction 2-c, the observed shift is even smaller than would be expected. Performance on this test might have been more clearly depressed if the test had been given earlier in the session; it was the last test of Session A, administered 50-60 minutes postintox, and the level of intoxication for most subjects (as indicated by pulse and subjective high ratings) had begun to drop somewhat.

Table 3

Relative Shifts: Effect of Marihuana on Indices of Cognitive Style

Index	Adjusted Means			Significance Level
	Intox	Nonintox	Difference	
A/P Ratio*	1.183	0.943	0.240	p < .05
A-P Balance*	1.068	-2.749	3.817	p < .005

* See text for definition

Table 4

Absolute Shifts: Effect of Marihuana on Cognitive Ability Scores

Score	Adjusted Means			Percent change from Nonintox	Significance level
	Intox	Nonintox	Difference		
Verbal Composite	11.921	13.565	-1.644	-12.12%	$p < .05$
Closure Composite	12.989	10.817	+2.172	+20.08%	$p < .05$
Disembedding	4.083	4.174	-0.090	-2.15%	n.s.
Visualization Composite	71.092	75.954	-4.862	-6.40%	n.s.

The result for the visualization composite score is not consistent with our original predictions. We originally thought that visualization tests would tap mostly appositional functions (since they are nonverbal and spatial); therefore, we predicted that such scores would be higher in the intoxicated state. Instead, the visualization composite score showed a small (nonsignificant) de-decrease with intoxication (see Table 4 and Figure 1).

In light of these results, we have reexamined the specific tasks used to test visualization and searched out further neuropsychological data on their lateralization. A simple, though post hoc, explanation has emerged: our "visualization" tasks are in fact cognitively complex, and although some of the cognitive abilities involved may be enhanced (e.g., visualization), other abilities involved in performing the same tasks are impaired (e.g., sequential memory). Thus, the effect of marihuana on these visualization tasks is seen as consistent with prediction 2-c. (Evidence for this interpretation is summarized briefly below.)

Results for individual cognitive tests. Data for the individual cognitive ability tests are summarized in Table 5 and Figure 2. With the small number of subjects tested in this study, it is difficult to demonstrate significant changes in "higher level" cognitive abilities by means of single tests rather than composite scores (see Appendix 1, "Problems of sample size"). Thus, it is interesting to note that despite this handicap, two of the individual cognitive ability tests show a significant difference between nonintox and intox conditions. Further, the pattern of shifts demonstrated by these two tests supports both the relative and absolute cognitive shift predictions. Scores on the Inference Test, an analytical-verbal test, are significantly lower in the intox condition, while those for the Harshman Figures, a holistic-nonverbal test, are significantly higher. Most of the other tests show trends in the predicted directions. Several of the individual tests, however, do not show the expected trends, and thus warrant further discussion.

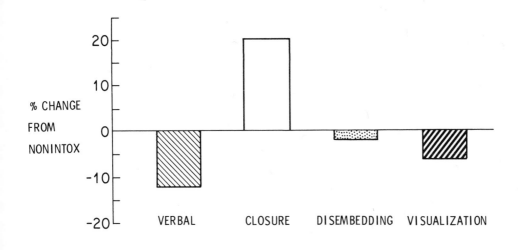

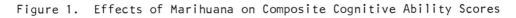

Figure 1. Effects of Marihuana on Composite Cognitive Ability Scores

Table 5

Effects of Marihuana on the Individual Tests of Cognitive Abilities

Test Name	Adjusted Means			Percent change from Nonintox	Significance Level
	Intox	Nonintox	Difference		
Nonsense Syllogisms	5.359	6.128	- .770	-12.55%	n.s.
Inference Test	6.563	7.438	- .875	-11.76%	p <.02
Street Test	3.009	3.093	+ .006	+ 0.21%	n.s.
Gestalt Completion Test	7.979	8.080	- .104	- 1.29%	n.s.
Harshman Figures	8.025	6.963	+1.060	+15.25%	p <.02
Gollin Figures (errors)	6.114	7.322	-1.210	+16.50%*	n.s. (p <.10)
Hidden Figures Test	4.084	4.174	- .090	- 2.15%	n.s.
Form Board Test	45.522	52.003	-5.580	-10.54%	n.s.
Surface Development Test	19.497	18.752	+ .744	+ 3.97%	n.s.
Paper Folding Test	5.073	5.198	- .025	- 2.41%	n.s.

* Sign changed to indicate enhanced performance due to drop in errors.

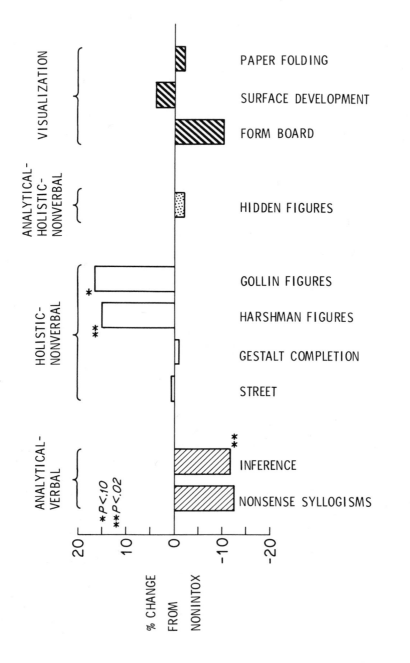

Figure 2.   Effects of Marihuana on Individual Cognitive Ability Tests

While two of the four closure tests show substantial improvements with intox, the other two (the Street and Gestalt Completion tests) show essentially no change (Table 5). There are several possible distinguishing characteristics of these latter two tests which might account for their failure to show an enhancement. These include psychometric flaws, differences in timing procedures, differences in effective level of intoxication (due to place in the testing schedule), and possible differences in test content.[6] The fact that subtle differences in these closure tests may have substantial effects on the observed performance with marihuana points out the difficulties of obtaining reliable measures of the effects of marihuana on "higher" cognitive functions. (Multiple tests of a given ability become almost essential.

Results for the visualization tests present a more complicated picture. Performance on the Surface Development Test improved with intoxication, but the change was small. The Paper Folding Test showed a very slight decrease, and the Form Board Test showed a larger decrease in performance with intoxication (Table 5, Figure 2). We now interpret these varied results as due to the cognitive complexity of the tasks used in this study to test visualization. The small observed shifts are interpreted as resulting from the incomplete cancellation of opposing effects of marihuana intoxication on different aspects of the tasks. The direction of shift for a particular test reflects the relative importance of marihuana effects on the analytic vs. holistic processing components of that task. While this interpretation is admittedly post hoc, it is supported by three types of independent evidence: (a) factor analysis of task content (for example, French, 1951), (b) performance data from split-brain patients performing similar tasks (for example, D. Zaidel, personal communication, 1975), and (c) complex and statistically significant patterns of correlations between the change scores on the visualization tasks and the change scores on other cognitive tests.

Perceptual Ability Tests

The perceptual ability tests (which we presume to not be dependent upon "higher level" cognitive functions of a given hemisphere but rather to tap more preliminary levels of lateralized data processing) are relevant for the evaluation of the second "hemisphere shift" hypothesis, dependent upon how generally this hypothesis is stated. Exploring in more detail our functional models of the hypothesized changes in interhemispheric relationships during marihuana intoxication, it is possible to distinguish between certain functional models which would predict and others which would not predict that marihuana will cause hemisphere-related shifts in performance on lateralized perceptual tasks.

Perhaps the simplest model of a shift in hemispheric participation in cognition is the "general activation" model which predicts a systematic shift in performance on lateralized perceptual tasks. Thus, the general level of

cortical activation of the right hemisphere is increased while the left is decreased during marihuana intoxication. If there is a generalized shift in relative cortical activation, performance shifts would be expected in both cognitive and perceptual lateralized tasks.

Table 6 summarizes the perceptual task data. All of the perceptual
tasks remain unaffected by marihuana intoxication.

The data do not show any evidence of a systematic hemisphere-related
shift in perceptual abilities; thus, they do not support the "generalized hemispheric activation" model. We might ask, then, what sort of model would be
consistent with a selective cognitive or "higher level" shift.

One possible model consistent with these data hypothesizes an "altered
locus of executive control" after marihuana intoxication. This model postulates
that for most nonintoxicated persons, the "locus of executive control" of attention and cognition is usually in the left hemisphere. Thus, the left hemisphere
often interferes with the ability of the right hemisphere to carry out more complex cognitive processing by retaining control of attention and inserting interfering verbal and analytic stimulus transformations into the incoming stimulus
field. During marihuana intoxication, however, the right hemisphere is (hy-
pothetically) given a greater degree of "executive" control, allowing attention

Table 6

Effects of Marihuana on Tests of Perceptual Abilities

Left Lateralized Tests (dichotic listening)	Adjusted Means			Percent change from Nonintox	Significance Level
	Intox	Nonintox	Difference		
Matched Syllables					
Left Ear	16.584	17.479	-0.895	- 5.12%	n.s.
Right Ear	19.170	19.399	-0.229	- 1.18%	n.s.
Matched Words					
Left Ear	13.213	13.582	-0.369	- 2.72%	n.s.
Right Ear	16.928	17.110	-0.182	- 1.06%	n.s.
Right Lateralized Tests					
Timbre Test	41.857	41.655	+0.202	+ 0.48%	n.s.
Arc-Circle Test (errors)					
Circles	1.694	1.708	-0.014	- 0.82%	n.s.
Large Arcs	2.139	2.194	-0.055	- 2.51%	n.s.
Small Arcs	6.444	5.639	+0.805	+14.28%	n.s.

to be focused (or defocused) for a longer period of time in a manner appropriate to holistic higher level processing, with less intruding verbal or analytic processing from the left hemisphere.

This model would attribute the selective effects of marihuana on "higher level" cognitive processing to the relatively greater dependence of such "higher level" processing on appropriate executive control. Simple sensory or perceptual processing (such as would be involved in recognizing two tones or two curvatures as similar) would take place so quickly and involve so few mental operations that it would be relatively unaffected by frequent interruptions from the left hemisphere, even in the nonintoxicated state. Thus, with marihuana intoxication it would not show a significant improvement. Conversely, dichotic syllable recognition would be simple and quick enough so that the intoxicated subject could complete his left hemisphere processing before a return of control to the right hemisphere would interfere with performance. Thus, he would not show significant impairment with intoxication.

On the other hand, longer analytic sequences (such as those required by the Inference Test or Nonsense Syllogisms Test) would be frequently disrupted by episodes of right hemisphere control more characteristic of the marihuana intoxicated state. Thus, such activities would be impaired by marihuana intoxication. However, increased right hemisphere executive control would be advantageous for tasks requiring "higher level" holistic interpretive processing (e.g., closure), since this type of processing is "blocked" as long as the left hemisphere maintains control and imposes an analytic framework on the incoming perceptual field.

It should be emphasized that an "executive control" model of marihuana's effects is not here proposed as a final or complete interpretation of the data from this study. (For one thing, it is not clear how it can account for the transformations of perceptual experience which are reported by intoxicated persons, for example, enhancement of subjective depth.) Nonetheless, it provides an example of the more complex type of model which may be necessary to account for some of the selective effects of marihuana on "higher level" lateralized cognitive functions.

Other implications. The stability of the perceptual task scores demonstrates a relative lack of subject or procedural bias in favor of either intoxication or nonintoxication conditions. These nonsignificant shifts in scores are particularly significant in any consideration of possible biasing in motivation. The dichotic task is particularly difficult and frustrating and yet subject scores remained approximately the same in both conditions.

Preference and Other Tests

Since the three preference tests and questionnaire data are less crucial to the major experimental hypotheses, results will be only briefly noted. Intoxication produced the following results: (1) on a verbal vs. spatial sorting task (Galin Grouping Test), subjects tended to make more spatial and fewer verbal choices (p < .10); (2) there was no change on the Design Judgment Test, a measure of aesthetic preference or judgment; (3) conjugate lateral eye movement measurements of preferred cognitive mode showed a paradoxical result contrary to expectation. There was an increase in right movements (indicating more left hemisphere preference). However, this increase in right eye movement to reflective questions was from an extremely strong left-looking, right-hemispheric eye movement pattern in the normal condition and shifted to a less consistent, more bilateral pattern when intoxicated. This shift was much less apparent in those subjects who showed low lateralization according to dichotic listening (see below). While not well understood, these latter findings give credence to a marihuana-induced reduction in functional asymmetry in highly lateralized subjects.

Relation of These Results to Previously Published Findings

Verbal-analytical tests. The decrease in verbal-analytical cognitive ability is consistent with other published results (Clark et al, 1970; DeLong and Levy, 1973; Drew et al, 1972; Melges et al, 1970; Miller and Drew, 1972; Weil and Zinberg, 1969).

Closure tests. Previously published data on closure ability during mari-huana intoxication have been inconclusive. Pearl et al (1973), combining the Gestalt Completion Test items with another closure test, found no impairment at a moderate dose level (5 – 15 mg THC depending upon subject's intake) yet found impairment of certain verbal tasks. At a high dose level (10 – 30 mg THC) they found a significant decrease in performance. To determine high dose level subjects were encouraged to smoke until they felt too "high," which resulted in negative side effects in some subjects. Barratt, Beaver, White, Blakeney, and Adams (1972) used the parallel forms of a closure test from the Moran battery (Moran and Mefferd, 1959). The observed trend (improvement with marihuana) was not significant, and was confounded with learning effects since the same five subjects were repeatedly tested. However, there was a significant increase in variability of closure scores when subjects were intoxicated, suggesting that some effect of marihuana was present.

The data which are perhaps most comparable to ours come from an informal pilot study by Marsh and Chemtobe (personal communication, 1973). They used the Street Test, but with a method of administration which differed from ours. While we split this test into two parallel halves, they gave the entire test, intoxicated half of their subjects, and then readministered the test and measured the improvement. Their 12 intoxicated subjects showed significantly greater improvement than 12 nonintoxicated controls.

Visualization tests. Barratt et al (1972) tested visualization using forms from the Moran battery (Moran and Mefferd, 1959) and found a nonsignificant trend toward enhancement with marihuana. But, as with their closure results, this finding was difficult to interpret because of confounding with learning effects and the small sample size (5 subjects).

Disembedding test. The decrease on the Hidden Figures Test, if reliable, is also consistent with previously published results for this test. Significant impairment on Hidden Figures during marihuana intoxication was observed by Carlin, Bakker, Halpern, and Post (1972) and a nonsignificant decrease was reported by Meyer, Pillard, Shapiro, and Mirin (1971). On similar
tests of disembedding, decreases were noted by Pearl, Domino, and Rennick
(1973) and Hollister and Gillespie (1970).

A marihuana-induced decrement in disembedding is consistent with
our hypotheses concerning marihuana's action and current evidence as to the
lateralization of this type of test. The relatively small amount of decrease
might be attributable to the involvement of both hemispheres in the task (Poeck,
1973; Teuber and Weinstein, 1956; Zaidel, 1973), while the presence of decrease rather than enhancement might be attributable to the particular sensitivity of the task to language-related processes (Poeck, 1973; Teuber and Weinstein, 1956) and to the greater relative involvement of the left hemisphere in
performance (Zaidel, 1973). (This description of the components contributing
to the disembedding performance is also consistent with factor analytic descriptions of the test, for example, Thurstone, 1944; French, 1951.) It should be
noted that at higher dose levels performance disruption may be due more to
interference with attention and motivation than with cognitive style shifts,
since this is a difficult test requiring prolonged concentration.

Perceptual tests. The lack of perceptual effects reported here is consistent with other studies which also failed to find changes on "low level"
perceptual tests when moderate doses were used. Like the present findings,
Klonoff, Low, and Marcus (1973) found no change on the Timbre Test while
reporting significant impairments of motor performance and verbal-analytical
ability at dose levels of 13.6 mg THC.

RESULTS AND DISCUSSION II:
FURTHER TESTING FOR A "HEMISPHERIC SHIFT"

The evidence presented previously provides indirect support for the
hypothesis of altered hemispheric participation in cognition during marihuana
intoxication. By comparing the performance level of left lateralized and
right lateralized functions, we are indirectly comparing the performance of
the two hemispheres, and any shift in the ratio or balance of these scores suggests a shift in the relationship between the hemispheres. However, other
mechanisms might also cause such a shift in performance, and therefore more
"direct" tests of the activity of the two hemispheres are needed.

EEG Data

Perhaps the best measure would have been EEG data on the activity
of the two hemispheres, collected while subjects were performing the tasks
used in this study. Such data are not available. Nonetheless, we were

gratified to learn that preliminary results of EEG analyses on some of the same marihuana subjects were conducted by John Hanley, Eleanore Tyrrell, and Pierre Hahn (see Cohen, 1975a) and appeared to show an increase in left hemisphere alpha activity and a decrease in right hemisphere alpha activity after intoxication. Subsequent statistical analysis by Hanley et al (see Cohen, 1975b) indicated that these differences, while substantial, were not statistically significant because of large inter-subject variability. Still, the direction of these trends is interesting, since this same pattern of alpha amplitude shift is seen when nonintoxicated subjects are deliberately moved from propositional to appositional processing by the use of spatial tasks (see, for example, Galin and Ornstein, 1972). Since reduction in alpha amplitude is usually associated with greater arousal or "mental activity," the observed shift indicates a shift toward greater relative proportion of cerebral processing in the right hemisphere, as would be predicted by our second experimental hypothesis.

This relative alpha shift was only found in the temporal-frontal placement, not in the parietal-occipital placement. Such a pattern is suggestively analogous to our result that "higher level" functions were selectively affected by marihuana. Once again, the "general hemisphere activation" interpretation is not supported. Of course, any identification of these different recording placements with "higher" vs. "lower" functions is certainly oversimplified, but perhaps has some value as a stimulus to more precise investigation.

If these preliminary EEG trends are replicated, using larger samples or more specific mental tasks to stabilize inter-subject variations (subjects were recorded in the eyes-closed resting state), they could provide important support for the "hemispheric shift" hypothesis of this study.

Dichotic Listening Data

The most direct measure of asymmetrical hemispheric functioning in our study is provided by comparing the accuracy of the right and left ears during the dichotic listening task. While several factors seem to influence performance on this task, a well-established result is that verbal stimuli are usually better perceived by the right ear while musical, environmental, and certain other nonverbal stimuli are usually better perceived by the left ear (see Kimura, 1967, for a discussion of these results). These ear asymmetries are reversed in individuals with reversed cerebral dominance as tested by intra-carotid injection of sodium amytal (Kimura, 1961).

It is a consequence of the mechanisms presumed to underlie dichotic listening (see Kimura, 1967, for discussion) that the right ear advantage for verbal stimuli is a function of (a) the degree of left hemisphere specialization for the type of verbal perception involved, and (b) the degradation of the left ear's sensory information as it passes from the right hemisphere across the cerebral commissures to reach the specialized processing "centers" in the left hemisphere. Thus, ear asymmetry scores, on the average, provide some indication of the degree of lateralization of verbal perception in a group of individuals, although other factors will also affect the scores.

Dichotic listening scores were collected on both test and retest for all but one subject. Scores for each condition were based on two sets of stimuli: (a) 30 pairs of syllable-contrastive nonsense stimuli (for example, pa vs. ka, ba vs. ta); and (b) 30 pairs of monosyllabic words ending in "ought" (for example, "pot" vs. "cot," "bought" vs. "tot"). See Appendix 4 for a more detailed description. These 60 stimuli were presented twice, with earphones reversed for the second presentation, providing 120 dichotic pairs in all, and thus providing a fairly stable measure of the subject's performance on this task.

The effect of marihuana on dichotic listening scores would depend on its mode of action in the brain. If, for example, it altered the information transfer properties of the corpus callosum, then it should have affected the left ear scores. A decrease in callosal transfer would have selectively lowered left ear scores, raising dichotic ear asymmetries. An increase in callosal transfer would have had the opposite effect, raising the left ear score and bringing the two ears closer together. If marihuana seriously interfered with the perception of consonants by the left hemisphere, the right and left ear scores should both have been lowered (in fully lateralized individuals for whom this task is performed, for both ears, by the left hemisphere).

The results are shown in Table 6. Marihuana did not have an appreciable effect on the performance of either ear, although there is a small, non-significant drop in left ear performance and an even smaller drop in right ear performance.

To further examine the effects of marihuana on ear asymmetry, we computed for each subject an intox and nonintox score using each of the various standard ratio and difference indices of ear asymmetry: POE = the left ear's errors divided by the total errors; Phi = the correlation between accuracy and side of presentation across trials; POC = the right ear's correct divided by total correct; R-minus-L = the difference between the percent accuracy of the two ears. None of these measures shows a significant or appreciable difference between nonintox and intox conditions.

These results suggest that marihuana does not produce a substantial blockage or facilitation of the transmission of auditory sensory information across the cerebral commissures. If marihuana does affect callosal information transfer, it would appear that it acts on pathways other than those used for transmission of (pre-phonetic) auditory information from the right to the left hemisphere.

Differing Marihuana Effects Related to Subject Lateralization

If one of the ways that marihuana produces the observed cognitive and preference shifts is by affecting the functional relationship between the cerebral hemispheres, then individuals who have reduced or atypical hemispheric specialization might be expected to show reduced or atypical responses to marihuana.

In order to further explore the relationship between marihuana's effects and hemispheric lateralization of function, the total subject sample was divided into two groups of 12 subjects each, on the basis of a median split of their non-intox dichotic listening POE lateralization scores (dichotic data was missing on one subject, so he was omitted from the analysis). Separate analyses were then performed to determine the drug effects on those subjects who were above the median (the "high lateralization" group) as compared to those subjects who were below the median (the "low lateralization" group). The results are summarized in Figure 3.

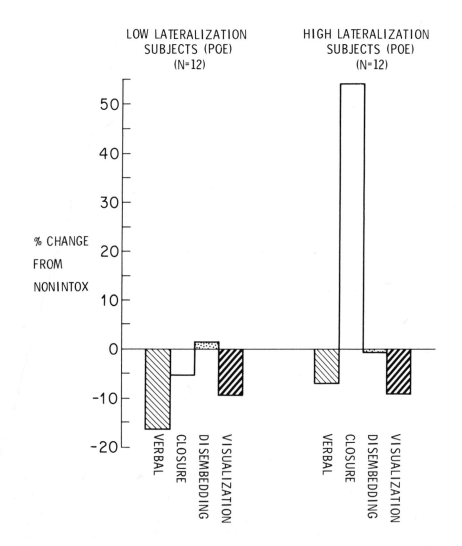

Figure 3.   Marihuana Effects for High vs. Low Lateralized Subjects

These two groups of subjects show different patterns of response to mari-huana intoxication. "Low lateralization" subjects show a stronger impairment of verbal-analytical abilities and show no improvement of closure when intoxi-cated. "High lateralization" subjects show a smaller impairment of verbal-analytical abilities and a strong enhancement of closure ability when intoxi-cated. Despite the small $\underline{N}$ of 12, the "high lateralization" group's closure enhancement was statistically significant ($\underline{p}<.05$, for 10 d.f., 2Q). None of the "low lateralization" group's changes was statistically significant, al-though the depression of verbal-analytical performance approached significance ($.05<\underline{p}<.10$). The results obtained using POC to measure lateralization were similar, but not quite as dramatic. (When the subjects were divided at the median POC score, one subject in the POE "low" group changed to the POC "high" group, and one in the POE "high" group changed to the POC "low" group.)

To test the statistical significance of the relationship between laterali-zation and response to marihuana, correlations were computed between size of drug effect and degree of lateralization. (Size of drug effect was measured by intox minus nonintox difference scores, and lateralization was measured by $\underline{nonintoxicated}$ dichotic listening scores. Partial correlations, with the effects of treatment order partialed out, were used to test these hypotheses in order to minimize contamination from learning or marihuana-learning inter-action effects.)

Several significant correlations were found (Table 7). The partial correlation between lateralization and enhancement of closure during intoxi-cation is approximately .36 ($\underline{p}<.05$, 1Q). More lateralized subjects show significantly more enhancement of closure ability when intoxicated. While no other $\underline{linear}$ correlation involving composite variables is significant, inspec-tion of scatter diagrams for these relationships suggested that systematic non-linear relationships might be present. This impression was strengthened by separate analysis of the "middle" vs. "extreme" lateralization groups. The sample was divided into four quartiles on the basis of lateralization scores (POE) and a separate analysis was performed for the middle two vs. the extreme two quartiles.

The most striking result was obtained with respect to visualization. The "middle lateralization" group showed a 10 percent $\underline{increase}$ in visualiza-tion performance when intoxicated, although this increase was not statistically significant. On the other hand, the "extreme lateralization" group showed a 24 percent $\underline{decrease}$ in visualization performance when intoxicated, and this change was highly significant ($\underline{p}<.002$, for 10 d.f., 2Q).

To test these trends, $\underline{nonlinear}$ correlations were computed. (Laterali-zation scores were transformed into parabolic functions, symmetric about the mean, according to the relation: $nonlin = (lin-mean)^2$). As Table 7 shows, highly significant $\underline{nonlinear}$ correlations were obtained between lateralization

Table 7

Effect of a Subject's Lateralization on His Response to Marihuana:
Partial Correlations between Intox-minus Nonintox Cognitive Change Score and
Nonintox Dichotic Listening Lateralization Scores (Controlling for Treatment Order)

Variable	Dichotic Listening Lateralization Scores (d.f. = 21)					
	POE	Phi	POC	$(POE-mean)^2$	$(Phi-mean)^2$	$(POC-mean)^2$
I-N Change in Verbal Composite	.21	.23	.22	.33	.32	.29
I-N Change in Closure Composite	.38*	.37*	.35*	-.17	-.26	-.31
I-N Change in Visualization Composite	-.16	-.12	-.08	-.28	-.15	-.06
I-N Change in A/P Ratio	.15	.13	.12	-.42**	-.48**	-.50**
I-N Change in A-P Balance	.19	.17	.16	-.39	-.47**	-.49**

* N = 24; p<.05; one-tailed test
**N = 24; p<.05; two-tailed test

Explanations of Dichotic Listening Lateralization scores given in Method section.

and shifts in cognitive style. The nonlinearity of these effects on cognitive style indices is apparently due mainly to the nonlinearity of the effects on the verbal components entering into them, although the verbal change scores showed only a nonsignificant trend toward nonlinearity when considered by themselves (combined linear-nonlinear polynomial regression produced a correlation of around .45, which had borderline significance, .05<p<.10, 2Q). On the other hand, despite the apparent trends in the scatter diagrams and in the middle vs. extreme group analyses, the nonlinear relationship between visualization drug effects and lateralization was not statistically significant when tested by this technique.

The reason for the nonlinearity of cognitive style correlations with lateralization is not clear, but it might, in part, reflect differences in drug response arising from differences in nonintoxicated ability. These subjects showed a significant nonlinear relationship between nonintoxicated verbal-analytical performance (verbal composite scores) and degree of lateralization (polynomial regression showed a p<.025, 2Q). Further, those subjects who do best nonintoxicated show the largest drop when intoxicated (partially, perhaps, a regression toward the mean). This may induce a nonlinearity into the change scores. On the other hand, no relationship -- linear or nonlinear -- was found between nonintoxicated closure performance and degree of lateralization. Possibly as a consequence, the relationship between closure drug effects and lateralization was a simple linear one, with increasing drug effects correlating, as expected, with increasing lateralization.

The relationships between degree of lateralization and drug effects, as tentatively suggested by these data, are diagrammatically summarized in Figure 4.

These correlational results should, of course, be viewed as highly tentative and preliminary until replicated. This is particularly true of the linear correlations. While all nonlinear correlations were tested using a two-tailed test, the linear correlations were tested with one-tailed tests. It might be argued, however, that our prediction of a greater drug effect for more lateralized subjects was too tentative to justify the use of a one-tailed test. According to such a highly conservative approach, the closure-change-vs.-lateralization correlations become only "borderline" in significance (.05<p <.10), and the evidence for statistically significant relationships between

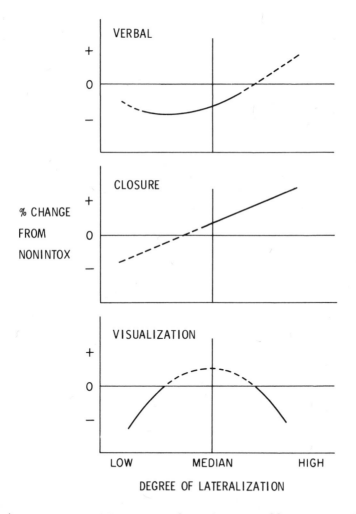

Figure 4.   Patterns of Change of Marihuana Effects as a Function of Subject's Lateralization Score

drug effect and lateralization rests more heavily on the surprising nonlinear correlations between lateralization and cognitive style shifts.

Nonetheless, the overall pattern of results (for example, Figure 3) is strikingly consistent with the hypothesis that some of marihuana's effects are related to hemispheric lateralization. With our small sample size, we are at a handicap in trying to demonstrate statistical significance, and so the border-line nature of some of these correlations (and the nonsignificance of others) should not be too surprising or discouraging. Many more "significant" corre-lations between lateralization and drug response have been found than would be expected by chance with these data, and therefore we are encouraged to look further into this type of relationship. The possibility of finding a physio-logical basis for some of the individual differences in responses to marihuana provides strong motivation for continuing the investigations.

CONCLUSION

The data of this study tend to support both the hypothesis of a cogni-tive style shift and the hypothesis of a shift in hemispheric participation in cognitive processing during marihuana intoxication. These results must be replicated, however, before they can provide firm support for any interpreta-tions concerning the effects of marihuana on cognitive functioning. Further-more, it is not yet known whether the pattern of enhancement will extend to include better ("purer") tests of visualization and to additional right hemi-sphere functions; further studies of the generality of these effects are needed.

In this study, the types of cognitive tests which showed the clearest shifts during intoxication were those which are the most clearly lateralized according to published neuropsychological evidence, and scores on these tests shifted in the predicted directions. Additional support for the hypothesis that marihuana alters the relationship between the left and right cerebral hemi-sphere was provided by the contrasting patterns of drug effects exhibited by "low" vs. "high" lateralized subjects.

We are not yet ready to propose specific models of the brain mecha-nisms that might underlie these observed effects. Many aspects of these data suggest that marihuana causes a change in interhemispheric communication, but the stability of dichotic lateralization scores across nonintox and intox conditions would seem to argue against this (unless only a selective effect on certain callosal pathways is involved). Any neurological model proposed to explain these data would have to more clearly specify, for example, the hy-pothesized nature of the reduced lateralization in "low lateralized" subjects. Perhaps future findings will lead us closer to a concrete model of marihuana's effects on hemispheric functioning, along with a more detailed model of indi-vidual differences in patterns of hemispheric specialization of the human brain.

APPENDIX 1

Statistical Procedures:
Definitions, Methods, and Rationales

The basic statistics computed for this report were (a) "adjusted means" for the intox and nonintox conditions, (b) a difference score across conditions, (c) a "percent change from nonintox" score, (d) a statistical significance level for the observed change, based on (e) a repeated measures analysis of variance.

The rationale, interpretation, and computing procedures (or programs) used for these analyses are explained in the following paragraphs. In addition, there is a discussion of the issue of sample size.

Adjusted means. Test performance is summarized by the use of "adjusted means" for the nonintox and intox conditions. These means are "adjusted" in order to correct for unequal $\underline{N}$'s in the two treatment-order groups. Instead of weighting each subject equally, the 12 subjects in the intox-first treatment order are given the same total weight as the 13 subjects in the nonintox-first treatment order. (This is done by simply averaging the two treatment order submeans.) In practice, this adjustment has only a slight effect on the mean values.

Percent change from nonintox. For each pair of adjusted means, a difference between conditions is computed (intox minus nonintox), and this performance difference is then expressed as a percentage of the normal (nonintox) performance level for that task. This provides a percent change in performance level "due to" intoxication, perhaps the most meaningful expression of the size of the marihuana effect for a given task. This percentage is computed as follows: $PC = ((I-N)/N) \times 100$.

Significance level. The statistical significance of the observed change with intoxication is evaluated on the basis of the $\underline{F}$ value for the main effect of drug condition in the analysis of variance, described below. One-tailed tests (1Q) are used for all main effects of condition where the direction of change was predicted by the experimental hypotheses. Two-tailed tests are used for all other comparisons.

Analysis of Variance. The statistical significance of differences among the means for a given test was evaluated (initially) by performing a repeated measures analysis of variance. Two main effect terms and one interaction term were extracted from the data.

The main effect term for drug condition was used to test the significance of marihuana effects, i.e., overall differences between nonintox and intox scores on a given task.

The main effect term for order was used to test overall differences between the scores of the intox-first group of subjects and the nonintox-first group. (Such a difference might arise, for example, if the disadvantages of performing a given task in the intox condition on first test carried over to the nonintox retest and lowered scores there also. Presumably, this would indicate an effect of marihuana on learning as well as on simple performance.) Normally, this term is not expected to be significant. When it is, interpretation is not simple, and depends on the particular case in question. However, this main effect term arises as a natural consequence of the experimental and analysis design and provides the basis for generating the condition-by-order interaction term, which does have a straightforward interpretation.

The condition-by-order interaction term was used to test for overall differences between test and retest scores on a given task. Usually, a significant interaction occurred when the intox scores were better in order 1 than 2, whereas nonintox scores were better in order 2 than 1. Since in order 1 the intox was on retest, and in order 2 the nonintox was on retest, this interaction pattern reflects a generally superior performance on retest compared to test, that is, a simple task learning effect. However, since parallel forms rather than identical tests were used for retest, any learning effect was not due to memory of test content, but instead -- and more interestingly -- to learning of successful performance strategies for that type of cognitive or perceptual task. These results have not been discussed in any detail here, but a number of significant learning effects were observed. Plots of the means suggested that some tests also showed marihuana-learning interactions.

As a precaution, we also performed analyses of variance incorporating an additional main effect term for test form (and, as a consequence, interaction terms for form with condition, form with order, and a three-way interaction of form with order with condition). These analyses were done on all tests employing two parallel forms (that is, cognitive ability and preference tests; the perceptual tests did not have a memorizable content, and thus did not have parallel forms). Although there was an occasional significant two- or three-way interaction term, it was usually neither interpretable nor informative. Therefore, these more complicated analyses are not discussed here.

All analyses of variance were performed at the UCLA Campus Computing Network, using the BMD P2V computer program from the P-series Biomedical Computer Programs (Dixon, 1975). This program performs repeated measures analysis of variance with unequal N's and complex designs. (In BMD terminology, the design used for the analyses in this study was "1G,2 (nY)".) For more details on the program, see Dixon (1975).

Problems of sample size. In this study, it was difficult to demonstrate the statistical significance of an observed pattern of changes in mean scores because of the small number of subjects tested. This may seem at first implausible since other published marihuana studies, and a number of medical studies in the 94-day project, worked successfully with a sample almost as small. However, it is important, when evaluating the size of a subject sample, to keep in mind the type of data obtained, the reliability of the measures involved, and the amount of uncontrollable variability to be expected in relation to the size of the systematic effects one wants to detect.

While it is true that published physiological studies sometimes use 20 or fewer subjects, published psychological studies of mental traits, particularly correlational multivariate psychometric studies, almost always use at least 50 and often several hundred subjects. One reason for the larger N's in psychological studies is that techniques of measurement for psychological variables are often less reliable than for physiological variables. Larger N's are needed to "average out" fluctuations due to larger errors of measurement. Furthermore, psychological variables are often affected by a greater number of influences difficult to control experimentally. Specifically, the effect of marihuana on cognitive functions is quite variable from individual to individual and from one occasion to the next, much more so, for example, than its effect on pulse rate. A great number of personality and mood variables can influence a particular cognitive response to marihuana. To study or control for the interrelations of these many factors, more complicated experimental designs are required, which need a larger number of subjects to fill all their "cells." Even the simple counterbalanced design of this study required dividing the subjects into two groups of 12 and 13 subjects each (not counting the further division into groups taking Form A on intox vs. Form B on intox in each group). This counterbalancing further restricted our effective N's for many comparisons.

The handicap of a small number of subjects (for the type of data and experimental design involved) was partially overcome by the use of several tests of each important cognitive ability being examined, and by looking at broad patterns of change across several variables rather than concentrating on changes on a single test. These broader comparisons, more appropriate for the type of hypotheses involved, were accomplished through the use of composite variables.

APPENDIX 2
Analyses of Variance for Composite Variables

Table A2-1

A/P Ratio (Closure Composite/Verbal Composite)

Source	Degrees of Freedom	Mean Square	F	Prob. F Exceeded
Mean	1	56.3795	80.3996	0.000
Order	1	0.0073	0.0105	0.919
Error	23	0.7012		
Condition	1	0.7211	3.0054	0.048 (1Q)
Condition x Order	1	0.2571	1.0717	0.311
Error	23	0.2399		

Table A2-2

A-P Balance (Closure Composite minus Verbal Composite)

Source	Degrees of Freedom	Mean Square	F	Prob. F Exceeded
Mean	1	35.2622	0.2823	0.600
Order	1	18.7814	0.1503	0.702
Error	23	124.9113		
Condition	1	181.7795	8.2394	0.004 (1Q)
Condition x Order	1	46.8408	2.1231	0.159
Error	23	22.0619		

Table A2-3

Verbal Composite Score

Source	Degrees of Freedom	Mean Square	F	Prob. F Exceeded
Mean	1	8106.8984	209.3654	0.000
Order	1	5.7617	0.1488	0.703
Error	23	38.7212		
Condition	1	33.7390	2.9732	0.049 (1Q)
Condition x Order	1	4.5793	0.4035	0.532
Error	23	11.3473		

Table A2-4

Closure Composite Score

Source	Degrees of Freedom	Mean Square	F	Prob. F Exceeded
Mean	1	7072.7968	81.6027	0.000
Order	1	45.3474	0.5232	0.477
Error	23	86.6735		
Condition	1	58.8901	3.2609	0.042 (1Q)
Condition x Order	1	80.7128	4.4694	0.046
Error	23	18.0589		

Table A2-5

Disembedding (Hidden Figures Test)

Source	Degrees of Freedom	Mean Square	F	Prob. F Exceeded
Mean	1	782.8522	36.7787	0.000
Order	1	1.0605	0.0498	0.826
Error	21	21.2854		
Condition	1	0.0928	0.0111	0.458 (1Q)
Condition				
x Order	1	7.7015	0.9272	0.347
Error	21	8.3057		

Table A2-6

Visualization Composite Score

Source	Degrees of Freedom	Mean Square	F	Prob. F Exceeded
Mean	1	269847.1250	318.7741	0.000
Order	1	23.0234	0.0272	0.870
Error	23	846.5148		
Condition	1	294.9397	1.8119	0.191 (2Q)
Condition				
x Order	1	1384.9626	8.5082	0.008
Error	23	162.7791		

APPENDIX 3

Instructions and Sample Items from Representative Cognitive Tests

Gestalt Completion Test -- Cs-1

This is a test of your ability to perceive a whole picture even though it is not completely drawn. You are to use your imagination to fill in the missing parts.

Look at each incomplete picture and try to see what it is. Write on the line beneath it a word or a few words telling what the picture is. You need not describe it in detail; just name the picture or its important parts.

Try the sample pictures below.

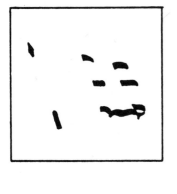

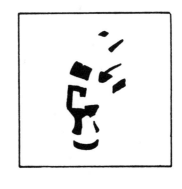

A _____   B _____

Picture A is a flag and picture B is a hammer head.

Your score on this test will be the number of pictures identified correctly. Even if you are not sure of the correct identification, it will be to your advantage to guess. Work as rapidly as you can without sacrificing accuracy.

You will have <u>3 minutes</u>. There are <u>2</u> pages of items.

DO NOT TURN THIS PAGE UNTIL ASKED TO DO SO.

B

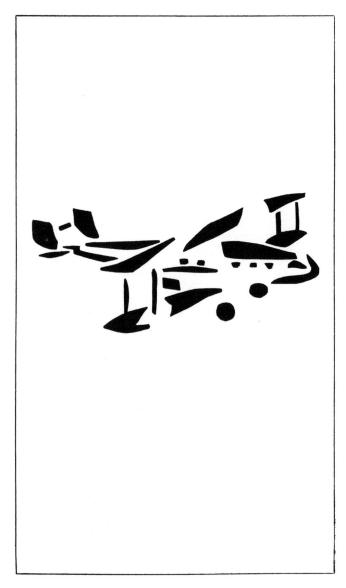

Sample item from the Street Test

Inference Test -- Rs-3

In each item on this test you will be given one or two statements such as you might see in newspapers or popular magazines. The statements are followed by various conclusions which some people might draw from them. In each case, decide which conclusion can be drawn from the statement(s) without assuming anything in addition to the information given in the statement(s). There is only one correct conclusion.

Mark your answer by putting an X through the number in front of the conclusion that you select.

Consider the following sample item:

Bill, a member of the basketball team, is 6 feet, 2 inches tall and weighs 195 pounds. To qualify for the team, a person must be at least 5 feet, 10 inches tall.

    1-The larger a man is, the better basketball player he is.
    2-Basketball players are often underweight.
    3-Some players on the team are more than 6 feet tall.
    4-Bill is larger than the average man.
    5-The best basketball players come from the ranks of larger-
      than-average men.

Only conclusion 3 may be drawn without assuming that you have information or knowledge beyond what the statements give. The statements say nothing about how good different players are, nothing about whether they are underweight, and nothing about average or taller-than-average men.

Your score on this test will be the number marked correctly minus some fraction of the number marked incorrectly. Therefore, it will not be to your advantage to guess unless you are able to eliminate one or more of the answer choices as wrong.

You will have 6 minutes. There are 3 pages, with a total of 10 items.

DO NOT TURN THIS PAGE UNTIL ASKED TO DO SO.

Form Board Test -- Vz-1

This is a test of your ability to tell what pieces can be put together to make a certain figure. Each test page is divided into two columns. At the top of each column is a geometrical figure. Beneath each figure are several problems. Each problem consists of a row of five shaded pieces. Your task is to decide which of the five shaded pieces will make the complete figure when put together. Any number of shaded pieces, from two to five, may be used to make the complete figure. Each piece may be turned around to any position but it cannot be turned over. It may help you to sketch the way the pieces fit together. You may use any blank space for doing this. When you know which pieces make the complete figure, mark a plus (+) in the box under ones that are used and a minus (–) in the box under ones that are not used.

In Example A, below, the rectangle can be made from the first, third, fourth, and fifth pieces. A plus has been marked in the box under these places. The second piece is not needed to make the rectangle. A minus has been marked in the box under it. The rectangle drawn to the right of the problem shows one way in which the four pieces could be put together.

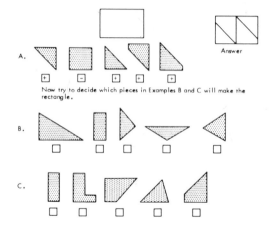

A.

Now try to decide which pieces in Examples B and C will make the rectangle.

B.

C.

In Example B, the first, fourth, and fifth pieces are needed. You should have marked a plus under these three pieces and a minus under the other two pieces. In Example C, the second, third, and fifth pieces should be marked with a plus and the first and fourth with a minus.

Your score on this test will be the number marked correctly minus the number marked incorrectly. Therefore, it will not be to your advantage to guess unless you have some idea whether or not the piece is correct.

You will have 8 minutes for this test. It has 2 pages.

DO NOT TURN THIS PAGE UNTIL ASKED TO DO SO.

APPENDIX 4

Test Descriptions and/or References, Plus References on Test Lateralization

Cognitive Tests

ETS Tests. Most of the cognitive tests were taken from the Kit of Reference Tests for Cognitive Factors published by the Educational Testing Service. Tests from this source are followed by the notation (ETS) in Table 2. Descriptions and bibliographies for each of these tests can be found in French, Ekstrom, and Price (1963). Instructions and sample items for these tests can be found in Appendix 3. These tests were administered according to the time limits and instructions found on the tests themselves, except that these instructions were modified to reflect the fact that only one of the two parallel parts of each test was administered in a given session. The tests were scored as recommended in French, Ekstrom, and Price (1963).

Lateralization of these tests was determined on the basis of similar tests which have been administered to brain damaged subjects. For lateralization of verbal tests, see Newcombe (1969) and Weisenburg and McBride (1935). For lateralization of closure tests, see Bogen, DeZure, TenHouten, and Marsh (1972); DeRenzi and Spinnler (1966); Lansdell (1970); Newcombe (1969); Warrington and James (1967). For a discussion of lateralization of visualization, see Footnote 6, and for a discussion of lateralization of disembedding, see "Relation of These Results to Previously Published Findings" in this chapter.

Street Test. Our version was based on the version by Street (1931). From his original 13 pictures, two parallel forms were constructed as follows: Form A consisted of items 1, 3, 5, 9, 11; Form B consisted of items 2, 4, 6, 8, 10. Items 7, 12, and 13 were discarded (largely because of factor-analytic evidence that they were poor measures of closure, see TenHouten, 1973). After examining a sample item, subjects were given a booklet containing five pictures and were asked to identify as many as possible on an answer sheet in 90 seconds. Score = number correct (maximum: 5).

For specific data on lateralization of the Street, see Bogen, DeZure, TenHouten, and Marsh (1972) and DeRenzi and Spinnler (1966).

Harshman Figures. Two parallel sets of 11 items each were selected from a larger set of preliminary items. The subject was shown each item for 20 seconds, followed by five seconds of no stimulus in which he could record his identification on an answer sheet. Score = number correct (maximum: 11).

Gollin Figures. Our version was based on a test described by Gollin (1960). There are five versions of each picture, each version including more of the picture than the last. To increase difficulty, we presented each picture for only five seconds, followed, if necessary, by five seconds of no picture, so that the subject could record his answer. On the basis of preliminary testing, two parallel forms were constructed as follows: Form A consisted of items a, g, h, i, m, n, o, p, s, t; Form B consisted of items b, c, d, e, f, j, k, l, q, r. Subjects were shown an example before testing (Example III for Form A, Example II for Form B). Score = number of errors (maximum: 50).

For specific data on lateralization of the Gollin Figures, see Warring-ton and James (1967).

Perceptual and Preference Tests

Timbre Test. For a detailed description, norms, etc., see the test manual (Seashore, Lewis, and Saetveit, 1960). This test consists of 50 pairs of complex tones. The subject must decide whether the two tones in each pair are the same or different. Score = number correct (maximum: 50).

For specific data on lateralization of the Timbre Test, see Milner (1962).

Matched Syllables. The original tape was provided by Charles Berlin, Kresge Laboratories, Louisiana State University. This test consists of two presentations of Berlin's dichotic tape. The tape contains 30 pairs of dichotic monosyllables, comprising all of the different combinations of distinct mono-syllables from the set /pa, ta, ka, ba, da, ga/. Stimuli are presented over earphones; one monosyllable of each pair is presented to the right ear while a different monosyllable is presented to the left ear. The subject is instructed to write down both monosyllables (guessing if necessary) in either order, with-out regard to ear of presentation. Prior to the test, sample stimuli are presented both monotically and dichotically to familiarize the subject with the task.

Matched Words. This tape was provided by Peter Benson, University of California at San Diego. This test is similar to the matched syllables, ex-cept that each syllable ends with the consonant "t," transforming it into an approximation of a meaningful English word. The thirty pairs consist of every combination of distinct words from the set /"pot," "tot," "cot," "bought," "dot," "got"/.

Test Sequence. The timbre and dichotic tests were assembled into a standardized test tape which included subject instructions, stimulus examples, etc. Each test is presented twice on this tape in order to provide greater re-liability, with the earphones and test sequence reversed between presentations to counterbalance possible sources of error (see Table 2). Thus, each subject received a total of 120 dichotic stimulus pairs, and 100 Timbre Test items during a given testing session.

For a discussion of lateralization and the right ear advantage, see "Dichotic Listening Data" of this chapter; also see Berlin, Lowe-Bell, Cullen, Thompson, and Loovis (1973), and Kimura (1967, 1973).

Arc-Circle Test. This test is based on the test developed by Nebes (1971). The subject must find the correct circle, out of three circles, which matches the circle or fragment of a circle which he is presented with. Both the three target circles and the fragment are behind a curtain so that the task is performed by touch alone. In addition to fragments of four different sizes, whole circle control items are also included. In our version, three sets of 15 stimuli are presented in pseudo-random order. Seven training items preceed test items. Scores = number of errors (maximum: 45), subscores for circle-circle comparisons (maximum: 18), circle-large arc comparisons (maximum: 9); circle-small arc comparisons (maximum: 18). Lateralization is discussed in Appendix 5.

Design Judgment Test. This test was developed by Matland Graves (1948) and consists of pairs (or occasionally triples) of pictures or simple designs. The subject picks out the one which he prefers from each set. To construct parallel forms, odd items were used for Form A and even items for Form B. Score = number correct (maximum: 45). Results are discussed in Cohen (1975b, pages 31-34).

Galin Grouping Test. This test was developed by David Galin, and is briefly described in Galin and Ornstein (1974). It consists of sets of three items from which one can be eliminated on the basis of words, and a different item can be eliminated on the basis of pictures. For a more detailed discussion of the test, as well as the results obtained, see Cohen (1975b, pages 28-31).

Reflective Eye Movements (CLEM). For a discussion of the rationale and procedure, as well as results obtained with this test, see Cohen (1975b, pages 34-39). For a discussion of the relation between eye movements and lateralization, see Bakan (1969), Day (1964), Galin and Ornstein (1974), and Kinsbourne (1972).

APPENDIX 5

The "Perceptual" vs. "Cognitive" Classification
of the Arc-Circle and Dichotic Listening Tasks

It is a question of interpretation whether the Arc-Circle Test (and, to a lesser extent, the dichotic listening tests) should be classified as "perceptual" or "cognitive." Thus, our decision to classify these tests as perceptual requires further explanation.

Dichotic Listening Tests

The dichotic listening tests require the subject to distinguish and identify two syllables, differing only in initial consonant. These syllables are presented simultaneously, one to each ear. There is evidence that this identification task involves a "feature processor" located in the left hemisphere. However, such identification is restricted to the rapid discrimination among a small fixed set of elements, in terms of a small number of features, and thus might be considered perceptual rather than cognitive. In the dichotic task used in this study, there were six consonants (p, t, k, b, d, g) which linguists usually classify in terms of two features, "voicing" and "place of articulation"; these consonants are usually identified very quickly. In contrast, the closure tasks appear to involve a greater degree of processing. They require the interpretive integration of a large number of simultaneously presented elements, and result in identification of objects or scenes from an "infinitely" large set of possibilities. Further, closure seems to require a number of seconds of processing time for all but the easiest pictures (although subjects cannot usually verbalize any distinctive phases of the processing that transpired during that period, and final solution appears to the subject to resemble a sudden insight). Likewise, the Inference Test and Nonsense Syllogisms Test appear to involve a greater degree of processing than the dichotic task, since they involve extended logical analysis, interpretation of verbal material, and use of conceptual relationships.

Arc-Circle Test

The Arc-Circle Test poses the most serious problem of interpretation with respect to classification as either "perceptual" or "cognitive." R. D. Nebes, who developed the test (see Nebes, 1971), specifically intended it to be a test of "part-whole matching." He interpreted "part-whole matching" as a cognitive ability distinct from simple curvature perception and similar to closure. His "split-brain" subjects showed a specific right hemisphere (left hand) superiority on the arc-to-circle matching task which was not shown on two control tasks of circle-to-circle and arc-to-arc matching. This evidence provided strong support for his interpretation of this task as a "higher level" part-to-whole matching task, rather than a simple curvature matching task.

When our subjects performed this task, however, they did not seem to be comparing each arc to the complete circles. Rather, they would feel the arc and then feel a similar sized <u>portion</u> of each circle. This strategy, seen repeatedly with our subjects, transformed the "part-whole" task into a simple arc-arc comparison task. Perhaps, for these subjects, the further aspect of mentally projecting the arc into a circle and then feeling the whole comparison circle was more of a distraction than a help. (The accuracy level of our subjects was about 75 percent on the arc-circle comparisons and 90 percent on the circle-circle comparisons. This is comparable to Nebes' subjects on the arc-circle comparisons, but distinctly better on the circle-circle comparisons.)

But if this arc-circle task is best performed as a simple curvature comparison task, then why did the "split-brain" subjects fail to perform much above chance on the arc-circle task when they used their right hand? Why couldn't the right hand (left hemisphere) of a "split-brain" subject simply use the same curvature comparison ability on the arc-circle task which it had used so successfully on the arc-arc matching task? By matching curvatures (on the arc-arc task), the right hand of these subjects achieved a correct identification rate comparable to that obtained by the left hand on the arc-circle task, and comparable to that obtained by either hand on the circle-circle task. Nebes' interpretation of his data does not (to us) appear to provide an adequate explanation for the puzzling failure of his subjects to resort, when necessary, to a curvature-matching strategy, particularly since this strategy seemed to be actually preferred by many of our subjects in situations where both this and the part-whole strategy were available. Nonetheless, it is just this paradoxical failure of performance for the right hand which Nebes relies on to establish his "cognitive" interpretation of the results.

A further check on the closure or part-whole interpretation of the arc-circle task is provided by examining its correlation with the closure tasks in our battery. Nebes' interpretation might predict almost as high a correlation between closure tasks and the arc-circle task as among closure tasks themselves. However, analysis of our nonintox data shows only low (.1 to .2) and nonsignificant correlations between the Arc-Circle scores and closure scores, compared to moderately high (.5 to .65) correlations among the half-length closure tasks themselves (except for the half Street Test, which is particularly unreliable; see Appendix 4). This evidence is further supported by a factor analysis of nonintox scores. All the closure tests came out on a common closure factor (the Street less clearly). The Arc-Circle did not load on this factor but instead on a different right hemisphere factor with some other right lateralized perceptual tests.

On the basis of the various types of evidence described above, from Nebes' study, from our observations of our own subjects, and from our preliminary correlational and factor analytic results, we concluded that the Arc-Circle Test was best classified as a perceptual task. However, this was not a firm classification. As is apparent from the discussion above, the data do not yet allow the status of the Arc-Circle Test to be clearly resolved.

Footnotes

[1]The same (or generally similar) hypotheses have been independently deduced, on similar grounds, by others, including John Marsh and Claude Chemtobe (personal communication, 1973), Richard Stillman (personal communication, 1975), Robert Ornstein (1974), and Stephen Szara (personal communication, 1975). Earlier, Joseph Bogen made closely related suggestions about possible implications of lateralization and the function of the corpus callosum for the study of psychopharmacological agents (see Bogen, 1970). Since this article was written, a study by Weckowicz et al (1975) has been published which is directed at similar hypotheses.

[2]In interpreting differential shifts, it is important also to consider the effects of factors such as impairment of attention, which might be more crucial for some tests than others. However, impairment of attention might also encourage a shift into a more parallel processing mode, and this corresponds to a cognitive style shift.

[3]Pharmacological Effects of Cannabinoids in Man, principal investigator Dr. Sidney Cohen.

[4]Because of the likely bilaterality of disembedding, the long length of the available tests, and the availability of previous data on the effects of marihuana on these tests, it was decided to include only one disembedding test in the battery.

[5]It should be noted that the shifts predicted in (2) could also come about by some mechanisms other than a shift in relative hemisphere participation (for example, selective stimulation of certain types of neural tissues and depression of other types of neural tissues, regardless of hemisphere). Conversely, a shift in relative hemisphere participation could occur without causing the absolute performance shifts predicted in (2) (for example, if there were also an overall depression of performance in addition to the hemisphere shift, this would mask the enhancement of right hemisphere functions, making them appear as merely less depressed than those of the left hemisphere; such an effect might be likely at higher doses of marihuana). Nonetheless, if the pattern of performance shifts predicted in (2) were observed, it would provide additional support for the second ("hemispheric") hypothesis of this study.

[6]The Gestalt Completion Test suffered from a "ceiling effect" because it was too easy for our subject population. Almost one third of all subjects made a perfect score in the nonintox condition, and many others scored 80 percent or higher, leaving little room for improvement with intoxication. The Street Test suffered from a different psychometric flaw -- poor reliability (as suggested by correlation analysis). This was probably due to the small number of items in each form (five) and the fact that, of these five items, several were either too easy or too difficult to discriminate among levels of ability.

Timing procedures were different for these tests; the Street and Gestalt Completion Tests were timed as a whole, and the subjects could move back and forth freely among items, whereas each item on the Harshman and Gollin Tests had its own time limit, and subjects could not "go back" to look at past items again.

The Street and Gestalt Completion were the first two tests administered (see Table 2), thus they came immediately after intoxication, whereas the Gollin and Harshman Figures were eighth and ninth in the session, placing them at least 25-35 minutes after intoxication. The effective levels of intoxication (or type of drug effects) may have been different at these two points in the post-intox response curve.

The four closure tests may not have been measuring exactly the same abilities. (It is interesting to note, for example, that the change scores (Intox minus Nonintox) for the Street Test correlate +.65 with those for the Surface Development Test, whereas the Harshman Figure change scores show only a very low correlation with those of the Surface Development Test.) Perhaps the Street Test (in particular) may tap some other abilities in addition to closure (this interpretation is also suggested by factor analytic data on the Street; see, for example, French, 1951).

Acknowledgements

The authors would like to thank Sidney Cohen for placing this study in the 94 day program, Roger Remington and Karen Niemi for assistance in the early phases, particularly with construction of tests and running pilot subjects, and Joseph Bogen and Stephen Krashen for valuable suggestions. We are also very grateful for the help and cooperation of the staff of the 94 day project: Phyllis Lessin, Michael Hofman, Carol Brach, Jeannine Frank, Patty Majcher, Jerry Marsh, Perry Nelson, Bob Nowlan, Jim Tehan, and Olga Wright. We particularly want to thank Sheri Berenbaum for helping by contributing scientific insights and assisting in the data analysis, pointing out errors and fuzzy arguments in earlier versions, correcting English style, typing the manuscript, and staying up many nights to see that it all got done.

References

Anonymous. The effects of marijuana on consciousness. In C. T. Tart (Ed.), Altered states of consciousness. New York: Wiley, 1969.

Bakan, P. Hypnotizability, laterality of eye-movements and functional brain asymmetry. Perceptual and Motor Skills, 1969, 28, 927-932.

Barratt, E., Beaver, W., White, R., Blakeney, P., & Adams, P. The effects of the chronic use of marijuana on sleep and perceptual motor performance in humans. In M. F. Lewis (Ed.), Current research in marijuana. New York: Academic Press, 1972.

Berlin, C. I., Lowe-Bell, S. S., Cullen, J. K., Thompson, C. L., & Loovis, C. F. Dichotic speech perception: An interpretation of right ear advantage and temporal offset effects. Journal of the Acoustical Society of America, 1973, 53, 699-709.

Black, F. W. Memory and paired-associate learning of patients with unilateral brain lesions. Psychological Reports, 1973, 33, 919-922.

Blakemore, C., Iverson, S. D., & Zangwill, O. L. Brain functions. Annual Review of Psychology, 1972, 23, 413-456.

Bogen, J. E. The other side of the brain II: An appositional mind. Bulletin of the Los Angeles Neurological Societies, 1969, 34, 135-162.

Bogen, J. E. The corpus callosum, the other side of the brain and pharmacologic opportunity. In W. L. Smith (Ed.), Drugs and cerebral function. Springfield: Charles C. Thomas, 1970.

Bogen, J. E., & Gordon, H. W. Musical test for functional lateralization with intracarotid amybarbital. Nature, 1971, 230, 524-525.

Bogen, J. E., DeZure, R., TenHouten, W. D., & Marsh, J. F. The other side of the brain IV: The A/P ratio. Bulletin of the Los Angeles Neurological Societies, 1972, 37, 49-61.

Carlin, A. S., Bakker, C. B., Halpern, L., & Post, R. D. Social facilitation of marijuana intoxication: Impact of social set and pharmacological activity. Journal of Abnormal Psychology, 1972, 80, 132-140.

Clark, L. D., & Nakashima, E. H. Experimental studies of marijuana. American Journal of Psychiatry, 1968, 125, 379-383.

Clark, L. D., Hughes, R., & Nakashima, E. H. Behavioral effects of marihuana. Archives of General Psychiatry, 1970, 23, 193-198.

Cohen, B. D., Berent, S., & Silverman, A. J. Field-dependence and lateralization of function in the human brain. Archives of General Psychiatry, 1973, 28, 165-167.

Cohen, B. D., Noblin, C. D., & Silverman, A. J. Functional asymmetry
of the human brain. Science, 1968, 162, 475-477.

Cohen, S. Pharmacological effects of cannabinoids in man (Progress Report).
Los Angeles: UCLA Neuropsychiatric Institute, June, 1975. (a)

Cohen, S. Pharmacological effects of cannabinoids in man (Final Report).
Los Angeles: UCLA Neuropsychiatric Institute, September, 1975. (b)

Crawford, H. J. Effects of marijuana on primary suggestibility. Unpublished
dissertation, University of California, Davis. Dissertation Abstracts
International, 1974, 35 (6); order no. 74-29, 298.

Darley, C. F., Tinklenberg, J. R., Roth, W. T., Hollister, L. E., & Atkinson, R. C. Influence of marihuana on storage and retrieval processes
in memory. Memory and Cognition, 1973, 1, 196-200.

Day, M. E. An eye-movement phenomenon relating to attention, thought,
and anxiety. Perceptual and Motor Skills, 1964, 19, 443-446.

DeLong, F. L., & Levy, B. I. Cognitive effects of marihuana described in
terms of a model of attention. Psychological Reports, 1973, 33, 907-
916.

DeRenzi, E., & Spinnler, H. Visual recognition in patients with unilateral
cerebral disease. Journal of Nervous and Mental Disease, 1966, 142,
515-525.

Dimond, S. J., & Beaumont, J. G. (Eds.) Hemisphere function in the human
brain. New York: Wiley, 1974.

Dinnerstein, A. J. Marijuana and perceptual style: A theoretical note.
Perceptual and Motor Skills, 1968, 26, 1016-1018.

Dixon, W. J. (Ed.) BMD-P: Biomedical computer programs. Berkeley:
University of California Press, 1975.

Dornbush, R. L., Fink, M., & Freedman, A. M. Marijuana, memory, and
perception. American Journal of Psychiatry, 1971, 128, 86-89.

Drew, W. G., Kiplinger, G. F., Miller, L. L., & Marx, M. Effects of
propranolol on marihuana-induced cognitive functioning. Clinical
Pharmacological and Therapeutics, 1972, 13, 526-533.

Dumas, R., & Morgan, A. EEG asymmetry as a function of occupation, task, and task difficulty. Paper presented at the annual conference of the Society of Clinical and Experimental Hypnosis, Newport Beach, California, April, 1973.

Ekstrom, R. B. Cognitive factors: some recent literature (ETS PR-73-30). Princeton: Educational Testing Service, 1973.

French, J. W. The description of aptitude and achievement tests in terms of rotated factors. Psychometric Monographs, 1951, No. 5.

French, J. W., Ekstrom, R. B., & Price, L. A. Manual for kit of reference tests for cognitive factors (revised 1963). Princeton: Educational Testing Service, 1963.

Galin, D., & Ornstein, R. Lateral specialization of cognitive mode: an EEG study. Psychophysiology, 1972, 9, 412-418.

Galin, D., & Ornstein, R. Individual differences in cognitive style-1. Reflective eye movements. Neuropsychologia, 1974, 12, 367-376.

Gollin, E. S. Developmental studies of visual recognition of incomplete objects. Perceptual and Motor Skills, 1960, 11, 289-298.

Gordon, H. W., & Bogen, J. E. Hemispheric lateralization of singing after intracarotid sodium amylobarbitone. Journal of Neurology, Neurosurgery, and Psychiatry, 1974, 37, 727-738.

Graves, M. Design judgment test 1948 manual. New York: Psychological Corporation, 1948.

Gur, R. C., & Gur, R. E. Handedness, sex and eyedness as moderating variables in the relation between hypnotic susceptibility and functional brain asymmetry. Journal of Abnormal Psychology, 1974, 83, 635-643.

Hollister, L. E., & Gillespie, H. K. Marihuana, ethanol, and dextroamphetamine. Archives of General Psychiatry, 1970, 23, 199-203.

Jones, R. T., & Stone, G. C. Psychological studies of marijuana and alcohol in man. Psychopharmacologia, 1970, 18, 108-117.

Kimura, D. Cerebral dominance and the perception of verbal stimuli. Canadian Journal of Psychology, 1961, 15, 166-171.

Kimura, D. Left-right differences in the perception of melodies. Quarterly Journal of Experimental Psychology, 1964, 16, 355-358.

Kimura, D. Functional asymmetry of the brain in dichotic listening. Cortex, 1967, 3, 163-178.

Kimura, D. The asymmetry of the human brain. Scientific American, 1973, 228(3), 70–78.

Kimura, D., & Durnford, M. Normal studies on the function of the right hemisphere in vision. In S. J. Dimond & J. G. Beaumont (Eds.), Hemisphere function in the human brain. New York: Wiley, 1974.

Kinsbourne, M. Eye and head turning indicates cerebral lateralization. Science, 1972, 176, 539–541.

Kinsbourne, M. Direction of gaze and distribution of cerebral thought processes. Neuropsychologia, 1974, 12, 279–281.

Klonoff, H., Low, M., & Marcus, A. Neuropsychological effects of marijuana. Canadian Medical Association Journal, 1973, 108, 150–156.

Lansdell, H. Relation of extent of temporal removals to closure and visuomotor factors. Perceptual and Motor Skills, 1970, 31, 491–498.

Levy, J. Possible basis for the evolution of lateral specialization of the human brain. Nature, 1969, 224, 614–615.

Levy, J. Lateral specialization of the human brain: Behavioral manifestations and possible evolutionary basis. In J. A. Kiger Jr. (Ed.), The biology of behavior. Corvallis, Oregon: Oregon State University Press, 1973.

Levy, J. Psychobiological implications of bilateral asymmetry. In S. J. Dimond & J. G. Beaumont (Eds.), Hemisphere function in the human brain. New York: Wiley, 1974.

Melges, F. T., Tinklenberg, J. P., Hollister, L. E., & Gillespie, H. K. Marijuana and temporal disintegration. Science, 1970, 168, 1118–1120.

Meyer, R. E., Pillard, R. C., Shapiro, L. M., & Mirin, S. M. Administration of marijuana to heavy and casual marijuana users. American Journal of Psychiatry, 1971, 128, 198–204.

Miller, E. Handedness and the pattern of human ability. British Journal of Psychology, 1971, 62, 111–112.

Miller, L., & Drew, W. G. Effects of marijuana on recall of narrative material and Stroop colour-word performance. Nature, 1972, 237, 172–173.

Milner, B. Laterality effects in audition. In V. Mountcastle (Ed.), Interhemispheric relations and cerebral dominance. Baltimore: Johns Hopkins Press, 1962.

Milner, B. Brain mechanisms suggested by studies of temporal lobes. In C. H. Millikan & F. L. Darley (Eds.), Brain mechanisms underlying speech and language. New York: Grune and Stratton, 1967.

Milner, B. Interhemispheric differences in the localization of psychological processes in man. British Medical Bulletin, 1971, 27, 272-277.

Moran, L. J., & Mefferd, R. B., Jr. Repetitive psychometric measures. Psychological Reports, 1959, 5, 269-275.

Nebes, R. D. Superiority of the minor hemisphere in commissurotomized man for the perception of part-whole relations. Cortex, 1971, 7, 333-349.

Nebes, R. D. Perception of spatial relationships by the right and left hemispheres in commissurotomized man. Neuropsychologia, 1973, 11, 285-289.

Newcombe, F. Missile wounds of the brain. London: Oxford University Press, 1969.

Ornstein, R. The psychology of consciousness. New York: Viking Press, 1972.

Pearl, J. H., Domino, E. F., & Rennick, P. Short term effects of marijuana smoking on cognitive behavior in experienced male users. Psychopharmacologia, 1973, 31, 13-24.

Poeck, K., Kerschensteiner, M., Hartje, W., & Orgass, B. Impairment in visual recognition of geometric figures in patients with circumscribed retrorolandic brain lesions. Neuropsychologia, 1973, 11, 311-317.

Seashore, C. E., Lewis, D., & Saetveit, J. G. Seashore measures of musical talents: Manual. New York: Psychological Corporation, 1960.

Siegel, S. Nonparametric statistics for the behavioral sciences. New York: McGraw-Hill, 1956.

Solomon, D. (Ed.) The marihuana papers. New York: Bobbs-Merrill, 1966.

Street, R. F. A gestalt completion test. Contributions to education no. 481. New York: Columbia University Teachers College, 1931.

Tart, C. T. On being stoned: A psychological study of marijuana intoxication. Palo Alto, California: Science and Behavior Books, 1971.

TenHouten, W. D. Cognitive styles and the social order. Final report, part II, OEO Study BOO-5135, "Thought, Race and Opportunity," Los Angeles, California, 1971.

TenHouten, W. D., & Kaplan, C. Science and its mirror image. New York: Harper & Row, 1973.

Teuber, H. L., & Weinstein, S. Ability to discover hidden figures after cerebral lesions. A.M.A. Archives of Neurology and Psychiatry, 1956, 76, 369-379.

Thurstone, L. L. A factorial study of perception. Chicago: University of Chicago Press, 1944.

Thurstone, L. L., & Jeffrey, T. E. Closure speed test administration manual – revised, 1966. Chicago: Industrial Relations Center, University of Chicago, 1966.

Tyler, L. E. The psychology of human differences. New York: Appleton-Century-Crofts, 1965.

Warrington, E., & James, M. Disorders of visual perception in patients with localized cerebral lesions. Neuropsychologia, 1967, 5, 253-266.

Waskow, I. E., Olsson, J. E., Salzman, C., & Katz, M. M. Psychological effects of tetrahydrocannabinol. Archives of General Psychiatry, 1970, 22, 97-107.

Weckowicz, T. E., Fedora, O., Mason, J., Radstaak, D., Bay, K. S. & Yonge, K. A. Effect of marijuana on divergent and convergent production cognitive tests. Journal of Abnormal Psychology, 1975, 84, 386-398.

Weil, A. T., & Zinberg, N. E. Acute effects of marihuana on speech. Nature, 1969, 222, 434-437.

Weil, A. T., Zinberg, N. E., & Nelsen, J. M. Clinical and psychological effects of marihuana in man. Science, 1968, 162, 1234-1242.

Weisenburg, T. H., & McBride, K. E. Aphasia: A clinical and psychological study. New York: Commonwealth Fund, 1935.

Witkin, H. A., Lewis, H. B., Hertzman, M., Machover, K., Meissner, P. B., & Wapner, S. Personality through perception. New York: Harper, 1954.

Witkin, H. A., Dyk, R. B., Faterson, H. D., Goodenough, D. R., & Kays, S. A. Psychological differentiation. New York: Wiley, 1962.

Zaidel, E. Linguistic competence and related functions in the right cerebral hemisphere of man following commissurotomy and hemispherectomy. Doctoral dissertation, California Institute of Technology, 1973. (University Microfilms No. 73-26, 481)

CHAPTER 16

SUBJECTIVE BENEFITS AND DRAWBACKS OF MARIHUANA AND ALCOHOL

Walton T. Roth
Jared R. Tinklenberg
Bert S. Kopell

Department of Psychiatry and Behavioral Sciences
Stanford University School of Medicine
Stanford, California
and
Veterans Administration Hospital
Palo Alto, California

NOTE: This work was supported by National Institute for
Mental Health grants DA 00854 and AA 00397 and the Veterans
Administration. The authors wish to express their appreciation
to M. J. Rosenbloom and P. L. Murphy for their assistance.

INTRODUCTION

How can the broader spectrum of drug action be assessed in a way to determine the valence of effects of these agents from the standpoint of the user? We report here findings from a questionnaire that enumerated some of the reputed benefits and drawbacks of marihuana and alcohol and asked users which of these they agreed with, based on their own experience. This method is extremely naive in a sense, since behaviorists and psychoanalysts alike agree that it is futile to ask people why they do things. One reason is that what they say in different situations is often inconsistent. For example, there is evidence that people report their moods as more positive when they know the experimenter is trying to evaluate the effects of marihuana cigarettes smoked half an hour before (Mendelson, Rossi and Meyer, 1974), as compared to mood reports when the subject is unaware of the experimenter's purpose. Even if people could give an accurate account of why they like things while unintoxicated, both marihuana (Darley, Tinklenberg, Roth, Hollister and Atkinson, 1973) and alcohol (Overton, 1972) distort the memory of what happened during intoxication. For example, alcoholics persist in saying that they expect alcohol to relieve feelings of anxiety and depression, while both of these moods are actually increased during experimental intoxication of alcoholics (Mello, 1972).

However, in spite of the limitations of subjective reporting, there are reasons not to discount this method entirely, at least as a starting point for more objective studies. In the case of marihuana, users responding to questions in a 220-item questionnaire were quite consistent in identifying many diverse effects as characteristic of marihuana intoxication (Tart, 1971). Some of these effects have already been objectively confirmed in laboratory studies. For example, we (Roth, Rosenbloom, Darley, Tinklenberg and Kopell, 1975) found that Thematic Apperception Test stories written under the influence of marihuana show a timeless, non-narrative quality, with greater discontinuity in thought sequence, more frequent inclusions of contradictory ideas, and more novelty. The raters, blind to whether the story was written under marihuana or placebo, verified the cognitive changes often reported by users. In addition, asking people what desirable and undesirable effects they experience from drugs may help us to assess the potential benefits and drawbacks of these drugs in terms of the values of society. Valuable information about which drugs lead to violence has been obtained by interviews with youthful offenders who have used various drugs (Tinklenberg, Murphy, Darley, Roth and Kopell, 1974). In the same way, clues to drug benefits that are psychotherapeutic in a broad sense may be gleaned from the testimonials of drug users.

Several surveys of reasons why people use marihuana have been made in the past ten years. McGlothlin, Arnold, and Rowan (1970) interviewed people who had volunteered for an LSD experiment ten years before. In that study, the top-ranked reasons for taking marihuana were to produce a feeling of well-being, to relax, to relieve tension, and to increase enjoyment of plays and movies. This sample, however, was quite special, limiting the generalizability of the findings. The specific mention of plays and movies may have come from the fact that about half of the sample worked in art or entertainment fields. Mizner, Barter, and Werme (1970) surveyed college students and reported their answers to an open-ended question about why they continued marihuana use after the first occasion. The most common answer was the unrevealing and non-specific response that smoking marihuana is fun (68%), while the second largest category of response was that marihuana produces insight into one's self (7%). Rouse and Ewing (1972; 1973) also surveyed college students, asking them to rate the desirability of various hypothetical mental states and "what risk were you willing to take to achieve these feelings with marihuana?" Users rated "sensory awareness" first and "rapid, logical thought" second as desirable mental states that they would be willing to take moderate risks to achieve. Unfortunately, the students were posed hypothetical questions about effects that in some cases, like the second mentioned, are not common marihuana effects. Tart (1971) asked 150 users of marihuana and alcohol to compare their effects and their desirability in various situations. Marihuana was credited with enhancement of sensory perception and appreciation, while alcohol was said to dull the senses. Both drugs were said to be equally able to produce relaxation and a happy mood. The subjects indicated that alcohol produced liveliness in large groups, while marihuana was better for small intimate groups. Tart's informants were decidedly anti-alcohol and pro-marihuana: 43% of them stated that they would never use alcohol in the future.

Recently, a questionnaire has been developed by members of the Navy Medical Neuropsychiatric Research Unit in San Diego, California, that lists 31 reasons for using psychoactive drugs and 39 possible risks associated with such drugs. The items are generally quite specific and comprehensive and have allowed the determination of specific patterns of subjective benefits (Nail, Gunderson and Kolb, 1974) and risks (Kolb, Gunderson and Nail, 1974) that users expect from such drugs as marihuana, LSD, heroin, amphetamines, and barbiturates. Their subjects attributed a number of desirable properties to marihuana: a feeling of well-being, a relief of tension, an increased sensitivity to tastes and to music, and a relief of boredom and depression. Many users admitted to social reasons: they used it to be "in" with a certain group. Undesirable effects included sleepiness, dulled thinking, and paranoid thoughts.

The study that we are reporting used a questionnaire similar to that of the San Diego group, except that we added a number of new and more specific items. Instead of asking users about a variety of psychoactive drugs, we concentrated exclusively on marihuana and alcohol, the latter drug having been omitted in the San Diego studies. In many ways, alcohol is the standard to which pleasure-giving drugs must be compared, just as chlorpromazine is the standard for major tranquilizers. We also sampled a different group of young people. The San Diego group studied patients in Navy drug rehabilitation programs. Of these patients, 30% had been expelled from high school more than once and 38% had been arrested for other than traffic offenses. Our sample was largely professional and pre-professional students assoc ted with Stanford University, a group who display more outward conformity with society and who have been very successful in school.

METHODS

Our questionnaire had three parts. The first part asked questions about the age and social status of the respondents and how often they used marihuana and alcohol; the second part asked them about 38 possible effects that could be reasons for taking these drugs; and the third part asked about 34 potential drawbacks of these drugs. The following are examples of questions and the possibilities for reasons:

Part 2: Reasons for taking the drug	Alcohol	Marihuana
(22) Increases my enjoyment of food	N O 12 I A	N O 12 I A
(23) Relieves anxiety or tension	N O 12 I A	N O 12 I A

and so forth.

Part 3: Drawbacks of the drug   Alcohol   Marihuana

(69) Makes me unable to work   N O 12 I A   N O 12 I A

(70) Increases my feelings of   N O 12 I A   N O 12 I A
     hostility

and so forth.

Subjects were to circle N if they had not experienced this effect, O if they
had experienced it but it was not a reason for or against taking the drug, 1 if
they had experienced it and it was a minor reason for taking the drug (part 2)
or a minor drawback (part 3), and 2 if they had experienced it and it was a
major reason for taking the drug (part 2) or major drawback (part 3). Subjects
were also to circle I if the effect was immediate (present during intoxication)
or A if the effect was an after-effect. There were spaces at the end of the
second and third parts for writing in additional reasons and drawbacks.

We placed our questionnaires in the mail-boxes of an entering class of
first-year law students and of medical students and house officers in the
University Hospital. In addition, a few of the questionnaires were distributed
among research personnel in our department. Respondents were not to write
their names and were to fill out the questionnaires regardless of their level of
alcohol or marihuana use. However, the data reported here are based on the
51 people who has used both drugs with a frequency of greater than once a
month for some six-month period of their life. In this way, we were able to
compare opinions about the two drugs in people who had had enough experience
to have informed opinions. About a quarter of the questionnaires were returned
within ten days and about a third of the respondents met our frequency of use
criteria. Table 1 summarizes the demographic characteristics of our sample
and their frequency of drug use. The sample is young, in professional training,
predominantly male and unmarried, and of mixed religious preferences.
(Almost everyone who replied met the criterion for alcohol use, and most of
the respondents who did not meet the criteria failed on the basis of insufficient
marihuana experience.) Even though the sample had approximately equal
exposure to alcohol and marihuana during the six-month period of peak use,
during the last six months the sample used alcohol more frequently than
marihuana.

RESULTS

Tables 2 and 3 list the effects that are reasons for using alcohol and
marihuana. The effects are listed in rank order of their desirability. Some
effects are similar for both drugs, while others are produced more often by
one drug than by the other. Marihuana is sought after for its ability to
enhance sensory appreciation. This is reflected in items about sights and
sound, "experiencing ordinary objects in a new way," sexual sensation, and
the enjoyment of food. These effects are all more prominent with marihuana

Table 1
Characteristics of the Sample (N=51)

Age	%	Sex	%	Marital status	%
20–25	59	Male	81	Single	73
26–30	25	Female	19	Married	21
31–35	12			Divorced	6
> 35	4				

Religion	%	Occupation	%
Jewish	31	Law student	67
Protestant	28	Medical student or house officer	25
Catholic	4	Other	8
Other or none	37		

Length of use	Marihuana %	Alcohol %
< 1 year	2	0
1–3 years	13	4
4–10 years	79	66
>10 years	6	30

Frequency of use during the six months of most frequent use		
At least once a day	22	6
> once a week	43	73
> once a month	35	21
< once a month	0	0
Never	0	0

Frequency of use during the last six months		
At least once a day	2	0
> once a week	16	49
>once a month	37	43
< once a month	29	6
Never	16	2

Table 2

Effects that are Reasons for Taking Marihuana (in % of total number)

Effect	Major reason	Minor reason	Not a reason	Not an effect	Comparison with alcohol
1. Increases enjoyment of sights and sounds	45	37	10	8	M > A **
2. Enables me to experience a different state of consciousness	40	28	20	12	M > A *
3. Makes me feel elated or euphoric	31	33	16	20	NS
4. Enables me to go along with my friends	26	31	26	37	NS
5. Enables me to experience ordinary objects in a new way	24	30	20	26	M > A **
6. Enhances sexual sensation	18	52	18	12	M > A **
7. Relieves anxiety or tension	18	35	27	20	A > M *
8. Enhances my sense of humor	16	41	23	20	NS
9. Increases my feeling of sociability	16	39	22	23	A > M *
10. Makes me less inhibited in thinking, saying or doing certain things	12	41	29	18	NS
11. Makes me less inhibited sexually	12	31	18	39	NS
12. Enables me to think more creatively	12	23	18	47	M > A **
13. Enables me to get insight into myself	12	21	23	44	M > A **
14. Enables me to fall asleep more quickly or to sleep more soundly	10	22	41	27	NS
15. Enables me to have unusual thoughts	10	22	37	31	M > A **
16. Relieves boredom	8	39	24	29	NS
17. Enables me to focus on the "now" rather than the past or future	8	22	23	47	NS
18. Enables me to express my feelings	8	21	16	55	NS
19. Enables me to stop worrying	8	19	18	55	NS
20. Enables me to get psychological insight into others	8	12	15	65	M > A *
21. Makes me less self-conscious	6	27	20	47	NS
22. Enables me to accept contradiction	6	2	23	69	NS
23. Increases my enjoyment of food	4	49	37	10	M > A **
24. Alleviates depression	4	21	18	57	NS
25. Provides philosophic or religious insights	4	21	16	59	M > A **
26. Decreases a tendency to overanalyze or think too much	4	16	19	61	NS

* p < .01

**p < .001

Table 3

Effects that are Reasons for Drinking Alcohol (in % of total number)

Effect	Major reason	Minor reason	Not a reason	Not an effect	Comparison with marihuana
1. Increases my feeling of sociability	37	41	18	4	A >M *
2. Relieves anxiety or tension	26	47	27	0	A >M *
3. Makes me feel elated or euphoric	24	35	23	18	NS
4. Makes me less inhibited in thinking, saying or doing certain things	18	45	35	2	NS
5. Enables me to go along with my friends	18	31	22	29	NS
6. Enables me to experience a different state of consciousness	16	22	25	37	M >A *
7. Makes me less inhibited sexually	14	33	27	26	NS
8. Enables me to stop worrying	10	41	14	35	NS
9. Alleviates depression	10	22	20	50	NS
10. Makes me less self-conscious	6	41	26	27	NS
11. Enables me to fall asleep more quickly or to sleep more soundly	6	32	42	20	NS
12. Decreases a tendency to overanalyze or think too much	6	27	22	45	NS
13. Enhances my sense of humor	4	45	33	18	NS
14. Enables me to express my feelings	4	24	29	43	NS
15. Enhances sexual sensation	4	22	23	31	M >A **
16. Makes me more open and less critical of others	4	18	27	51	NS
17. Increases my enjoyment of food	4	14	29	53	M >A **
18. Makes me feel more attractive to others	4	13	12	71	NS

* $p < .01$

** $p < .001$

than with alcohol. Cognitive changes, such as the ability to think more
creatively, psychological and philosophical insights, and the ability to have
unusual thoughts, are experienced more with marihuana than with alcohol.
These are reported by fewer respondents than the sensory effects and are less
valued. More non-specifically, marihuana is taken to produce a different
state of consciousness, a property that alcohol has as well, albeit to a lesser
degree. Alcohol is ranked highest for its socializing properties and its use as
an anti-anxiety agent. In both cases, these effects are also mentioned as
marihuana effects, but they are more common with alcohol. Alcohol's
socializing properties are also indicated by the ranking of items about less
inhibition, less self-consciousness, more attractiveness to others, and being
more open and less critical. Both drugs are ranked high on the ability to
produce euphoria. Other mood changes attributed to both drugs are decreased
anxiety and, in about half the subjects, relief of depression. Relief from
worry and from a tendency to overanalyze are attributed to both drugs,
although many subjects do not experience these effects or consider them of
only minor importance. About 80% of the sample have experienced an
increased sense of humor with both marihuana and alcohol, and over half of
these people consider this effect to be at least a minor reason for taking the
drugs.

Tables 4 and 5 list the drawbacks attributed to marihuana and alcohol
use. Both drugs have the same three top-ranked drawbacks: "makes me unable
to work," "dulls my thinking," and "makes me liable to motor accidents."
The inability to work was seen as persisting after the period of intoxication
for both drugs in about half of the people reporting this effect. Other
complaints about both drugs were "makes me sleepy" and "makes me feel I
am losing control." Also some users worry about possible long-term side
effects and cost. Because of the law, marihuana draws some special complaints
in that users worry about being arrested when using marihuana and find it
difficult to get. In addition, marihuana made some of our sample become
suspicious or paranoid, become withdrawn socially, or feel that their memory
was worse. These effects are seen as immediate except in the case of the
effect of marihuana on memory, which is perceived as continuing after the
period of intoxication. Alcohol is disliked for its propensity to produce
headaches after intoxication has worn off.

The most common write-in responses were enjoyment of the taste as a
reason for using alcohol (especially wine) and irritation of the respiratory
tract as a drawback of marihuana smoking.

DISCUSSION

The greatest value of marihuana, according to our subjects, is
increased enjoyment of sights and sounds. This and related sensory changes
are often mentioned in surveys, but since these changes are more in the
apperception of stimuli than in simple perception, they have not been amenable
to experimental confirmation. The second-ranked benefit was experiencing a
different state of consciousness, which Weil (1972) believes is the primary

Table 4

Effects that are Drawbacks to Taking Marihuana (in % of total number)

Effect	Major draw-back	Minor draw-back	Not a draw-back	Not an effect	Comparison with alcohol
1. Makes me unable to work	30	26	28	18	NS
2. Makes me liable to motor accidents	22	16	20	44	NS
3. Dulls my thinking	20	26	28	28	NS
4. The drug is too expensive for me	19	32	12	48	NS
5. Makes my memory deteriorate	19	24	24	44	M > A *
6. I worry about danger of arrest	18	32	18	34	M > A **
7. Makes me sleepy	14	28	40	20	NS
8. Makes me feel suspicious or paranoid	10	24	24	44	M > A **
9. Makes me withdraw socially	10	24	22	46	M > A *
10. Use of the drug causes disapproval by people I respect	10	16	14	61	NS
11. Makes me less ambitious	8	28	26	36	NS
12. Gives me a headache	8	10	18	66	NS
13. I have difficulty getting a supply of the drug	6	28	26	42	M > A **
14. I worry about other possible long-term adverse effects	6	18	12	66	NS
15. Makes me feel I am losing control of myself	6	14	24	56	NS
16. Makes me more anxious and tense	6	8	16	72	NS
17. It is contrary to my religious or moral principles	6	4	4	94	NS
18. Makes me feel depressed	4	14	16	68	NS

* p < .01
** p < .001

Table 5

Effects that are Drawbacks to Taking Alcohol (in % of total number)

Effect	Major draw-back	Minor draw-back	Not a draw-back	Not an effect	Comparison with marihuana
1. Makes me liable to auto accidents	46	18	14	24	NS
2. Dulls my thinking	28	34	28	12	NS
3. Makes me unable to work	24	32	32	14	NS
4. Makes me sleepy	16	26	46	14	NS
5. Gives me a headache	14	20	20	48	NS
6. Makes me poorly coordinated	10	40	40	10	A > M **
7. Makes me feel I am losing control of myself	8	16	20	58	NS
8. I worry about possible drug dependence	8	12	6	74	NS
9. Makes my memory deteriorate	8	6	14	74	M > A *
10. Makes me lose contact with reality	6	4	16	76	NS
11. The drug is too expensive for me	4	22	12	64	NS
12. Makes me dizzy	4	22	22	52	NS
13. I worry about other possible long-term adverse physical effects	4	20	6	72	NS
14. Makes me feel physically weak	4	14	14	70	NS
15. Use of the drug causes disapproval by people I respect	4	6	8	84	NS

* p < .01

** p < .001

motivation for taking mind-altering chemicals. For our subjects, elation or euphoria was in third place, although in other studies it was first (McGlothlin et al., 1970; Mizner et al., 1970). Twenty percent of our subjects did not experience elation with marihuana. Its effects as an anxiety reducer were also variable: 20% did not experience this effect and 28% experienced increases in anxiety. Users gave marihuana poor marks as an anti-depressant, though 4% cite this as a major reason for taking it. These replies about marihuana influences on affect are consistent with the laboratory findings of Mendelson et al. (1974), who found that dysphoric moods were often intensified. Its failure as an anti-depressant in depressive illness was noted in an early study by Stockings (1947) and confirmed more recently by Kotin (1973).

The reasons given for drinking alcohol are consistent with what is commonly observed in social situations and in the laboratory (Ekman, Frankenhaeuser, Goldberg, Bjerver and Jarpe, 1963; Ekman, Frankenhaeuser, Goldberg, Hagdahl and Myrsten, 1964). Our subjects found alcohol an excellent anxiety-tension reducer, which is discrepant from the findings of Mello (1972) that alcohol produced an increase in anxiety in alcoholics. Evidently alcoholics differ in their response to alcohol from our subjects who, from their reports of drinking frequency, are not alcoholics.

There is a healthy realism in the three top-ranked drawbacks for marihuana and alcohol. The cognitive and performance deficits produced by marihuana have often been demonstrated in the laboratory (Kiplinger, Manno, Rodda and Forney, 1971; Klonoff, Low and Marcus, 1973; Pearl, Domino and Rennick, 1973; Roth, Tinklenberg, Whitaker, Darley, Kopell and Hollister, 1973; Evans, Martz, Brown, Rodda, Kiplinger, Lemberger and Forney, 1973; Darley, Tinklenberg, Roth, Hollister and Atkinson, 1973).

Similar deficits are well-known in alcohol intoxication (Idestrom and Cadenius, 1968; Jones and Vega, 1972). Klonoff (1974) has documented the impairment in driving produced by marihuana. Our subjects find that marihuana intoxication interferes with their work, which is reasonable in view of the subjects' occupations. In Jamaica, users take marihuana to make themselves work better (Rubin and Comitas, 1975). However, their daily work is not intellectual, but tedious manual labor which marihuana somehow makes more tolerable without unduly decreasing its efficiency.

Do these questionnaire responses suggest any psychotherapeutic uses for these drugs? Inferences that can be made from a sample of non-patients are limited in terms of mental disease. Yet, if mental health is defined as better psychological functioning in general, rather than the absence of disease, the responses of our subjects can be relevant.

Marihuana is valued as a drug for experiencing and thinking about things in a new way. Since much of psychotherapy is based on helping people to achieve new perspectives and insights, marihuana might be considered as an aid for psychological problem solving and growth. There is ambivalence among therapists about the use of drugs for this purpose for a number of reasons.

The drug-induced insights may not hold up as valid in the unintoxicated state, if indeed they can be remembered. Naranjo (1973) has reported gains he obtained by treating patients with psychedelic drugs in the context of psychoanalytic or gestalt therapy, but the relative importance of the drugs and the therapy is unclear. Many therapists who advocate special states of consciousness prefer to achieve them via drug-free methods such as meditation, hypnosis, or biofeedback, thus avoiding the possibility of physical or psychological dependence on a chemical agent. However, non-drug pathways to altered consciousness are arduous and long, and if their worth is demonstrated, we should hold open the possibility of chemical facilitation. Many drugs in the psychedelic category besides marihuana would also have to be considered (Hollister, 1968) and their relative risks weighed.

One special therapeutic application for marihuana, as suggested by reports from our sample and elsewhere, is enhancement of sexual sensation. Marihuana might be used as an adjunct in the therapy of sexual dysfunction, a therapeutic use long a part of traditional Hindu medicine (Chopra and Chopra, 1957). When performance anxiety leads to male impotence or female frigidity, marihuana might enhance sexual sensation, permitting enough success to break out of the vicious circle of failure leading to anxiety leading to further failure.

Our informants seem to use alcohol as an over-the-counter minor tranquilizer. It is rapid-acting, with a short half-life in comparison with benzodiazepines. These tranquilizing effects are used by some to approach phobic situations such as an airplane flight or for reducing social anxiety at a party with strangers. Since learning under alcohol is partly state-dependent, these methods of coping may seem to require continued drug use. However, the experience of behavior therapists in using barbituates to aid in the desensitization of phobias indicates that mastery of the phobic situation may continue without the drug (Brady, 1972). Yet, what physician would prescribe alcohol over the benzodiazepines? The risks of dependence and physical damage with alcohol are well known, and even its social lubricating effects often overshoot the mark, making the intoxicated person obnoxiously uninhibited in the eyes of his companions.

Questionnaire studies like ours are hardly the last word on marihuana and alcohol uses, but are only starting points for more detailed research. Clearly marihuana and alcohol are taken for effects that seldom have been submitted to experimental test, partly because of the difficulty in finding appropriate tests. Most experimental studies have concentrated on drug-produced deficits that are only a fraction of the total psychic effects of these drugs, and these deficits provide little insight into why people use the drugs. Hopefully, we can widen our research horizons and sharpen our methodology to attack some of these difficult but highly relevant problems.

REFERENCES

Brady, J.P. Systematic desensitization. In W.S. Agras (Ed.), Behavioral modification: Principles and clinical applications. Boston: Little, Brown, 1972, 127–150.

Chopra, I.C., & Chopra, R.N. The use of cannabis drugs in India. U.N. Bulletin on Narcotics, 1957, 9, 4–29.

Darley, C.F., Tinklenberg, J.R., Roth, W.T., Hollister, L.E., & Atkinson, R.C. Influence of marihuana on storage and retrieval processes in memory. Memory and cognition, 1973, 1, 196–200.

Ekman, G., Frankenhaeuser, M., Goldberg, L., Bjerver, K., Jarpe, G., & Myrsten, A.L. Effects of alcohol intake on subjective and objective variables over a five-hour period. Psychopharmacologia (Berlin), 1963, 4, 28–38.

Ekman, G., Frankenhaeuser, M., Goldberg, L., Hagdahl, R., & Myrsten, A.L. Subjective and objective effects of alcohol as functions of dosage and time. Psychopharmacologia (Berlin), 1964, 6, 399.

Evans, M.A., Martz, R., Brown, D.J., Rodda, B.E., Kiplinger, G.F., Lemberger, L., & Forney, R.B. Impairment of performance with low doses of marihuana. Clin. Pharmacol. Ther., 1973, 14, 936–940.

Hollister, L.E. Chemical psychoses: LSD and related drugs. Springfield: C. Thomas, 1968.

Idestrom, C.M., & Cadenius, B. Time relations of the effects of alcohol compared to placebo. Psychopharmacologia (Berlin), 1968, 13, 189–200.

Jones, B.M., & Vega, A. Cognitive performance measured on the ascending and descending limb of the blood alcohol curve. Psychopharmacologia (Berlin), 1972, 23, 99–114.

Kiplinger, G.F., Manno, J.E., Rodda, B.E., & Forney, R.B. Dose-response analysis of the effects of tetrahydrocannabinol in man. Clin. Pharmacol. Ther., 1971, 12, 650–657.

Klonoff, H. Marijuana and driving in real-life situations. Science, 1974, 186, 317–324.

Klonoff, H., Low, M., & Marcus, A. Neuropsychological effects of marihuana. Can. Med. Assoc. J., 1973, 108, 150–156.

Kolb, D., Gunderson, E., & Nail, R.L. Perception of drug abuse risks in relation to type of drug used and level of experience. J. of Community Psychology, 1974, 2, 380–389.

Kotin, J., Post, R.M., & Goodwin, F.K. Delta-9-tetrahydrocannabinol in depressed patients. Arch. Gen. Psychiat., 1973, 28, 345-348.

McGlothlin, W.H., Arnold, D.O., & Rowan, P.K. Marihuana use among adults. Psychiatry, 1970, 33, 433-443.

Mello, N.K. Behavioral studies of alcoholism. In B. Kissin & H. Begleiter (Eds.), The biology of alcoholism, Vol. 2: Physiology and behavior. New York: Plenum Press, 1972, 219-291.

Mendelson, J.H., Rossi, A.M., & Meyer, R.E. The use of marihuana: A psychological and physiological inquiry. New York: Plenum Press, 1974.

Mizner, G.L., Barter, J.T., & Werme, P.H. Patterns of drug use among college students: A preliminary report. Amer. J. Psychiat., 1970, 127, 15-24.

Nail, R.L., Gunderson, E., & Kolb, D. Motives for drug use among light and heavy users. J. of Nervous and Mental Diseases, 1974, 159, 131-136.

Naranjo, C. The healing journey: New approaches to consciousness. New York: Ballantine Books, 1973.

Overton, D.A. State-dependent learning produced by alcohol and its relevance to alcoholism. In B. Kissin & H. Begleiter (Eds.), The biology of alcoholism, Vol. 2: Physiology and behavior. New York: Plenum Press, 1972, 193-217.

Pearl, J.H., Domino, E.F., & Rennick, P. Short-term effects of marijuana smoking on cognitive behavior in experienced male users. Psychopharmacologia (Berlin), 1973, 31, 13-24.

Roth, W.T., Tinklenberg, J.R., Whitaker, C.A., Darley, C.F., Kopell, B.S., & Hollister, L.E. The effect of marihuana on tracking task performance. Psychopharmacologia (Berlin), 1973, 33, 259-265.

Roth, W.T., Rosenbloom, M.J., Darley, C.F., Tinklenberg, J.R., & Kopell, B.S. Marihuana effects on TAT form and content. Psychopharmacologia (Berlin), 1975, 43, 261-266.

Rouse, B.A., & Ewing, J.A. Marihuana and other drug use by graduate and professional students. Amer. J. Psychiatry, 1972, 129, 415-420.

Rouse, B.A., & Ewing, J.A. Marihuana and other drug use by women college students. Amer. J. Psychiatry, 1973, 130, 486-491.

Rubin, V., & Comitas, L. Ganja in Jamaica: A medical anthropological study of chronic marihuana use. The Hague: Mouton, 1975.

Stockings, G.T. New euphoriant for depressant mental states. Brit. Med. J., 1947, 1, 918-922.

Tart, C.T. On being stoned: A psychological study of marijuana intoxication. Palo Alto: Science and Behavior Books, 1971.

Tinklenberg, J.R., Murphy, P.L., Darley, C.F., Roth, W.T., & Kopell, B.S. Drug involvement in criminal assaults by adolescents. Arch. Gen. Psychiatry, 1974, 30, 685-689.

Weil, A.T. The natural mind. Boston: Houghton Mifflin, 1972.

CHAPTER 17

MARIHUANA AND HUMAN COGNITION: A REVIEW OF LABORATORY

INVESTIGATIONS

Loren L. Miller

Department of Psychiatry
University of Kentucky Medical Center
Lexington, Kentucky

NOTE: Preparation of this paper was supported in part
by grant DA00879-02 from the National Institute on
Drug Abuse.

INTRODUCTION

Beginning with the elegant characterization of hashish intoxication
on human mental functioning by Moreau in 1845, interest in cannabis preparations and their behavioral manifestations has waxed and waned over many
decades. However, at the present time, the elucidation of behavioral alterations produced by cannabis remains a scientific as well as a social concern
mainly because of its widespread use in our society. The use of cannabis has
burgeoned at such a rate that it is doubtful that research efforts will keep pace
with the discovery of new social consequences concerning its abuse. In addition, political and moral considerations have in some instances clouded the
issue of determining in a systematic and objective manner the effects of cannabis not only on human behavior but its medical consequences. Specious
conclusions concerning the actions of cannabis become magnified as proponents
for or against its legalization seize upon early data returns to support their
contentions. When vacuous scientific findings become publicized, they are
also more scrutinized and hence confusing to the public. It is the job of scientists to wade through the morass of conflicting opinions both social and scientific. Perhaps the moderating social climate toward cannabis use or at least reduced criminal penalties will contribute to this goal.

Description of the behavioral and pharmacological effects of cannabinoids has involved a myriad of disciplines. Psychologists, pharmacologists,
physicians, and physiologists as well as other scientists have all contributed to

a basic description of the medical and behavioral actions of cannabinoids. Unfortunately, attempts to synthesize these points of view have been sparse; findings often appear to exist independently of one another. We seem to be faced with another case of the blind men and the elephant with the biases of each discipline determining which part of the elephant will be seen.

The goal of this paper is to present an overview of the cognitive effects of cannabinoids in man, with special emphasis on synthesizing much of the existing data in an attempt to determine specificity of action of this class of compounds on behavior.

SUBJECTIVE PSYCHOLOGICAL EFFECTS

Experienced marihuana smokers describe the effects of the drug in terms of a "high," reporting euphoria and exhilaration. However, this state of arousal is a mutable one, giving way to feelings of relaxation and drowsiness late in the intoxication period. Occasionally anxiety and dysphoria are felt. These effects become more prominent as the dosage of delta-9-tetrahydrocannabinol (delta-9-THC) contained in the marihuana increases.

Sensory and perceptual experiences are often enhanced so that, for example, hearing becomes more acute or colors become more vivid. Increased visual imagery and a readiness to engage in fantasy also are common effects. Accompanying these perceptual changes are altered thought processes. These may consist of "racing thoughts" or "flighty ideas." With high doses of delta-9-THC, these effects become intensified so that rapidly changing emotional states, including feelings of depersonalization and derealization, become coupled with disjointed thinking and the intrusion of irrelevant associations. These perceptual and cognitive changes may have a wave-like character resembling an LSD-like experience. Mental set and environmental setting can often determine the direction of subjective reactions even at moderate doses. Thus, observable behavioral reactions to marihuana are always a product of a number of factors, both pharmacological and psychological.

PSYCHOMOTOR PERFORMANCE AND SIMPLE COGNITIVE FUNCTIONS

A plethora of research studies have assessed the effects of cannabinoids on a variety of tests measuring psychomotor ability and simple cognitive functions. Performance has been sampled on a diversity of tasks, including tests of immediate memory such as digit span or story recall, simple and complex reaction time, pursuit rotor and tracking, driver simulation, digit symbol substitution, free association, speech, continuous performance tests, vigilance, speed and dexterity tests, and problem solving and concept formation tests.[1]

Although the results of many of these investigations appear to be straightforward, a number of inconsistent reports exist in this area. Disparate findings may be attributable to a number of methodological variables including dosage, route of administration, task parameters, amount of task practice, sensitivity of specific measures, and previous history of drug use.

To illustrate the complexity of results in these studies, comparisons can be made across investigations employing common performance measures. Three of the most commonly employed measures are digit span, digit symbol substitution (DSST), and pursuit rotor or tracking performance. Each task is thought to measure a slightly different function. Digit span is a classic measure of immediate memory while DSST is a measure of psychomotor speed and ability to shift set in which geometric symbols are matched with numerical digits. Pursuit rotor performance involves keeping the tip of a stylus in contact with a metal disk which is embedded in a moving turntable. All three tasks have been widely used in psychology and psychiatry and each is fairly standardized.

The effects of cannabinoids on digit span performance or recall of digits have been assessed in no fewer than eleven studies. Doses have ranged from 0.7 to 18 mg THC by smoking and up to 60 mg THC orally. The two earliest of these studies found little or no effect of cannabinoids on digit span (La Guardia report, 1944; Williams et al, 1946) employing smoked marihuana or pyrahexyl. Of 9 other studies, 4 have found reduced performance under smoked marihuana or oral THC (Galanter et al, 1973; LeDain Commission Report, 1972; Melges et al, 1970; Weingartner et al, 1972) while five have found no evidence of impaired performance (Cappell and Pliner, 1973; Casswell and Marks, 1973; Tinklenberg et al, 1972; Rafaelsen et al, 1973; Waskow et al, 1970). An examination of these studies suggests that no single variable can alone account for the differing results. Positive and negative results are found across different routes of administration, dosage, whether casual or heavy users were employed, and whether warm-up or practice was or was not given. Some studies have reported effects with doses as low as 6.2 mg THC while doses as high as 12 mg by smoking and 20 mg by the oral route have produced no detrimental performance. Since some laboratories are more likely to find the effect than others, perhaps unspecified procedural differences may exist which determine the direction of the effect. What these procedures may be remains elusive at this point.

Another popular standardized measure is the DSST which has been used in at least 8 studies. This measure appears to be somewhat more sensitive than digit span to the effects of marihuana. Four studies have reported decrements on this task which appears to be largely a function of dosage (Borg et al, 1972; Vachon et al, 1974; Weil et al, 1968). Four studies have found no effect (Dornbush et al, 1972; Jones and Stone, 1970; Hollister and Gillespie, 1970; LeDain Commission Report, 1972; Meyer et al, 1971). The one exception to this rule is the study by Hollister and Gillespie (1970) who reported no decrement following a 32 mg dose orally. Borg et al (1975) also showed that even though a decrement in DSST performance occurred which was dose-related, intoxicated subjects were able to improve their scores with practice. Task variables may also be important since Vachon et al (1974) reported more profound changes employing an automated version of the DSST which allowed evaluation of additional parameters such as response speed. Thus, task sensitivity may be an important factor in terms of magnitude of decrement.

Another task which has been widely employed by marihuana researchers involves some form of pursuit tracking. This may be the traditional pursuit rotor, or a pursuit tracking task. Employing the traditional pursuit rotor task, three studies have shown no detrimental effect of marihuana (Barratt et al, 1972; Carlin et al, 1972; Meyer et al, 1971), while two studies demonstrated negative performance (Cappell et al, 1973; Weil et al, 1968). It is difficult to attribute these divergent findings to dosage since the Carlin et al (1972) study found no performance deficit with a 15 mg dose by smoking. However, on more complex tracking tasks significant deficits have been found (Manno et al, 1974; Roth et al, 1973). Manno et al (1974) found pronounced effects with low doses administered by inhalation and a very sensitive tracking procedure.

The results of the studies discussed under each of the three tasks illustrate the difficulty many investigators as well as legislators have faced with regard to interpreting these findings and making decisions on their basis with respect to the possible hazards marihuana might have on everyday functioning. One problem with the approach of a number of these studies is that while gross performance measures on a large number of tasks give us an overall view of the behavioral effects of marihuana, they minimize the possibility that a specific locus of action will be revealed. The demonstration of a general impairment following any drug treatment is not a sufficient condition for understanding its action; rather selective-impairment is the sine qua non of behavioral pharmacology. In recent years, concern for the latter has become more apparent in the published literature on marihuana. For this reason, recent studies have shifted from the "shotgun" approach to the assessment of specific questions concerning the effects of cannabis. Three general areas which have lent themselves well to this approach are the areas of memory, state-dependent learning, and perception, especially the perception of time. Research of mainly a behavioral nature in both humans and infrahumans has shed light on mechanisms which may be common to a variety of behaviors as well as possible central nervous system mediators.

MEMORY

Descriptions of the acute intoxication syndrome under hashish by Moreau (1845) are replete with accounts of lapses in recall and speeded-up thought processes. Ames (1958) spoke of fragmentation of thought processes, and interruptions in the stream of thought so that what was said a few seconds earlier was forgotten. According to an early study by Bromberg (1934), "Speech is rapid, flighty...ideas flow quickly...these flighty ideas are not deep enough to form an engram that can be recollected -- hence, the confusion that appears on trying to remember what was thought." Objective substantiation of some of these observations has been gained in recent studies employing known doses of delta-9-THC in smoked marihuana or orally ingested delta-9-THC.

Although earlier studies sometimes employed potent cannabis preparations which produced extreme reactions (panic states, hallucinations, and delusions), consistent cognitive alterations are found with low to moderate doses of THC. However, while many investigators have shown that marihuana has some gross effect on memory, they have failed to specify what aspects of memory are particularly affected by marihuana.

For a number of years, scientists of divergent disciplines have debated the question of whether there is a single mechanism involved in memory or whether there are two mechanisms which have different capacities for storing information. The issue of whether a "unitary" or "dualistic" theory is most appropriate has never been resolved. However, evidence gathered over the last fifteen to twenty years which is based on psychological, neurophysiological, and neuroanatomical observations has supported the validity of viewing memory as a two-component process containing a short-term and long-term component (Shiffrin and Atkinson, 1969; Kesner, 1973). The model proposed by Shiffrin and Atkinson has three basic aspects: a sensory register, a short-term memory store, and a long-term memory store. The sensory register acts to hold sensory information in an unaltered form for a few milliseconds while analysis, identification, and encoding take place. The short-term memory store is an individual's working memory. It is responsible for holding the trace of the external stimulus and at the same time matching the memory trace of the stimulus with a previously encoded representation of the stimulus from the long-term storage component. The short-term store and long-term store differ mainly in both information capacity and duration. Only a small number of items can be maintained in the short-term store at any given time. Maintainance can be increased by various control processes including rehearsal, imagery, or use of mnemonics. When information resides in short-term storage for a reasonable period of time, it is transferred to long-term memory. The long-term store is a permanent repository for information.

A number of studies have investigated the actions of marihuana on different aspects of memory employing this model. The experimental paradigm consists of a free recall task involving lists of words. The basic dependent variable is the probability of recall as a function of position of word in the list or its "serial position." A bimodal U-shaped function relating probability of recall to serial position of an item can be plotted. Since the beginning and end of the serial position curve respond differently to a range of experimental variables, the positions are thought to represent output from different storage mechanisms. The probability of recall for both early and late items is higher than for middle items. These two effects are termed, respectively, the primacy and recency effects.

A study by Darley, Tinklenberg, Roth, Hollister, and Atkinson (1973) demonstrated the effects of orally administered delta-9-THC (20 mg) on the different aspects of memory proposed by this model. Subjects were presented with 10 lists of 20 words, each of which was followed by an immediate recall test. Immediately following the last list, half the subjects ingested a 20 mg dose of delta-9-THC, the other half placebo. One hour later, subjects were given a delayed recall and recognition test. Then the whole sequence of list presentation, immediate delayed recall, and recognition were repeated. The results indicated that if THC was administered after list presentation but be-fore recall, no effects were noted which were different from placebo, sug-gesting that retrieval processes were not influenced.

When THC was administered prior to list presentation, performance during immediate recall testing was depressed except for those items in the terminal list positions, suggesting that some aspect of storage was disrupted. However, items appeared to enter the sensory register and short-term store equally well. Since recall of THC-treated subjects was lower for both delayed recall and recognition, it was suggested that transfer of information from short-term to long-term memory did not take place. One possible reason for the lack of transfer is that subjects do not rehearse incoming information, a pro-cess necessary for transfer to take place (Abel, 1971b). However, Darley and Tinklenberg (1974) found that drugged subjects still displayed impaired recall when amount of rehearsal was fixed in both groups. It was felt that there was a reduced level of attention to list items probably because of in-creased competition during the intoxicated state from the subjects' own thoughts which might account for the inadequate transfer. Another possibi-lity is that items residing in the short-term store are lost more quickly and this results in the transfer deficit. A study by Dornbush, Fink, and Freedman (1971) supports this proposition. In that study, subjects were presented with a series of 3-letter trigams and attempted to recall each after a delay of 0, 6, 12, or 18 seconds. The delay interval was occupied by an interfering task. Results indicated that marihuana (22.5 mg-THC) produced a deficit in delayed recall but not at the 0 delay. Neither a low dose of marihuana (7.5 mg) or placebo had any effect on recall. The results of Darley et al (1973) have been confirmed in a number of other studies employing smoked marihuana (Dornbush, 1974; Abel, 1971b) and orally administered THC (Dittrich, Bat-ting and von Zeppelin, 1973), but have not been found when digits were em-ployed as stimuli (Galanter et al, 1973).

An interesting aspect of a number of studies in this area is the report of an increased incidence of what might be termed inclusive errors. In recall experiments, these usually involve the introduction of intralist or extralist intrusions (Cappell and Pliner, 1973; Dornbush, 1974; Darley et al, 1973), the introduction of unrelated, extraneous material during the recall of prose (Miller et al, 1972) or an increase in false alarms rather than misses in recog-nition memory tasks (Abel, 1971b; Zeidenberg et al, 1972). According to Dornbush (1974), a subject may lose his ability to discriminate between old and new material, lowering his criterion of acceptability. Thus, it is possible that at least some of the memory loss found with cannabis may be due to en-hanced imagery or thought flow which potentiates interference (due to intrusion of irrelevant associations), a phenomenon which has been shown in a number of studies to be a primary mediator of forgetting (Underwood, 1957). How-ever, why enhanced thought flow and imagery would not produce interference with retrieval processes is not clear.

In infrahuman organisms, memory deficits are less easily specified. Nevertheless, data which do exist generally support the human findings. The most commonly employed method is the delayed matching to sample task. In the simplest variant of delayed matching, a subject is situated in front of three response keys. A press on the center key produces a visual stimulus (usually presented above the key). This stimulus remains on for a given period of time and then after a delay period the sample is projected above one of the side keys. The subject's task is to remember the sample stimulus and press the outer key which contains that stimulus and not to respond on the other key above which is projected an incorrect stimulus. The delay between stimulus sample offset and presentation of comparison stimuli specifies the length of short-term memory.

Zimmerberg, Glick, and Jarvik (1971) studied the effect of smoked marihuana on the performance of monkeys on a delayed matching task. Two monkeys were given access to 30 marihuana cigarettes a day (0.5 mg) during a 4-hour matching session. Delay intervals of 0, 5, and 30 seconds were employed. On control days, monkeys smoked regular cigarettes. Results showed that monkeys performed no differently during marihuana and control sessions at the 0 delay but were impaired at the other delay intervals.

In a second experiment, 4 monkeys were trained on an oddity problem having to choose the odd color among three colors presented. Four delay conditions were employed, 0, 2, 8, and 32 seconds. 0.5, 1, and 2 mg/kg THC were administered orally. Accuracy of performance was impaired in a dose-related manner across delays. These results have generally been confirmed by Ferraro and Grilly (1973). It should be noted that the effects of marihuana in these studies was independent of any deleterious motor effects. The latter is certainly a consideration in any study employing psychomotor measures of performance, since higher doses of cannabinoids have definite depressant qualities.

Deficits in performance on numerous other behavioral tasks have been found under cannabinoids (Miller and Drew, 1974). All of these effects are certainly not attributable to memory deficits in infrahuman organisms. Other performance variables probably play a role in producing behavioral impairment in animals and presumably play a role in human deficits as well.

DISSOCIATION OR STATE DEPENDENT LEARNING

The term dissociation has been most often used with reference to various psychopathological states including hysterical neurosis or psychoses such as schizophrenia. For example, Janet (1907) spoke of dissociation of consciousness which occurs during episodes of hysteria, while William James (1890) suggested that different states of consciousness could coexist in disturbed personalities. An extreme form of dissociated personalities has been aptly portrayed in the recent book "Sybil" and the movie "The Three Faces of Eve." Hysterical fugue states which are frequently precipitated by emotional experiences of a traumatic nature provide another interesting example of dissociation.

On a more pharmacological level, the alcohol-induced "blackout"

constitutes a state of dissociation. Alcohol appears to be capable of inducing a dose-related deficit in memory registration such that permanent en-
grams are not formed. During the blackout period, immediate memory appears
to be intact so that an individual can follow simple instructions or answer
questions but events are rapidly forgotten. Memory for events occurring
during the blackout are absent when recall is attempted in the sober state.

Why is the study of drug-induced dissociation under marihuana as
well as other drugs important?

First of all, we can classify various agents in terms of their ability to
produce dissociation. It has been shown that anesthetics, alcohol, and anti-
muscarinics reliably produce dissociation, while phenothiazines, convulsants,
stimulants, and muscarinics do not (Overton, 1973). Secondly, classifying
drugs in this manner may enable one to elucidate the common biochemical
as well as behavioral mechanisms of action.

Interestingly, Overton (1973) has noted a positive correlation between abuse potential and the dissociative effects of drugs. Data of this sort
would certainly seem relevant to establishing the abuse potential of numerous
agents and therefore dissociation experiments may be a necessary method in
the arsenal of drug-screening devices.

The two basic procedures employed to study the dissociative effects
of drugs are transfer methods and drug discrimination paradigms (Overton,
1974). In the transfer design four groups of subjects are placed into the cells
of a 2 X 2 factorial design (Miller, 1957). Two groups of subjects acquire
some response under drug or no-drug conditions and then, after a given interval of time (usually 24 hours), are split into two subgroups and retested
in the drug or no-drug state. Dissociation is said to have occurred if the
state change groups perform more poorly during retest than the same state
groups. Evidence for dissociation is reflected in the interaction term of the
factorial. When dissociation occurs in both state change groups, it is referred to as symmetrical dissociation. When dissociation is found in the drug/
no-drug group but not the no-drug/drug group, asymmetrical dissociation is
said to have occurred.

Employing the transfer design, a number of human studies have reported
state dependency under cannabis (Darley and Tinklenberg, 1974; Eich, Weingartner, Stillman and Gillin, 1975; Hill, Schwin, Powell and Goodwin,
1972; Rickles, Cohen, Whitaker and McIntyre, 1973; Stillman, Weingartner,
Wyatt, Gillin and Eich, 1974). The simplest variant of the 2 X 2 design was
performed by Rickles et al (1973). Thirty-two male subjects were assigned
randomly to a marihuana group (14 mg THC) or a placebo group. Following
smoking, all subjects learned a list of 9 paired associate word pairs. Criterion of learning consisted of correctly anticipating all 9 words within a
single list sequence. Following criterion, 100% overtraining was given.
This procedure was instituted because marihuana subjects displayed initially
slower acquisition. To adequately determine the magnitude of the state dependent effect, equal performance in both drug and no-drug groups is needed

during acquisition. Otherwise, it would be difficult to distinguish between state dependent effects and performance deficits. Ten days later, a retention test was given which was followed by acquisition of a new list of paired associates. Marihuana impaired acquisition on both days, and dissociation was present in state change groups for recall of the day one list.

Other human studies have noted two important effects. First, dissociation produced by marihuana appears to be task dependent, and second, asymmetrical dissociation has been reported in at least two studies. Stillman et al (1974) ran male volunteers in the design shown in Table 1. Subjects were required to smoke marihuana (7 mg THC) or placebo in six consecutive sessions each separated by 3 to 4 days. In each session, subjects had to recall information from a previous session and then learn new material of the same nature. Tasks included recognition memory for pictures, free association for pictures, recall for words, and ordered arrangement and recall of pictures. State dependence was shown for picture recognition memory and was most pronounced for ordered arrangement of pictures. Dissociation was not found for the other tasks. These results confirmed the findings of Hill et al (1972).

Asymmetrical dissociation refers to the finding that learning which occurs in the drug state cannot be performed in the absence of drug, while learning in the non-drug state transfers to the drug state. It should be noted that this type of dissociation would not be predicted on the basis of a generalization decrement model because this model has to predict symmetrical dissociation. Eich et al (1975) demonstrated asymmetry in a free recall study. In a 2 X 2 factorial, recall of words and their categories was more complete in the marihuana-marihuana condition than marihuana-placebo condition. However, when category names were used as cues during recall, dissociation was not produced, suggesting that dissociation is mediated at least in part by inaccessibility of retrieval cues during recall.

Table 1. Design

Session	Group A	Group B
1 (Practice)	P/M	P/M
2	M	M
3	M	P
4	P	P
5	P	M
6	M	M

(P = placebo; M = marihuana)

In a number of instances, findings pertaining to dissociation in the animal literature parallel those found in the human cannabis literature. However, in animals dissociation under cannabis has been demonstrated with both transfer and drug discrimination paradigms. One of the first demonstrations of dissociation was obtained by Barry and Kubena (1971). An 8 mg/kg dose of delta-9-THC administered to rats over an 8-day period facilitated the acquisition of a bar press avoidance response. When THC-treated rats were switched to vehicle, the number of shocks received increased. However, rats trained under vehicle and switched to THC did not display impaired performance (asymmetrical dissociation).

The presence or absence of drug-induced dissociation in animals is also task dependent. Robichaud, Hefner, Anderson, and Goldberg (1972) have shown that the appearance of dissociation depends on the type of avoidance procedure employed. While dissociation was demonstrated for an active avoidance procedure, none was shown for pit avoidance, passive avoidance, or conditioned fear.

Another approach to the study of state dependence is through the use of drug discrimination procedures. The training method is similar to a sensory discrimination task. An organism learns one response under a given drug state and then learns another response in the non-drug state, under the influence of another drug, or with a different dose of the same drug. The basic dependent variable is the amount of training required to produce discrimination between the two states. The more rapid the discrimination the greater the dissociation. Subjects can also be trained to differentiate two drug states and then other drugs can be substituted to test for drug similarity.

The various tasks employed include T-maze discrimination procedures (Henriksson and Jarbe, 1972), two lever operant tasks (Bueno and Carlini, 1972; Ferraro, Gluck and Morrow, 1974), reversal learning (Jarbe and Henriksson, 1973). In a series of studies, Jarbe, Johansson, and Henriksson (1975) compared the discriminative properties of hashish, delta-8- and delta-9-THC, cannabidiol, cannabinol, as well as a number of other classes of drugs. The apparatus employed was a T-shaped water maze in which rats could escape from water by swimming into either of two arms.

In one study, it was shown that rats could learn a position discrimination between 5 mg/kg delta-9-THC and vehicle and between hashish smoke and placebo smoke. Discriminations were also established between pentobarbital, diazepam, atropine, and phencyctidine versus placebo and delta-9-THC. When each of the former drugs was substituted for THC or hashish smoke, predominantly control responses occurred. Transfer between hashish smoke and THC did occur, but not with cannabinol and cannabidiol. The results of this study generally confirm those of Kubena and Barry (1972). It should also be noted that tolerance development to THC retards the acquisition of a discrimination between THC and vehicle (Jarbe and Henriksson, 1973).

Studies of state dependent learning under cannabis may provide clues to its reinforcing properties. It is apparent that with continued cannabis use tolerance develops. This means that an increase in dose of THC may be necessary to produce the previous level of subjective effects (unconditioned reaction) or that certain emotional states or behavioral reactions induced by marihuana may become associated with the environmental cues linked with smoking (conditioned reaction). This may lead to what has been termed psychic dependence (Wikler, 1971, 1974). Therefore, certain behavior patterns and affective states deemed positive by the individual may become dependent on drug state for their appearance. For these reasons, laboratory studies of state dependent learning are a necessary step in evaluating the effects of cannabis on human behavior.

TIME PERCEPTION

Sensation and perception are known to be affected by a variety of chemical agents and are processes which are critical to understanding changes in cognitive processes.

According to Michon (1974), most introspective descriptions of drug-induced intoxications indicate that "thresholds for various stimuli are altered and that the invariants of perception which protect us from being overwhelmed by our perceptual environment seem to deteriorate."

One of the more consistently reported effects of cannabis is an alteration in the perception of time. Time often appears to stand still; a few minutes may seem like hours. This perceptual change may be responsible for impaired performance on the goal directed serial alternation task (GDSA), a task which requires a subject to serially coordinate and keep track of information in immediate memory. Adequate performance on this task depends on integrating current impressions with both preceding and subsequent experiences. Under marihuana, the time line extending from past to present appears discontinuous. This feeling of depersonalization appears to correlate highly with the deficit found on the GDSA which is termed temporal disintegration (Melges et al, 1970, 1971). It has been reasoned that marihuana speeds up an internal "pacemaker" or "clock" (Tinklenberg et al, 1972). This is often interpreted as meaning that there is an increase in the load of sensory information which reaches the central nervous system in a given period of "objective" time. Under marihuana an event which occurred recently in objective time is perceived as having occurred remotely in subjective time.

An evaluation of the process just described certainly suggests that objective measurement would be difficult. Measurement of sensation and perception in the behavioral sciences has of course been a topic of concern for the last 100 years or more (Boring, 1942) and has provided the major data base for much of psychological research. Yet, the application of psychological techniques in drug-perception studies has occurred infrequently.

According to Paton and Pertwee (1973), three techniques have been employed to study the effect of cannabis on time perception. These methods

differ in terms of whether "felt time" or "clock time" is the dependent variable. The former (method of estimation) involves giving an estimate of the
duration of a given interval while the latter (method of production) involves
asking a subject to generate a given time interval. The two estimates differ
in terms of whether the judgment is made before or after the passage of a time
interval. In the method of reproduction, the experimenter demonstrates a
given time interval (that is, by presenting a tone for 30 seconds) and the subject has to reproduce it. Employing the method of estimation, intoxicated
subjects tend to overestimate the passage of time (Clark et al, 1970; Jones
and Stone, 1970; Weil et al, 1968). For example, if 30 seconds has elapsed,
a subject might estimate the interval was 40 seconds in length. With time
production, intoxicated subjects underestimated the passage of time. Therefore, if a subject is asked to demonstrate when 30 seconds has elapsed, he
might produce 20 seconds. Actually, under normal conditions, subjects underestimate elapsed time. Under marihuana the underestimate is greater (Jones
and Stone, 1970; Tinklenberg et al, 1972; Williams et al, 1946). With either
time estimation or time production methods, the ratio of reported time to actual
elapsed time increased under marihuana. On time reproduction tasks, marihuana apparently has little effect (Dornbush et al, 1971).

In studying time perception in animals, more refined procedures have
been developed to assess timing efficiency, largely because of the lack of a
verbal repertoire. One procedure which has been used is a temporally controlled operant response or more specifically, a differential reinforcement of
low rate schedule (drl). Under a drl schedule, a response is reinforced only
after a specified interval of time has elapsed since the preceding response.
If an interresponse time (IRT) occurs which is shorter than the specified interval, no reward is given. All IRT's which exceed some minimum interval are
reinforced unless a limited hold condition is imposed. The limited hold sets
an upper limit on the amount of time that an organism can wait before responding and still be reinforced.

In chimpanzees, graded doses of delta-9-THC (0.125-4 mg/kg) decreased work output and reduced the number of reinforcements with increasing
doses on a multilink schedule which required the animal to respond on one
button and then wait at least 60 seconds (with a limited hold of 30 seconds)
before responding to a second. Five hundred responses on the second button
produced a reward. With low doses of THC, the chimpanzees became less
efficient by responding too early, thereby resetting the interval (they tended
to overestimate the passage of time) (Conrad, Elsmore and Sodetz, 1972).
Other studies have demonstrated biphasic dose response function for drl schedules in primates with low doses producing increased responding and high doses
a decrease (Ferraro and Billings, 1972; Ferraro, Grilly and Lynch, 1971).

A recent study with humans has generally confirmed the finding that a
dose-related increase in premature responding occurs on drl schedules. Graded
doses of marihuana (0, 2, 4, or 8 mg THC) and three doses of alcohol (0.48,
0.72, and 0.96 g/kg) were compared for their effects on this schedule. Results indicate that while alcohol produced little change in schedule controlled
responding, marihuana produced a dose related increase in premature responding

and a decrease in number of earned reinforcements.

Another approach to assess timing efficiency in infrahumans involves studying the discrimination of stimulus durations (Stubbs, 1968). The organism faces three response keys the middle of which produces a white light which can be varied in duration following a response. Stimulus durations can be defined as either long or short. With the offset of the sample stimulus, the two side keys can be illuminated with symbols such as X or 0. If a long stimulus light is on during sample presentation, a response to X is reinforced. If a short stimulus duration is in effect, a response to 0 is reinforced. If over-estimation of time is the rule under marihuana, the probability of choosing the X key would increase. Ferraro (1972) confirmed this prediction with chimpanzees employing 1 to 4 mg/kg doses of THC.

The significance of time sense disturbances under marihuana has yet to be elucidated. However, some interesting conjectures might be made at this point. According to Freud (1915), the sense of timelessness is a funda-mental aspect of primacy process thinking. Bleuler (1950) described schizo-phrenic thought disorder in terms of temporal aberrations. In neurological patients, lesions to the dorsomedial thalmus produces both transitory memory loss as well as time disorientation. In amnesic patients, permanent memory disorder can be accompanied by permanent time disorientation (Spiegel, Wycis, Orchinik, and Frees, 1955). These observations lend support to the view that memory content may be related to temporal experiences involving the concept of past, present, and future. Melges et al (1974) suggested that the induction of temporal disintegration produced by hashish is accom-panied by delusion-like ideation. Thus, changes in the rate and sequence of goal-directed thinking may produce unusual ideas about self and others.

These data as well as other literature suggest that most of the cogni-tive effects of marihuana may lie along a continuum of temporal experience ranging from temporal integration on one end to temporal disintegration on the other. With lower doses of THC, an amount of temporal disintegration occurs which is sufficient to produce small deficits in cognitive functions as well as some change in affect such as euphoria. As the amount of THC smoked or ingested increases, other more profound cognitive changes may take place, including severe depersonalization, emotional lability, sense distortions, hallucinations, and in some instances a toxic delirium. The latter is charac-terized by flight of ideas, psychomotor overreactivity, and paranoid delusions (Halikas, 1974).

The effect of marihuana on time perception may be related to a change in physiological parameters. For example, cannabinoids have been found to alter pulse rate, body temperature, blood pressure, and respiration. Lock-hart (1967) found that time judgments accompany changes in body temperature, but this may be an indirect effect since stress and discomfort also occur. Changes in heart rate and respiration might also serve mediators of time per-ception, but evidence for this has been less than convincing (Adam, 1971). In any event, the role of various physiological modulators should be explored in investigating this interesting phenomenon.

CANNABIS AND COGNITION:
IMPLICATIONS FOR THERAPEUTIC POTENTIAL

"The competent physician, before he attempts to give
medicine to his patient, makes himself acquainted not
only with the disease which he wishes to cure, but also
with the habits and constitution of the sick man." -- Cicero

The purpose of this conference is to explore the therapeutic potential
of cannabinoids. Any effort to modify the course of a disease with these
agents must take into account possible adverse reactions which may accompany
treatment. Many of the behavioral effects of cannabinoids described in this
presentation may be considered unwanted side effects of complications. The
frequency and severity or undesirable psychological reactions to cannabis are
dependent on a host of variables attributable to patient factors (personality,
physical health, attitudes, mental set, history of drug abuse, age), drug
factors (potency and type cannabinoid, route of administration, tolerance
development), and environmental factors (job requirements, stress). According
to Shader and DiMascio (1970), knowledge of these factors may enable the
physician to anticipate the impact that a given agent will have both behav-
iorally and medically.

Depending on the extent to which any one factor is influenced by
cannabis, some of its behavioral effects may seem innocuous, others annoying,
and some even dangerous. For example, marihuana might be used to stimulate
appetite in anorexia nervosa patients, but would only be of use in patients
with no pre-existing cardiac pathology. Unwanted side effects may be a drop
in blood pressure or severe tachycardia. Or marihuana might be successful
in treating glaucoma. However, a side effect might be mild perceptual impairment which could affect driving, especially at night.

Marihuana has been considered to have therapeutic potential for treating depression. However, if psychotherapy is instituted concomitantly, one
might be concerned whether learning, memory, and dissociative effects would
retard the efficacy of this process. Also, both paradoxical and pendular mood
alterations might occur. In the former case, mood changes in a direction opposite to a clinically desired one (that is, deepening of depression). In the
latter, an alteration in mood occurs in the desired direction but the resultant
affective state may be exaggerated (that is, manic episode). Another possibility is that the patient will display a disturbance not previously seen (that
is, delusions).

Therefore, the prediction of a drug response to marihuana appears to
be dependent on a variety of factors which seem ubiquitous and probably inter-
acting. Although the present paper has emphasized gross cognitive changes
produced by cannabis in controlled laboratory situations, the physician responsible for the welfare of patients has to accurately predict a drug response
with numerous patient and environmental factors largely uncontrolled. Thus,

the therapeutic potential of cannabis must be weighed against the probability of adverse behavioral and medical side effects.

NOTE

[1]See Abel (1970; 1971a); Barratt, Weaver, White, Blackeney, and Adams
(1972); Borg, Gershon, and Alpert (1975); Cappell, Kuchar, and Webster
(1973); Cappell and Pliner (1973); Carlin, Bakker, Halpern, and Post (1972);
Casswell and Marks (1972); Clark, Hughes, and Nakashima (1970); Clark and
Nakashima (1968); Dornbush, Clare, Zaks, Crown, Volavka, and Fink (1972);
Drew, Kiplinger, Miller, and Marx (1972); Galanter, Weingartner, Vaughn,
Roth, and Wyatt (1973); Hollister and Gillespie (1970); Hollister (1971); Jones
and Stone (1970); Klonoff and Low (1974); LaGuardia report (1944); LeDain
Commission (1972); Manno, Manno, Kiplinger, and Forney (1974); Melges,
Tinklenberg, Deardorff, Davies, Anderson, and Owen (1974); Melges, Tink-
lenberg, Hollister, and Gillespie (1970); Meyer, Pillard, Shapiro, and Mirin
(1971); Miller, Drew, and Kiplinger (1972); Moskowitz and McGlothlin (1974),
Pearl, Domino, and Rennick (1973); Rafaelsen, Christup, Bech, and Rafaelsen
(1973); Tart (1970); Tinklenberg, Kopell, Melges, and Hollister (1972);
Tinklenberg, Melges, Hollister, and Gillespie (1970); Vachon, Sulkowski,
and Rich (1974); Waskow, Olsson, Salzman, and Katz (1970); Weil, Zinberg,
and Nelson (1968); Weingartner, Galanter, Lemberger, Roth, Stillman,
Vaughn, and Wyatt (1972); Williams, Himmelsbach, Wikler, Ruble, and Lloyd
(1946); Zeidenberg, Clark, Jaffe, Anderson, Chin, and Malitz (1973); Zinberg and Weil (1969).

REFERENCES

Abel, E. L. Marihuana and memory. Nature, 1970, 227, 1151-1152.

Abel, E. L. Effects of marihuana on the solution of anagrams, memory and appetite. Nature, 1971a, 231, 260-261.

Abel, E. L. Marihuana and memory: acquisition or retrieval. Science, 1971b, 173, 1038-1040.

Adam, N. Mechanisms of time perception. T.I.T. Journal of Life Sciences, 1971, 1, 41-52.

Ames, F. A clinical and metabolic study of acute intoxication with Cannabis sativa and its role in the model psychoses. Journal of Mental Science, 1958, 104, 972-999.

Barratt, E., Beaver, W., White, R., Blakeney, P., & Adams, P. The effects of the chronic use of marijuana on sleep and perceptual-motor performance in humans. In M. F. Lewis (Ed.), Current research in marijuana. New York: Academic Press, 1972.

Barry, H., III, & Kubena, R. K. Repeated high doses of delta[1]-tetrahydrocannabinol enhance acquisition of shock avoidance by rats. Proceedings of the 79th Annual Convention of the American Psychological Association, 1971, 6, 747-748.

Bleuler, E. Dementia praecox or the group of schizophrenias. New York: International Universities Press, 1950.

Borg, J., Gershon, S., & Alpert, M. Dose effects of smoked marihuana on human cognitive and motor functions. Psychopharmacologia, 1975, 42, 211-218.

Bromberg, W. Marihuana intoxication. American Journal of Psychiatry, 1934, 91, 303-330.

Bueno, O. F. A. & Carlini, E. A. Dissociation of learning in marihuana tolerant rats. Psychopharmacologia, 1972, 25, 49-56.

Cappell, H., Kuchar, E., & Webster, C. D. Some correlates of marihuana self-administration in man: A study of titration of intake as a function of drug potency. Psychopharmacologia, 1973, 29, 177-184.

Cappell, H. D. & Pliner, P. L. Volitional control of marijuana intoxication: a study of the ability to "come down" on command. Journal of Abnormal Psychology, 1973, 82, 428-434.

Cappell, H. C. D., Webster, D. C., Herring, B. S., & Ginsberg, R. Alcohol and marihuana: A comparison of the effects on a temporally controlled operant in humans. _Journal of Pharmacology and Experimental Therapeutics_, 1972, 182, 195-203.

Carlin, A. S., Bakker, C. B., Halpern, L., & Post, R. D. Social facilitation of marijuana intoxication: Impact of social set and pharmacological activity. _Journal of Abnormal Psychology_, 1972, 80, 132-140.

Clark, L. D., Hughes, R., & Nakashima, E. N. Behavioral effects of marihuana: Experimental studies. _Archives of General Psychiatry_, 1970, 23, 193-198.

Clark, L. & Nakashima, E. Experimental studies of marihuana. _American Journal of Psychiatry_, 1968, 125, 379-384.

Conrad, D. G., Elsmore, T. F. T., & Sodetz, F. J. Delta-9-Tetrahydrocannabinol: Dose related effects on timing behavior in the chimpanzee. _Science_, 1972, 175, 547-550.

Darley, C. F. & Tinklenberg, J. R. Marijuana and memory. In L. L. Miller (Ed.), _Marijuana: Effects on human behavior._ New York: Academic Press, 1974.

Darley, C. F., Tinklenberg, J. R., Roth, W. T., Hollister, L. E., & Atkinson, R. C. Influence of marihuana on storage and retrieval processes in memory. _Memory and Cognition_, 1973, 1, 196-200.

Dittrich, A., Battig, K., & von Zeppelin, I. Effects of delta-9-Tetrahydrocannabinol (Delta-9-THC) on memory, attention and subjective state. _Psychopharmacologia_, 1973, 33, 369-376.

Dornbush, R. L. Marijuana and memory: Effects of smoking on storage. _Annals of the New York Academy of Sciences_, 1974, 234, 94-100.

Dornbush, R. L., Clare, G., Zaks, A., Crown, P., Volavka, J., & Fink, M. 21-day administration of marijuana in male volunteers. In M. F. Lewis (Ed.), _Current research in marijuana._ New York: Academic Press, 1972.

Dornbush, R. L., Fink, M., & Freedman, A. M. Marihuana, memory and perception. _American Journal of Psychiatry_, 1971, 128, 194-197.

Drew, W. G., Kiplinger, G. F., Miller, L. L., & Marx, M. Effects of propranolol on marihuana-induced cognitive dysfunctioning. _Clinical Pharmacology and Therapeutics_, 1972, 13, 526-533.

Eich, J. E., Weingartner, H., Stillman, R. C., & Gillin, J. C. State-dependent accessibility of retrieval cues in the retention of a categorized list. _Journal of Verbal Learning and Verbal Behavior_, 1975, in press.

Ferraro, D. P. Effects of delta-9-transtetrahydrocannabinol on simple and complex learned behavior in animals. In M. F. Lewis (Ed.), _Current research in marijuana_. New York: Academic Press, 1972.

Ferraro, D. P. & Billings, D. K. Comparison of the behavioral effects of synthetic delta-9-trans-tetrahydrocannabinol and marihuana extract distillate in chimpanzees. _Psychopharmacologia_, 1972, _25_, 169-174.

Ferraro, D. P. & Grilly, D. M. Lack of tolerance to delta-9-tetrahydrocannabinol in chimpanzees. _Science_, 1973, _179_, 490-492.

Ferraro, D. P., Grilly, D. M., & Lynch, W. C. Effects of marihuana extract on the operant behavior of chimpanzees. _Psychopharmacologia_, 1971, _22_, 333-351.

Ferraro, D. P., Gluck, J. P., & Morrow, C. W. Temporally-related stimulus properties of a delta-9-tetrahydrocannabinol in monkeys. _Psychopharmacologia_, 1974, _35_, 305-316.

Freud, S. The unconscious (1915). In _The complete psychological works of Sigmund Freud_. London: Hogarth Press, 1964.

Galanter, M., Weingartner, H., Vaughan, T. B., Roth, W. T., & Wyatt, R. J. Delta-9-transtetrahydrocannabinol and natural marihuana. _Archives of General Psychiatry_, 1973, _28_, 278-281.

Halikas, J. A. Marijuana use and psychiatric illness. In L. Miller (Ed.), _Marijuana: Effects on human behavior_. New York: Academic Press, 1974.

Henriksson, B. G. & Jarbe, T. U. C. Delta-9-tetrahydrocannabinol use as a discriminative stimulus for rats in position learning in a T-shaped water maze. _Psychonomic Science_, 1972, _27_, 25-26.

Hill, S. Y., Schwin, R., Powell, B., & Goodwin, B. W. State-dependent effects of marihuana on human memory. _Nature_, 1973, _243_, 241-242.

Hollister, L. E. Marihuana in man: Three years later. _Science_, 1971, _172_, 21-28.

Hollister, L. E. & Gillespie, H. K. Marihuana ethanol and dextroamphetamine. _Archives of General Psychiatry_, 1970, _23_, 199-203.

James, W. _Principles of psychology_. New York: Holt, 1890.

Janet, P. M. F. The major symptoms of hysteria. New York: McMillan, 1907.

Jarbe, T. U. C., & Henriksson, B. G. Effects of delta-8-THC and delta-9-THC on the acquisition of a discriminative positional habit in rats. Psychopharmacologia, 1973, 31, 321-332.

Jarbe, T. U. C., Johansson, J. O., & Henriksson, B. G. Delta-9-tetra-hydrocannabinol and pentobarbital as discriminative cues in the Mongolian gerbil (meriones unguiculatus). Pharmacology, Biochemistry and Behavior, 1975, 3, 403-410.

Kesner, R. A neural system analysis of memory storage and retrieval. Psychological Bulletin, 1973, 80, 117-203.

Klonoff, H., & Low, M. D. Psychological and neurophysiological effects of marijuana in man: an interaction model. In L. L. Miller (Ed.), Marijuana: Effects on human behavior. New York: Academic Press, 1974.

Kubena, R. K. & Barry, H., III. Stimulus characteristics of marihuana components. Nature, 1972, 235, 397-398.

LaGuardia Report: Mayor's committee on marihuana. The marihuana problem in the City of New York. Lancaster, Pa.: Jacques Cattell Press, 1944.

LeDain Commission. A report on the Commission of inquiry into the non-medical use of drugs. Ottawa: Information Canada, 1972.

Lockhart, J. M. Ambient temperature and time estimation. Journal of Experimental Psychology, 1967, 73, 286-292.

Low, M. D., Klonoff, H., & Marcus, A. The neurophysiological basis of the marihuana experience. Canadian Medical Association Journal, 1973, 108, 157-164.

Manno, J. E., Manno, B. R., Kiplinger, G. R., & Forney, R. B. Motor and mental performance with marijuana: Relationship to administered dose of delta-9-tetrahydrocannabinol and its interaction with alcohol. In L. Miller (Ed.), Marijuana: Effects on human behavior. New York: Academic Press, 1974.

Melges, F. T., Tinklenberg, J. R. Deardorff, C. M., Davies, N. H., Anderson, R. E., & Owen, C. A. Temporal disorganization and delusional-like ideation. Archives of General Psychiatry, 1974, 30, 855-861.

Melges, F. T., Tinklenberg, J. R., Hollister, L. E., & Gillespie, H. K. Marihuana and temporal disintegration. Science, 1970, 168, 1118-1120.

Melges, F. T., Tinklenberg, J. R., Hollister, L. E., & Gillespie, H. K. Marihuana and the temporal span of awareness. Archives of General Psychiatry, 1971, 24, 564-567.

Meyer, R. E., Pillard, R. C., Shapiro, L. M., & Mirin, S. M. Administration of marijuana to heavy and casual marijuana users. American Journal of Psychiatry, 1971, 128, 90-96.

Michon, J. A. Human information processing -- with and without drugs. Psychiatria. Neurologia. Neurocherurgia, 1973, 163-174.

Miller, L. L., & Drew, W. G. Cannabis: Review of behavioral effects in animals. Psychological Bulletin, 1974, 81, 401-417.

Miller, L., Drew, W. G. & Kiplinger, G. F. Effects of marijuana on recall of narrative material and Stroop colour-word performance. Nature, 1972, 237, 172-173.

Miller, N. E. Objective techniques for studying motivational effects of drugs on animals. In S. Garattini and V. Ghetti (Eds.), Proceedings of Internal Symposium and Psychotropic Drugs. Amsterdam: Elsevier, 1957.

Moreau, J. J. Du hachish et de l'alienation mentale: Etudes psychologiques 34, Paris: Libraire de Forten, Maison Paris, 1845.

Moskowitz, H. & McGlothlin, W. Effects of marihuana on auditory signal detection. Psychopharmacologia, 1974, 40, 137-145.

Overton, D. A. State-dependent learning produced by addicting drugs. In S. Fisher and A. M. Freedman (Eds.), Opiate Addiction: Origins and treatment. Washington, D. C.: V. H. Winston and Sons, 1973.

Overton, D. A. Experimental methods for the study of state-dependent learning. Federation Proceedings, 1974, 33, 1800-1813.

Paton, W. D. M., & Pertwee, R. G. The actions of cannabis in man. In R. Mechoulam (Ed.), Marijuana: chemistry, pharmacology, metabolism and clinical effects. New York: Academic Press, 1973.

Pearl, J., Domino, E. F., & Rennick, P. Short-term effects of marijuana smoking on cognitive behavior in experienced male users. Psychopharmacologia, 1973, 31, 13-24.

Rafaelsen, L., Christup, H., Bech, P., & Rafaelsen, O. J. Effects of cannabis and alcohol on psychological tests. Nature, 1973, 242, 117-118.

Rickles, W. H., Jr., Cohen, M. J., Whitaker, C. A., & McIntyre, K. E. Marijuana induced state-dependent verbal learning. Psychopharmacologia, 1973, 30, 349-354.

Robichaud, R. C., Hefner, M. A., Anderson, J. E., & Goldberg, M. E. Effects of delta-9-tetrahydrocannabinol (THC) on several rodent learning paradigms. Federation Proceedings, 1972, 31, 551.

Shader, R. I. & DiMascio, A. Psychotropic drug side effects: Clinical and theoretical perspectives. Baltimore: Williams and Wilkins, 1970.

Shiffrin, R. M. & Atkinson, R. C. Storage and retrieval processes in long term memory. Psychological Review, 1969, 76, 179-193.

Spiegel, E. A., Wycis, H. T., Orchinik, C. W., & Freed, H. The thalamus and temporal orientation. Science, 1955, 121, 771-772.

Stillman, R. C., Weingartner, H., Wyatt, R. J., Gillin, J. C., & Eich, J. State-dependent (dissociative) effects of marihuana on human memory. Archives of General Psychiatry, 1974, 31, 81-85.

Stubbs, A. The discrimination of stimulus duration by pigeons. Journal of the Experimental Analysis of Behavior, 1968, 3, 223-238.

Tart, C. T. Marihuana intoxication: common experiences. Nature, 1970, 226, 701-704.

Tinklenberg, J. R., Kopell, B. S., Melges, F. T., & Hollister, L. E. Marihuana and alcohol: Time production and memory functions. Archives of General Psychiatry, 1972, 27, 812-814.

Tinklenberg, J. R., Melges, F. T., Hollister, L. E., & Gillespie, H. K. Marihuana and immediate memory. Nature, 1970, 226, 1171-1172.

Underwood, B. Interference and forgetting. Psychological Review, 1957, 64, 49-60.

Vachon, L., Sulkowski, A., & Rich, E. Marihuana effects on learning, attention and time estimation. Psychopharmacologia, 1974, 39, 1-11.

Waskow, I. E., Olsson, J. E., Solzman, G., & Katz, M. M. Psychological effects of delta-9-THC. Archives of General Psychiatry, 1970, 22, 97-107.

Weil, A. T., Zinberg, N. E., & Nelson, J. M. Clinical and psychological effects of marihuana in man. Science, 1968, 162, 1234-1242.

Weingartner, H., Galanter, M., Lemberger, L., Roth, W. J., Stillman, R., Vaughn, T. B., & Wyatt, R. J. Effect of marijuana and synthetic delta-9-THC on information processing. Proceedings of the 80th Annual Convention of the American Psychological Association, 1972, 813-814.

Wikler, A. Present status of the concept of drug dependence. Psychological
        Medicine, 1971, 1, 377-380.

Williams, E. G., Himmelsbach, C. K., Wikler, A., Ruble, D. C., &
        Lloyd, B. J. Studies on marihuana and pyrahexyl compound. Public
        Health Reports, 1946, 61, 1059-1083.

Zeidenberg, P., Clark, W. C., Jaffe, J., Anderson, S. W., Chin, S.,
        & Malitz, S. Effect of oral administration of delta-9-tetrahydrocan-
        nabinol on memory, speech and perception of thermal stimulation:
        Results with four normal human volunteer subjects. Preliminary report.
        Comprehensive Psychiatry, 1973, 14, 549-556.

Zimmerberg, B., Glick, S. D., & Jarvik, M. E. Impairment of recent
        memory by marihuana and THC in rhesus monkeys. Nature, 1971,
        233, 343-345.

Zinberg, N. E. & Weil, A. T. A comparison of marijuana users and non-
        users. Nature, 1970, 226, 119-123.

DISCUSSION

Lemberger: I have a question for Dr. Harshman. Did you select these people based on their handedness?

Harshman: We did not. We took every subject who became a participant in Dr. Cohen's 94-day study. Most of these were right-handed, but there were some left-handed subjects.

Weiss: Did you see any difference between the left-handed and the right-handed subjects? Wouldn't the hemispheres be just the opposite?

Harshman: Left-handed is a very heterogeneous compilation. Perhaps a majority of them are just like right-handed people. Among the minority, you have some which are more bilateral, and a very small minority in which there is a sort of mirror image. We didn't have enough lefthanders to make any generalization in our study.

Miller: Do you have any idea how much marihuana was taken in?

Harshman: One marihuana cigarette first thing in the morning, and it contained approximately 19 mgs. of THC. That sounds like a lot, but these are chronic heavy users. We didn't impose on them the regimen of inhaling and holding for 30 seconds, and so on.

Cohen: Did they rate themselves as being very high?

Harshman: It varied. I think they had a conspiracy to rate the marihuana as being only moderately good, most of them anyway. They rated themselves as having a good, but not a spectacular high most of the time.

Cohen: I would like to ask Dr. Hanley or Harshman about the possibility of whether there was an EEG representation of this shift in laterality.

Hanley: We looked at that, and the problem is what measure do we choose? If you look at energy level, there certainly were differences that suggest some aspects of laterality, but the individual variations were so great, there really was no statistical significance.

Weiss: I would like to suggest something about the questionnaire study, something which is somewhat troublesome. I think that the sample you are taking is extremely biased because you are asking questions -- taking from a population of people who tend to return these types of questionnaires. On one piece of data there was "tends to make me more social," marihuana greater than alcohol. But this may be true of an extroverted person who would also be more likely to return a questionnaire of this nature.

Roth: It would be nice to have a personality test. It would be nice also to see who handed in questionnaires and who didn't. The percent response was about 60% and about one third of those had taken the drug in the requisite amount. The survey had to be anonymous; we couldn't identify individual people because of the illegal nature of marihuana.

Harshman: I think we can keep in mind that any of the data we are talking about in this conference comes from a nonrepresentative sample. I think this ranges from Dr. Rubin's study to my own to any of them. There is nothing so abnormal as the so-called normal volunteers when you compare them to the universe of people. For patient studies, the sort of patient who will volunteer to take marihuana for his or her glaucoma is apt to be quite atypical from other patients. It's something you can never overcome; it's something worth paying attention to.

Feeney: There was a study in the LaGuardia report which examined test scores when intoxicated vs. when not intoxicated. I don't remember the details, but one of the conclusions was that under the influence of marihuana there was a tendency to see the unusual in obvious things, which is one of the things that comes out in your questionnaire as well. I want to make this point in regard to the question we talked about earlier this morning -- the tremendous variability we see in the data under controlled conditions.

Roth: We actually have done a recent study on the responses to TAT cards by subjects intoxicated with marihuana and not intoxicated. These were scored by blind graders, and indeed there was more novelty, more unusualness in the kind of responses that people made. Whether that represents variability or a decline in organization is very difficult to know. It's difficult to define novelty or creativity in some satisfactory way, and that is the problem you describe.

Feeney: That brings up the question of why do people smoke marihuana when it is so difficult to get other species to take it. One possibility is that they are getting novel experiences from humdrum events. It has been documented that novelty itself is somewhat reinforcing, and if the drug is inducing stimulus change into a constant environment, that could be part of the reason of people seeking it out.

Roth: Right. Weil's The Natural Mind says that an altered state of consciousness is reinforcing in itself. People are bored with their humdrum state of consciousness after a little bit of life and they want to try something different regardless of what it is.

Stillman: We have some evidence in our laboratory which parallels that of Dick Harshman showing that the task which is shared by the two hemispheres seems to be taken over by the right hemisphere under the influence of marihuana. It has not been completely analyzed, but it's a different approach to the same thing. It would suggest there may be an inherent novelty, with just a different part of the brain assuming responsibility of processing the same data.

Braude: On your slide, Dr. Hanley, were the subjects under the influence of marihuana?

Hanley: Actually some years ago I did some studies with marihuana which showed a loss of energy in the EEG signal after marihuana, which is the opposite of what you see in epilepsy. Then more recently, as I showed this evening, there are quite large differences between phases of users of marihuana and nonusers. In fact, the differences are so great, it's possible to separate with a very high degree of success users and nonusers. The possibility of marihuana as a therapeutic tool in epilepsy when conventional medication doesn't do the job is worth considering. Energy reduction may be a good rationale for the utilization of the cannabinoids.

Vachon: I have a question which I would like to ask Dr. Hanley. After prolonged extensive use of marihuana for many days, was there any evidence of any kind of rebound like the way one would see with barbiturates?

Hanley: You had better explain what you mean by rebound.

Vachon: Well, if somebody is taking barbiturates and then they go off, you will see a high level of irritability, and so on.

Hanley: We did some testing on these subjects before they actually began the study, but within the study they were using the drug fairly constantly, and the only thing is that it's a lot harder to tell the difference between users smoking before and afterwards than it is to tell between a user and a nonuser, and it's harder to tell the difference between what for the purpose of this experiment is called a heavy user and a moderate. Things didn't change very much after they had been using the drug for quite a long time.

Tumor Problems

CHAPTER 18

ANALGESIC AND ANTITUMOR POTENTIAL OF THE CANNABINOIDS

Louis S. Harris

Department of Pharmacology
Medical College of Virginia
Health Sciences Division
Virginia Commonwealth University
Richmond, Virginia

NOTE: This work was supported, in part, by U. S. Dept.
of Health, Education and Welfare grants DA-00490,
CA 17840, CA 17551, the Alexander and Margaret Stewart
Trust Fund, and an American Cancer Society Institutional
Grant (IN 105A). The author wishes to acknowledge his
collaborators Drs. W. L. Dewey, A. E. Munson,
R. A. Carchman, and A. S. Bloom. Supplies of canna-
binoids used in this work were generously supplied by
Dr. Monique Braude of the National Institute on Drug Abuse
and Dr. Raj Razdan of the Sheehan Institute for Research.

There is an extensive folklore concerning the analgesic activity of
cannabis in man (Mikuriya, 1961). On careful examination, however, there
was no objective evidence for the efficacy of cannabis in this regard. With
the structural identity and synthesis of (-)-delta-9-tetrahydrocannabinol
(delta-9-THC) (Gaoni and Mechoulam, 1964), the major active principle of
cannabis, came reports of analgesic activity in laboratory animals. Indeed,
potency equal to morphine was reported for delta-9-THC (Grunfield and
Edery, 1968; Bauxbaum, Sanders-Bush and Efron, 1969).

Using the standard analgesic test procedures in our laboratory, we
have not had the same results (Dewey, Harris and Kennedy, 1972). In our
hands, delta-9-THC was inactive in the hot-plate and tail-flick tests at
doses below those that produced severe behavioral and psychomotor impairment. This may be due to the fact that we run a more stringent test procedure.
For instance, in the tail-flick test we use a normal reaction time of 2-4
seconds with a cutoff time of 10 seconds in mice and 20 seconds in rats

(Harris and Pierson, 1964; Harris, Dewey, Howes, Kennedy and Pars, 1969).
Using these criteria, until recently only the narcotic analgesics were active.
Indeed, there was such a good correlation between antinociceptive activity
in these tests and analgesics in man that we could accurately predict the
dose necessary to relieve pain in man. The development of the narcotic-
antagonist analgesics, which are inactive in the hot-plate and tail-flick
tests as we run them, caused a rethinking of our test procedures and led to
the extensive use of the "writhing" or "abdominal stretching" test (Hendershot
and Forsacth, 1959; Pearl and Harris, 1966; Pearl, Aceto and Harris, 1968).
This test did reveal activity for the narcotic antagonists. However, delta-9-
THC is again not active in this test unless doses are used which produce
behavioral and motor impairment. To date there have been four reports of
controlled analgesic studies with delta-9-THC in man (Noyes, Brunk, Baram
and Canter, 1975; Regelson, Butler, Schulz, Kirk, Peek, Green and Zakio
[in press]; Hill, Goodwin, Schwin and Powell, 1974; Roft, Gregg, Ghia
and Harris, pending). One of these reported good analgesic activity (Noyes
et al., 1975). Another reported no analgesic activity (Regelson et al., in
press) and two reported hyperalgesia (Hill et al., 1974; Roft et al., pending).
Thus, to date, the results with this compound are equivocal.

   Recently, a new cannabinoid 9-hydroxy-9-nor-hexahydrocannabinol
(HHC), with potent analgesic activity has been prepared by Wilson and May
(1974; also Wilson, May, Martin and Dewey, in press) (see Figure 1).

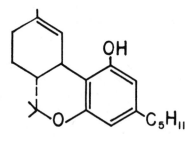
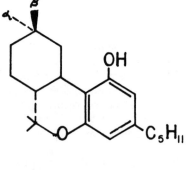

Δ^9-THC

	$\underline{\alpha}$	$\underline{\beta}$
9-nor-9α-OH-HHC	OH	H
9-nor-9β-OH-HHC	H	OH

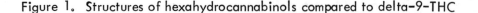

Figure 1. Structures of hexahydrocannabinols compared to delta-9-THC

This compound exists in the α- and β-form and diasterioisomers exist for each. We have found that potent antinociceptive activity is found in the β-isomer and that the β-1-isomer is approximately twice as potent as the racemic mixture in the hot-plate test and considerably more active in the tail-flick test (Table 1). This is the first compound closely related to the natural products which has shown potent antinociceptive activity in our test procedures.

In an attempt to determine whether β-HHC resembled the narcotic analgesics, we attempted to reverse its antinociceptive activity with naloxone. The results of one such experiment is shown in Table 2. While some antagonism of β-HHC could be obtained with naloxone, we were never able to completely reverse its antinociceptive activity. Another characteristic of narcotic analgesics is the cross-tolerance which occurs between members of this class of compounds. We attempted to determine whether cross-tolerance occurred between morphine and β-HHC. For this purpose, we used mice implanted with morphine pellets (Way, Loh and Shen, 1969). The results are shown in Table 3. While there is a marked tolerance to morphine, there is no cross-tolerance to β-HHC. Indeed, if anything, there is some enhancement of

Table 1. Antinociceptive Activity of Cannabinoids

Compound	Tail Flick Test (i.p.)	ED$_{50}$ mg/kg Hot-Plate Test (i.p.)	Abdominal Stretch Test (s.c.)
Delta-9-THC	NA[a]	NA	NA
(±)- α-HHC[b]	NA	NA	NA
(±)- β-HHC	7.1	2.9[c]	-
(-)- β-HHC	1.0	1.6[c]	0.03
Morphine SO$_4$	5.8	1.2[c]	0.56

[a] Not active at doses below 10 mg/kg.

[b] (±)- α-9-hydroxy-9-nor-hexahydrocannabinol.

[c] Wilson et al., J. Med. Chem.

Source: Martin, Dewey, Earnhardt, Adams, Harris, Wilson, May, and Razdan (pending).

Table 2. Reversal of the Effects of b-HHC on the Tail-Flick by Naloxone

Treatment	Tail-Flick % MPE
Vehicle	1
(±)- β-HHC, 20 mg/kg	85
(±)- β-HHC, 20 mg/kg + Naloxone 2 mg/kg	52

Source: Bloom, Dewey, Harris, and Brosins (1975).

Table 3. Tail-Flick Activity of Morphine and 9-nor-9β-OH-HHC in Placebo and Morphine Pellet Implanted Mice

	ED_{50} and 95% Confidence Limits mg/kg	
	Placebo Pellet	Morphine Pellet
Morphine	3.40 (1.20-9.64)	17.28 (9.21-32.44)
9-nor-9β-OH-HHC	7.20 (1.98-20.62)	3.83 (1.18-12.61)

Source: Bloom et al., 1975.

the antinociceptive effects. These results, coupled with data from the morphine-dependent monkey and the results with the heterocyclic derivatives presented later in this Symposium, give hope that a non-dependence-producing strong analgesic may emerge from the cannabis field.

The reports (Nahas, Suica-Foca, Armand and Marishima, 1974; Gupta, Grieco and Cushman, 1974; Munson, Levy, Harris and Dewey, in press) that marihuana and the naturally occurring cannabinoids interfered with certain immune systems prompted us to look at the effects of these compounds on some tumor systems. It was our hypothesis that since delta-9-THC to some degree inhibited the T-cell system, which is one of the body's few natural defenses against cancer, it would cause tumors to grow faster. The tumor system we first chose to study was the Lewis lung adenocarcinoma. In this system, 1×10^6 tumor cells were injected into the right hind gluteus muscle of C57BL/6 mice. Tumor size was measured weekly and converted to tumor weight by the method of Mayo (1972). The Lewis lung adenocarcinoma is a solid tumor and grows according to a Gompertzian function (Figure 2).

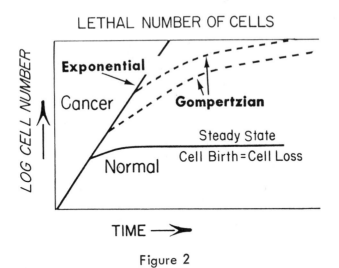

Figure 2

Although the tumor grows to a large mass, the animals do not die of the primary tumor but by metastases particularly to the lung. The results of our first experiment are shown in Figure 3. Much to our surprise, there was a marked inhibition of tumor growth and a significant increase in life span (Table 4) (Harris, Munson and Carchman, in press; Munson, Harris, Friedman, Dewey and Carchman, 1975). Of interest was the fact that the animals soon became tolerant to the behavioral effects of these rather large doses of delta-9-THC and did not lose weight, as is the case with most of the standard anti-tumor agents. This reflects the low toxicity of the cannabinoids relative to the standard anticancer drugs. Since these results were obtained with a 10-day treatment regimen, it was natural to try longer treatment schedules. When this was done, the early marked inhibition of tumor growth was overcome and there was no increase in life span. We have found that treatment every third day produces results as good as can be obtained but no better than our original regimen.

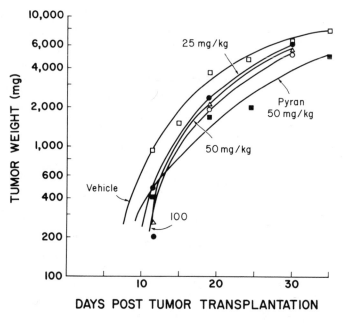

Figure 3

Table 4. Survival Time of delta-9-THC-Treated Mice
(10 Days) Hosting Lewis Lung Carcinoma[a]

Treatment	Dose (mg/kg)	Wgt.(g)[b]	Survival Time (Days)	% ILS[c]
Vehicle[d]	-	+1.0	25.8 ± 1.3	-
Pyran	50	-0.5	38.2 ± 1.5	48*
Delta-9-THC	25	+0.9	30.3 ± 2.0	17
Delta-9-THC	50	-0.3	27.4 ± 0.6	6
Delta-9-THC	100	-0.1	35.5 ± 1.1	36*

a. Group of mice inoculated with 10^6 Lewis lung cells and treated daily for 10 days. Control and delta-9-THC mice treated orally. Pyran injected i.p.

b. Whole body weight changes determined after 10 days of treatment.

c. Percent increased life span over control.

d. 0.01 ml/g of 7.5% bovine serum albumin.

* $p < .05$.

These studies have been expanded (Munson et al., 1975) to include a number of other tumor systems, such as the Friend leukemia virus-induced splenomegaly and the C3H mammary tumor where inhibitory activity is also seen. However, delta-9-THC is inactive in mice hosting the L-1210 murine leukemia. This tumor system grows rapidly and follows an exponential function.

A number of other natural cannabinoids have also been examined to ascertain their antitumor activity. Delta-8-THC is quite active (Figure 4), as is cannabinol, but cannabidiol produces a marked stimulation of tumor growth (Figure 5). To date, we have tested a wide variety of natural and synthetic cannabinoids as well as some heterocyclic analogs. None of these has proven to be either much more potent or efficacious than delta-9-THC.

To enhance our ability to examine large numbers of compounds and to attempt to determine mechanisms of action, we have turned to an in vitro system (Harris et al., in press; Munson et al., 1975). In this system, normal bone marrow or tumor cells are incubated with either the drug or drug vehicle and their ability to incorporate tritiated thymidine into DNA is examined.

Experiments with bone marrow and isolated Lewis lung cells incubated in vitro with delta-9-THC showed a dose-dependent inhibition of the incorporation of tritiated thymidine into DNA. Of great interest was an observed differential between the tumor and the bone marrow cells (Figure 6). The importance of this finding is twofold. First, few anti-tumor agents have such a selective effect. Second, if we can find an explanation for the differential effect we may discover some important difference between the tumor and normal cells which will allow a new rational approach to chemotherapy.

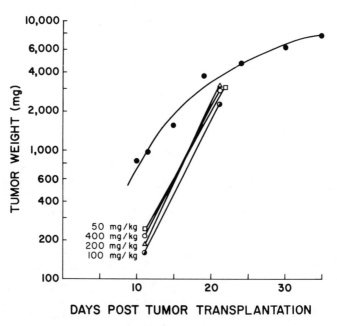

ACTION OF Δ8THC ON TUMOR GROWTH

Figure 4

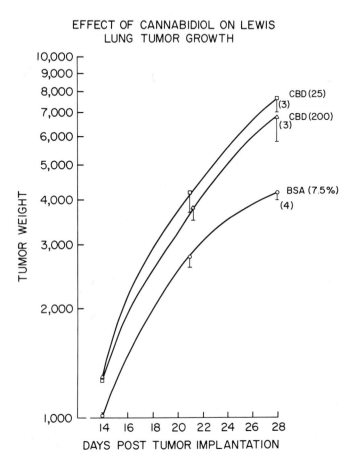

EFFECT OF CANNABIDIOL ON LEWIS
LUNG TUMOR GROWTH

Figure 5

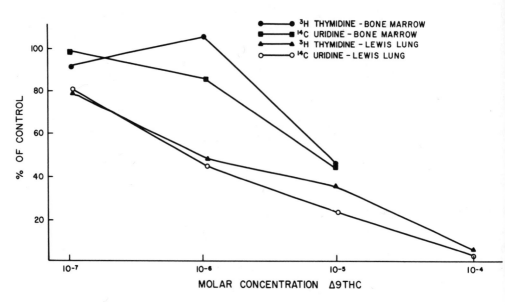

Figure 6

This in vitro system has allowed us to screen a wide variety of compounds as illustrated in Table 5. As can be seen, many compounds have inhibitory activity but none are much more potent than delta-9-THC. More importantly, none show the differential effect between tumor and normal cells that delta-9-THC does. It is also of interest to note that cannabidiol produces an enhancement of thymidine incorporation. This may reflect the mechanism for enhanced tumor growth observed in the in vivo system (Munson et al., 1975).

As to translation of these findings to tumor chemotherapy in man, there is a long way to go. We would like to have more efficacious compounds with greater potency than delta-9-THC and with little or no central nervous system activity. It may be that the cannabinoids will be useful only as adjuncts to other chemotherapy. We are currently investigating combination medication with a variety of antitumor agents and some of these appear promising. More important findings, however, will probably come from investigation of the basic mechanisms involved in the action of these drugs on tumor cells.

Table 5. The Effect of Cannabinoids and Cytosine Arabinoside on in vitro DNA Synthesis

Cannabidiol	3.37×10^{-5}M	*********	4.89×10^{-4}
ABN Cannabidiol	9.28×10^{-5}M	1.29×10^{-2}	5.51×10^{-6}
Cannabichromene	$>10^{-4}$M	$>10^{-4}$M	_____
$\epsilon\beta$, 11/di/OH Δ^9-THC	$>10^{-4}$M	$>10^{-4}$M	_____
Cannabicyclol	$>10^{-4}$M	_____	_____

DRUG	STRUCTURE	LEWIS LUNG	E.D. 50* L1210	BONE MARROW
Δ^9-THC		4.18×10^{-6}M	3.26×10^{-5}	2.06×10^{-5}
Δ^8-THC		2.99×10^{-6}M	8.70×10^{-6}	1.26×10^{-6}
ABN Δ^8-THC		1.48×10^{-6}M	5×10^{-6}M	3.56×10^{-6}
Cannabinol		2.3×10^{-6}M	2.2×10^{-6}	3.08×10^{-7}
ARA - C		1.36×10^{-7}	2.53×10^{-8}	1.57×10^{-7}M

Source: Carchman, R. A. et al. Cancer Res., 1976, 36, 95–100

REFERENCES

Bauxbaum, D., Sanders-Bush, E., & Efron, D. Analgesic activity of tetrahydrocannabinol (THC) in the rat and mouse. Fed. Proc., 1969, 28, 735.

Bloom, A. S., Dewey, W. L., Harris, L. S., & Brosins, K. Brain catecholamines and the antinociceptive action of ($\pm$)-9-nor-9-β-OH= hexahydrocannabinol. Neuroscience Abstracts, 1975, 9, 242.

Carchman, R. A., Harris, L. S., & Munson, A. E. The inhibition of DNA synthesis by the cannabinoids. Cancer Res., 1976, 36, 95-100.

Dewey, W. L., Harris, L. S., & Kennedy, J. S. Some pharmacological and toxicological effects of 1-trans-delta-8 and 1-trans-delta-9-tetrahydrocannabinol in laboratory rodents. Arch. int. Pharmacolog., 1972, 196, 133-145.

Gaoni, Y. & Mechoulam, R. Isolation, structure and partial synthesis of an active component of hashish. J. Amer. Chem. Soc., 1964, 86, 1646-1647.

Grunfield, Y. & Edery, H. Psychopharmacological activity of the active constituents of hashish and some related cannabinoids. Psychopharmacologia, 1968, 14, 200-210.

Gupta, S., Grieco, M. H., & Cushman, P., Jr. Impairment of rosette-forming T-lymphocytes in chronic marihuana smokers. New Eng. J. Med., 1974, 291, 874-877.

Harris, L. S., Dewey, W. L., Howes, J. R., Kennedy, J. S., & Pars, H. Narcotic-antagonist analgesics: Interactions with cholinergic systems. J. Pharmacol. Exp. Ther., 1969, 169, 17-22.

Harris, L. S., Munson, A. E., & Carchman, R. A. Anti-tumor properties of cannabinoids. Proceedings of the International Conference on the Pharmacology of Marihuana. Savannah: Raven Press, in press.

Harris, L. S., & Pierson, A. K. Narcotic antagonists in the benzomorphan series. J. Pharmacol. Exp. Ther., 1964, 143, 141-148.

Hendershot, L. C., & Forsacth, J. Antagonism of the frequency of phenylquinone-induced writhing in the mouse by weak analgesics and non-analgesics. J. Pharmacol. Exp. Ther., 1959, 125, 237-240.

Hill, S. Y., Goodwin, D. W., Schwin, R., & Powell, B. Marihuana: CNS depressant or excitant. Am. J. Psychiat., 1974, 131, 313-315.

Martin, B. R., Dewey, W. L., Earnhardt, J.T., Adams, M. D., Harris, L. S., Wilson, R. S., May, E. L., & Razdan, R. Submitted for publication.

Mayo, J. G. Biologic characterization of the subcutaneously implanted Lewis lung tumor. Cancer Chemother. Rep., 1972, 3, 325-330.

Mikuriya, T. H. Historical aspects of cannabis sativa in western medicine. New Physician, 1961, 18, 902-908.

Munson, A. E., Levy, J. A., Harris, L. S., & Dewey, W. L. Effects of delta-9-tetrahydrocannabinol on the immune system. Proceedings of the International Conference on the Pharmacology of Marihuana. Savannah: Raven Press, in press.

Munson, A. E., Harris, L. S., Friedman, M. A., Dewey, W. L., & Carchman, R. A. Antineoplastic activity of cannabinoids. J. Nat. Cancer. Inst., 1975, 55, 597-602.

Nahas, G. G., Suica-Foca, N., Armand, J. P., & Marishima, A. Inhibition of cellular immunity in marihuana smokers. Science, 1974, 183, 419-420.

Noyes, R., Jr., Brunk, S. F., Baram, D. A., & Canter, A. Analgesic effect of delta-9-tetrahydrocannabinol. J. Clin. Pharmacol., 1975, 15, 139-143.

Pearl, J., Aceto, M. D., & Harris, L. S. Prevention of writhing and other effects of narcotics and narcotic antagonists in mice. J. Pharmacol. Exp. Ther., 1968, 160, 217-230.

Pearl, J., & Harris, L. S. Inhibition of writhing by narcotic antagonists. J. Pharmacol. Exp. Ther., 1966, 154, 319-323.

Regelson, W., Butler, J. R., Schulz, J., Kirk, T., Peek, L., Green, M. L., & Zakio, O. Delta-9-THC as an effective anti-depressant and appetite stimulating agent in advanced cancer patients. Proceedings of the International Conference on the Pharmacology of Marihuana. Savannah: Raven Press, in press.

Roft, D. D., Gregg, J. M., Ghia, J., & Harris, L. S. Effects of intravenous delta-9-THC on experimental and surgical pain responses. J. Clin. Pharmacol. Submitted for publication.

Way, E. L., Loh, H. H., & Shen, F. H. Simultaneous quantitative assessment of morphine tolerance and physical dependence. J. Pharmacol. Exp. Ther., 1969, 167, 1-8.

Wilson, R. S., & May, E. L. 9-Nor-delta-8-tetrahydrocannabinol, a cannabinoid of metabolic interest. J. Med. Chem., 1974, 17, 475-476.

Wilson, R. S., May, E. L., Martin, B. R., & Dewey, W. L. The 9-nor-9-hydroxyhexahydrocannabinols. Synthesis, some behavioral and analgesic properties, and comparison with the tetrahydrocannabinols. J. Med. Chem. In press.

CHAPTER 19

TREATMENT EFFECTS OF DELTA-9-THC IN AN ADVANCED CANCER
POPULATION

Joel R. Butler
Leon A. Peek

North Texas State University
Denton, Texas

William Regelson
Mary M. Moore
Luise A. Lubin

Medical College of Virginia
Virginia Commonwealth University

Descriptions of the typical subjective effects of marihuana usage
abound in both popular and professional publications. For the most part,
these studies utilize sociological and anecdotal approaches (Weil, Zinberg and
Nelson, 1968). However, reports of systematic and objective research
efforts dealing with the effects of ingestion of marihuana or its active
ingredient, tetrahydrocannabinol (THC), on broad psychological cognitive
and physiological processes are almost nonexistent. This lack of relevant
research is attributable to a combination of legal, ethical, social, and
methodological problems.

Cannabis extracts were used in the United States as therapeutic agents
for the relief of pain during the nineteenth century; societal concern over the
drug's intoxicating properties and possible deleterious effects, and the subsequent establishment of severe legal penalties for its use, arose in the 1930's,
a development which served to make research in the area difficult (Task
Force on Narcotics, 1967). With the advances in the synthesis of one of
the active ingredients in marihuana, delta-9-tetrahydrocannabinol, and
increasing societal and medical/experimental use of this drug, it became
important, and more feasible than in the past, to investigate the question of
THC effect on an individual's function.

Prior to the investigation of Weil et al. (1968), there were only
three studies on human subjects performed by Americans in this area. The

313

results of these studies indicated that ingestion of marihuana had some negative effects on intellectual functioning, especially on tasks involving
numerical concepts. However, experienced users were negatively affected
less than non-users (Mayor's Committee on Marihuana, 1944; Williams,
Hienmelsbach, Wikler, Reble and Lloyd, 1946). Also, a decrease in
inhibitions, mild intoxication, hunger, and sleepiness were reported as
effects (Siler, Sheep, Bates, Clark, Cook and Smith, 1933).

Weil et al. (1968) reported that though 8 out of 9 naive subjects did
not report being "high" after smoking marihuana (equivalent to 18 mg of THC)
the group's overall performance on the Digit Symbol Substitution and rotor
pursuit tasks was impaired; experienced users, though reporting a subjective
state of intoxication, actually improved their performance on these tasks
while under the influence of the drug.

Ethical considerations in administering a drug with unknown long-term
effects have, in most cases, been dealt with by using experienced and
informed volunteers. This approach has difficulty in separating the effect of
the drug from the effect of each subject's set (Weil et al., 1968).

Results of research dealing with tolerance to marihuana, another
possible explanation for differences between naive and experienced subject
groups, are contradictory. Results of animal studies concerned with multiple
administration of delta-9-tetrahydrocannabinol have varied from indicating
development of a very marked tolerance to none at all (Carlini, 1968).
Human studies have emphasized the development of "reverse tolerance,"
that is, lower dose of marihuana being necessary to induce a "high" in an
experienced user (Lemberger, Silberstein, Axelrod and Kopin, 1970).

MOTOR PERFORMANCE AND SHORT-TERM MEMORY

Studies conducted to determine the effects of marihuana on memory
have found that the acquisition process was not hindered, and that performance
is not negatively affected, with doses of THC up to 7.5 mg (Abel, 1970,
1971a, 1971b; Caswell and Marks, 1973; Dornbush, Fink and Freedman,
1971; Waskow, Olsson, Solzman and Katz, 1970). Caswell and Marks
(1973) demonstrated that doses of 10 mg or less of THC smoked, and 20 mg or
less THC orally ingested, impair subjects' ability to remember and manipulate
symbols. Using higher doses of THC -- 20 mg, 40 mg, and 60 mg --
Tinklenberg, Melges, Hollister and Gillespie (1970) demonstrated impairment
in subjects' performance on the Digit Span when compared with the placebo
group, an effect which persisted for 3.5 hours. Very few controlled studies
have investigated the effect of THC on human motor performance. Manno,
Kiplinger, Haine, Bennett and Farney (1970) in an oscilloscope pattern
study found greater distractibility and susceptibility to interference from
external stimulation of subjects who have ingested THC.

Personality Variables

Marihuana, <u>Cannabis sativa</u>, has throughout history been a drug used as an agent for achieving euphoria (Harms, 1972). Pharmacologically, marihuana is in a class by itself, being neither a stimulant, tranquilizer, sedative, hallucinogen, nor narcotic, but sharing common properties with all of these (Pillard, 1970). Isbell (1967) suggests that there is a dose related response to THC. At low doses there is a relaxed euphoria; moderate doses, perceptual distortion; and at high doses, psychotomimetic effects.

As with many drugs, but especially so with marihuana, the effects are influenced by the user's character structure, expectation of the experience, previous experience with the drug, environmental (milieu) factors present at the time the drug was ingested, and the amount taken (Bialos, 1970; Jones, 1971).

Stockings (1947) found that marihuana could possibly be used for depressed patients. Kotin, Post and Goodwin (1973) did try THC on hospitalized depressed patients and found that although no global antidepressant effects occurred, there was a report of brief periods of feeling well, relaxation, and giddiness. Heath (1972) implanted electrodes in a depressed subject and found that with ingestion of marihuana, euphoria associated with high-amplitude slow wave activity focal in the septal region developed. Although this idiographic study does not lend itself to generalization, it does suggest that the nuclear sites in the septal region which are affected by marihuana could be the ones previously correlated with the pleasure response. In contrast, impaired activity of this region of the brain is correlated with dysphoria and aberrant emotional expression.

The studies conducted using oral doses of THC have produced mixed results. Using the Clyde Mood Scale, synthetic THC decreased unhappy scores (Melges et al., 1970). Hollister (1968) showed perceptual and psychic changes and indicated pronounced euphoria. McGlothlin (1970) reported on panicky psychotic states, with other subjects reporting a general feeling of euphoria. Doses of 20 to 60 mg THC ingested therefore tended to produce dominant euphoria, with these pleasant feelings tending to create positive reinforcement (Noyes, in press).

Hogan, Manaken, Conway and Gillespie (1970) classified subjects according to marihuana usage. The "user" classifications refer to persons who use drugs as recreational activities. Butler, Reed and Peek (1973) report that most occasional users also have some history of other drugs, drug-lifestyle, or marihuana in these data.

Those reports of clinical experience with marihuana users are based on that subset of users who develop psychiatric illness. Are the findings there reported due to marihuana or to the deviant personality? One study (Butler, Reid and Peek, 1973) reported trends suggesting two types of users: a recreational user and a deviant user. The latter type would probably be the psychiatric case.

Cancer Patients

The importance of psychological make-up (unconscious factors and symbolic meanings) in a person's particular response to his disease has been emphasized throughout the literature. Cancer and its treatment in almost every way constitutes a severe psychological stress for the individual. Often this stress takes the form of a depressive response. Because those who develop cancer appear so often to be tension-bound and starved for gratification and pleasure the use of a psychomotive drug might be of benefit as a means of providing relief from some of the many psychological threats which they face daily (Mastrovito, 1966).

Clinical studies of marihuana and/or its active derivative delta-9-THC have shown this agent to possess euphoriant properties. Current clinical studies of THC have been acute studies of short duration directed primarily to evaluation of euphoriant action. The need for chronic toxicity studies of THC in regard to providing data for the long-term physical and psychological effects of chronic marihuana toxicity is self-evident. The opportunity for some of this information to be obtained is justified by the possible therapeutic usefulness of THC in cancer patients. Preliminary appraisal of the chronic action of this marihuana-related drug should provide data as to the physiologic action of prolonged use of the parent compound while its clinical trial determines the potential medicinal value of this drug for very specific but important clinical objectives.

Analgesic effects for THC have been shown in mice, and appetite-stimulating properties are said to be characteristic in marihuana users (DHEW, 1971). There have been conflicting reports in regard to antiemetic activity. All these reported activities -- "euphoria, analgesia, appetite stimulation, and anti-emetic effects" -- would be of special value in cancer patients because they relate specifically to the problems of this patient population with its depression, related pain problems, anorexia, and disease- or drug-related nausea and vomiting. There has been a need to determine the role of THC in ameliorating symptoms in this population. A recent preliminary study of marihuana in 9 terminal cancer patients suggested that it may have clinical value in cancer for treatment of depression and appetite stimulation (DHEW, 1971).

The purposes of the present study were (1) to test the acute and chronic psychological and physiological correlates of delta-9-tetrahydrocannabinol on a selected population with limited life expectancy to establish dosage and toxicity; and (2) to evaluate the beneficial effects (for example, reverse depressive trends and anxious behavior, and to determine analgesic, anti-emetic, and appetite-stimulating effects) in inpatient cancer patients.

Preliminary Toxicity Study

Prior to the beginning of the main experimental study, an unblinded uncontrolled pilot study was done on 10 inpatient cancer patients. Based on the animal pharmacology and prior research with human subjects, a dosage range of 0. 10 to 0.34 mg/kg, p. o. q. i. d., was selected; the higher end was expected to be the toxic level.

No significant toxic changes were observed in other vital signs or laboratory values (CBC, platelet count, reticulocyte count and differential, urinalysis, and SMA-12) as an effect of THC. Significant side effects were reported with the 7 higher-dosage patients (somnolence, dizziness 2/7, feelings of drunkenness 2/7, nausea 1/7, headache 1/7). On the basis of this a dose of 0. 10 mg/kg, t. i. d., was determined to be acceptable for outpatient study.

METHOD

Subjects

The 54 subjects for this study were drawn from the Tumor and Radiation Therapy Clinics, Medical College of Virginia, Virginia Commonwealth University, private and service. All subjects had biopsy-proven cancer, for which there was no hope of cure by available modalities. The subjects were receiving chemotherapy and radiotherapy for this primary disorder. Patients having either primary or metastatic tumor activity in the CNS or those with severe deficiencies in gastric or renal function were excluded from study.

Drug

Delta-9-THC was supplied by the National Institute of Mental Health as 5 mg capsules. The THC was suspended in sesame oil and stored in a locked refrigerator in the hospital pharmacy. Comparable sesame oil placebo was also supplied and similarly stored.

Dosage was computed according to subjects' weight and the fixed 5 mg capsules. Dosage per kilogram body weight per day ranged from 0.30 to 0. 15 mg administered t. i. d. All patients were initially started on the 0.30 mg/kg, t. i. d., dosage. In those subjects showing significant untoward side effects an attempt to retain them in the study by halving their dosage was made. None of these attempts were successful.

Psychological Measures

The following psychological tests were routinely administered prior to study and at the end of each treatment condition: the Bender Gestalt test, the Eysenck Personality Inventory (EPI), the Zung Self-Rating Depression Scale (Zung or SDS), a depressive index (Mult) derived from the Minnesota Multiphasic Personality Inventory (MMPI), and form E of Cattell's Sixteen Personality Factor Inventory (16PF).

The Bender was objectively scored by the Butler method (1966) and provided a numeric score. The EPI provides scores on extroversion (EPI-E), neuroticism (EPI-N), and lie (EPI-L); forms A and B were alternately administered to each subject. The 16PH provides 16 scores; Table 1 gives the meanings of high and low values for each score.

The Zung was scored according to standard directions (Zung-Standard) as well as by two additional formats. The first format, Zung-Regular score, involved summing the raw scores from those items in which the subject had to affirm depressive symptoms, for instance, "I feel downhearted and blue." The other format, Zung-Reverse score, involved summing the raw scores for those items in which the subject had to deny the socially acceptable positive statement, for instance, "I feel hopeful about the future."

The Mult consisted of those items from the MMPI keyed on the L, F, K, or D scales. Further, these items were keyed over the Harris subscales for depression (D1 to D5; Harris and Lingoes, 1955).

Procedure

Clinic physicians referred subjects to the study group. The advised consent of the subject was obtained and the test battery was then administered, the prescription written for MCV 73A, and the subject was randomly assigned by the clinical pharmacist to be available for entry in the pre-randomized Latin squares used to balance position effect. Physicians, psychologists, examiners, and subjects were all blind as to whether a given subject was receiving drug or placebo during a given week.

The subjects were dispensed a week's supply of either delta-9-THC or placebo, and an appointment was made for them to return in one week. The subjects were re-administered the test battery, and the other treatment administered. At the end of the second week, the third battery administration was accomplished.

Those subjects whose performance status and reading ability permitted wrote their responses to the test battery. Other subjects had the battery orally administered to them.

Procedure: WAIS

Ten of the 54 subjects were, in addition to the standard test battery, administered modifications of the Wechsler Adult Intelligence Scale (WAIS) (Wechsler, 1958) at the end of the first and second treatment weeks.

At the end of the first week of treatment the odd-numbered items from the Information (I), Comprehension (C), Similarities (S), and Vocabulary (V) subtests were administered using standard instructions (discontinuation criteria were halved). The complete Digit Span (D) and Digit Symbol (DS)

Table 1

Meaning of 16PF Scores

Scale	Low Score (0)	High Score (10)
A	Reserved, Detached, Critical, Aloof, Stiff (Sizothymia)	Outgoing, Warmhearted, Easygoing, Participating (Affectothymia)
B	Less Intelligent, Concrete-thinking (Lower scholastic mental capacity)	More Intelligent, Abstract-thinking, Bright (Higher scholastic mental capacity)
C	Affected by feelings, Emotionally Less Stable, Easily Upset, Changeable (Lower ego strength)	Emotionally Stable, Mature, Faces Reality, Calm (Higher ego strength)
E	Humble, Mild, Easily Led, Docile, Accommodating (Submissiveness)	Assertive, Aggressive, Stubborn, Competitive (Dominance)
F	Sober, Taciturn, Serious (Desurgency)	Happy-go-lucky, Enthusiastic (Surgency)
G	Expedient, Disregards Rules (Weaker superego strength)	Conscientious, Persistent, Moralistic, Staid (Stronger superego strength)
H	Shy, Timid, Threat-sensitive (Threctia)	Venturesome, Uninhibited, Socially Bold (Parmia)
I	Tough-minded, Self-reliant, Realistic (Harria)	Tender Minded, Sensitive Clinging, Overprotected (Premsia)
L	Trusting, Accepting Conditions (Aloxia)	Suspicious, Hard-to-fool (Protension)
M	Practical, "Down-to-earth" Concerns (Proxemia)	Imaginative, Bohemian, Absent-minded (Autia)
N	Forthright, Unpretentious, Genuine but Socially Clumsy (Artlessness)	Astute, Polished, Socially Aware (Shrewdness)
O	Self-assured, Placid, Secure, Complacent, Serene (Untroubled adequacy)	Apprehensive, Self-reproaching, Insecure, Worrying, Troubled (Guilt proneness)
Q1	Conservative, Respecting Traditional Ideas (Conservatism of temperament)	Experimenting, Liberal, Free-thinking (Radicalism)
Q2	Group-dependent, a "Joiner" and Sound Follower (Group adherence)	Self-sufficient, Resourceful, Prefers Own Decisions (Self-sufficiency)
Q3	Undisciplined Self-conflict, Lax, Follows Own Urges, Careless of Social Rules (Low integration)	Controlled, Exacting Will Power, Socially Precise, Compulsive (High strength of self-sentiment)
Q4	Relaxed, Tranquil, Unfrustrated, Composed (Low ergic tension)	Tense, Frustrated, Driven, Overwrought (High ergic tension)

subtests were administered. Two of the four remaining performance subtests --
Picture Completion (PC), Block Design (BD), Picture Arrangement (PA), and
Object Assembly (OA) -- were administered on a predetermined random basis
so that each subtest had equal probability of being administered in the first
testing.

At the end of the second week of treatment the even-numbered items
of I, C, S, and V, the complete D and DS, and the other two then unadmin-
istered performance subtests were administered.

The raw scores on I, C, S, and V were doubled for each administration
and the Verbal IQ (VIQ) was calculated on these scores and the raw score
for Digit Span. The performance IQ (PIQ) score was prorated on the 3 of 5
subtests administered. The raw scores for digits forward, backward, and the
difference between them (F-B) were also retained for analysis.

Procedure: Clinical Observations

Clinical physicians as a part of their routine examination of the
subjects recorded observations of side effects -- weight, pain, and nausea
and vomiting. The recorded side effects had decreased probability of being
attributed to other medications.

The weight of 16 out of the 54 subjects was recorded upon entry into
the study and at the end of each treatment week.

For pain (N-27) and nausea and vomiting (N-22) the physicians gave
their subjective rating based upon their observations and the report of the
subject. Pain was rated on a seven-point scale; vomiting and nausea on a
three-point scale.

RESULTS

Table 2 summarizes the results of the psychological tests. The
comparisons of the means was accomplished with the use of analysis of
variance. Those scores showing drug effects and meeting or exceeding the
5% criterion are highlighted in the table.

The significant findings of interest to this report are those for the
16PF-I, 16PF-N, 16PF-Q3, and 16PF-Q4. The subjects showed significant
movement approaching the description of being more relaxed, tranquil, and
unfrustrated. The other scores for delta-9-THC subjects reflected movement
towards the standardization means, that is, away from being tender-minded,
clinging, over-protected, and sensitive; away from being shrewd, calculating,
worldly, and penetrating; and away from being controlled, socially precise,
and following self-image.

Table 2

Descriptive Statistics for Dependent Variables

Score	N Subjects	All Observations				Mean Placebo	Mean Drug	p of different med
		Mean	SD	Minimum	Maximum			
Bender	17	24.09	7.64	5	35	23.38	24.76	0.574
EPI-E	22	11.27	4.09	4	18	11.65	10.86	0.640
EPI-N	22	10.07	5.07	0	20	10.74	9.33	0.056
EPI-L	22	3.39	2.40	0	8	3.17	3.62	0.223
Zung-Standard	22	53.07	12.35	28	86	55.14	51.00	0.040*
Zung-Regular	22	19.16	6.49	10	40	20.95	17.36	0.050*
Zung-Reverse	22	23.61	6.56	10	39	23.91	23.32	0.683
Mult-L	22	5.32	2.61	0	10	4.95	5.68	0.135
Mult-F	22	8.07	6.71	1	32	8.23	7.91	0.550
Mult-K	22	13.89	4.20	6	21	14.45	13.32	0.273
Mult-D	22	27.23	7.33	11	43	27.41	27.04	0.791
Mult-D1	22	12.50	5.80	4	29	12.50	12.50	1.000
Mult-D2	22	7.16	2.60	2	13	7.14	7.18	0.912
Mult-D3	22	6.39	2.00	3	9	6.68	6.09	0.192
Mult-D4	22	5.50	3.36	1	15	5.32	5.68	0.539
Mult-D5	22	3.64	2.34	1	10	3.73	3.54	0.696
16PF-A	23	6.50	3.12	0	10	7.09	5.91	0.120
16PF-B	23	6.46	2.95	0	10	7.04	5.87	0.090
16PF-C	23	5.91	2.72	0	10	6.04	5.78	0.711
16PF-E	23	5.74	2.30	0	10	6.22	5.26	0.081
16PF-F	23	4.72	2.20	0	10	5.00	4.43	0.172
16PF-G	23	5.80	2.96	0	10	6.26	5.35	0.293
16PF-H	23	5.15	2.50	0	10	5.52	4.78	0.192
16PF-I	23	6.54	2.88	0	10	7.74	5.35	0.001*
16PF-L	23	5.15	2.14	0	10	5.61	4.70	0.154
16PF-M	23	6.70	2.88	0	10	7.43	5.96	0.085
16PF-N	23	6.65	2.73	0	10	7.61	5.70	0.006*
16PF-O	23	4.50	2.50	0	10	5.00	4.00	0.065
16PF-Q1	23	6.09	3.10	0	10	6.22	5.96	0.726
16PF-Q2	23	6.54	2.83	0	10	7.04	6.04	0.167
16PF-Q3	23	6.70	2.77	0	10	7.48	5.91	0.025*
16PF-Q4	23	4.30	2.33	0	10	5.00	3.61	0.008*

* These meet or exceed the 5% criterion.

The Zung-Standard and Zung-Regular scores showed a significant reduction in depression under THC. The Zung-Reverse failed to show much change. None of the MMPI adaptations showed any significant differences, although their movement was in the expected direction.

No significant differences were found for any of the WAIS scores. Table 3 contains the descriptive statistics for these scores.

Side Effects

Three patients each from the medication and placebo group were dropped due to distressing side effects of the "drug." Others discontinued for a variety of other reasons including death from cancer.

Table 3

Descriptive Statistics for Dependent Variables

Variable	Number Obs.	Mean	SD	Low	High
FSIQ	20	109.5	10.7	95.0	128.0
VIQ	20	116.9	13.7	100.0	143.0
PIQ	20	99.9	10.5	79.0	116.0
INFO	20	11.1	1.8	8.0	16.0
COMP	20	14.4	3.4	8.0	19.0
ARITH	20	11.0	2.8	7.0	17.0
SIM	20	9.8	3.0	3.0	15.0
DSPN	20	10.1	3.4	6.0	19.0
VOCAB	20	14.1	3.5	9.0	19.0
DSYM	20	6.3	2.6	2.0	12.0
DIGFWD	20	6.4	1.1	5.0	9.0
DIGBACK	20	4.6	1.4	3.0	8.0
DIGDIFF	20	1.7	0.9	0.0	4.0

Weight

Sixteen out of 54 patients were suitable for weight-change evaluation, that is, having no third space fluid accumulations and having recorded weight measurements for all three study periods including a baseline period and two following study weeks.

Looking at the total weight change for the entire group during the drug week, the group gained a total of 1 3/4 lb. During placebo week the same group lost a total of 21 1/4 lbs. During medication week 10 patients gained as a group a total of 21 lbs. while during placebo week only 3 patients gained a total of 4 lbs., the remaining lost weight or showed no change. This was statistically significant, p being less than .05 ($x^2 = 4.66$, p is less than 0.4).

Analyzing for position effect, we were unable to demonstrate that the position of medication vs. placebo made any difference in weight change ($x^2 = 0.02$, p is approximately equal to .85). A graphic representation of these data is presented in Figure 1.

Pain

Data for pain were available on 27 patients. In the drug group there was no change in 13 patients and 14 patients improved a total of 18 points. During the placebo week, 18 showed no change and 9 improved a total of 10 points. Worsening was not demonstrable in either case. The differences found were not statistically significant ($x^2 = 1.21$, df = 1, p is approximately equal to .25). However, 7 of the 9 patients who improved during placebo week were from the medication-first group and this position effect during placebo week for pain was significant ($x^2 = 4.22$, df = 1, p is less than .04).

Nausea and Vomiting

Data was available on 22 patients for evaluation of nausea and vomiting. In the drug period, there was no change in 12, and 2 were worse. During placebo week there was no change in 18: 1 grew worse 1 unit and 3 improved a total of 5 units. This was not statistically significant ($x^2 = 3.82$, df = 2, p is approximately equal to .22). However here again, the 3 patients who improved on placebo were all from the medication-first group and this position effect was statistically significant ($x^2 = 8.60$, df = 2, p is equal to .015).

DISCUSSION

The results, including both significant findings and trends, suggest that delta-9-THC, when administered as a "general tonic" to medically ill patients and within the context of their specific medical treatments (cancer

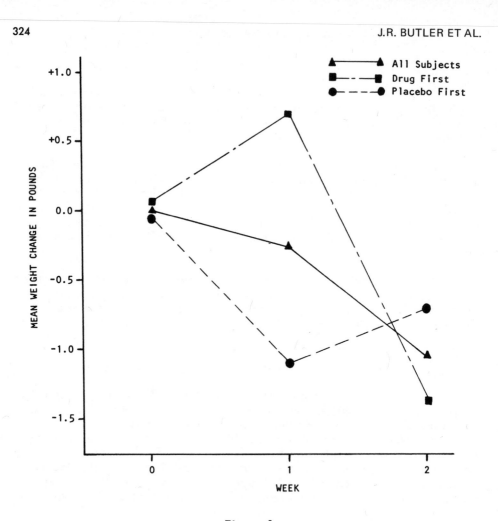

Figure 1.

chemotherapy), acts as both a mild tranquilizer and euphoriant. This conclusion is supported by prior results of the subjective effects of marihuana and
related compounds in other populations (Schwarz, 1969). Suspiciousness, as
reported elsewhere (Allentuck and Bowman, 1942; Ames, 1958), was not
observed in these data; in contrast, 16PF-L moved in a non-significant
($p = 0.154$) manner away from the description of suspicious, self-opinionated,
and hard-to-fool which characterizes prior reports. These differences in
characterization of those on delta-9-THC could be due either to the indication of suspiciousness arising from the illegal nature of recreational use in
prior studies in a non-cancer "user" population or to the masking of any
changes in suspiciousness because of the supportive experimental situation
itself which takes place in an environment of medical positivity where the
program is endorsed as having therapeutic benefit.

Emotional instability, as measured by the EPI-N scale, not only failed to rise under delta-9-THC but fell to a degree approaching significance (p = 0.056), thus indicating greater emotional stability. Additionally there was a nonsignificant reduction in the Mult F and K scales. This seems to support the position that the reported cases of marihuana-induced psychosis may have occurred in psychotics who used marihuana (Bialos, 1970).

The lack of change in the WAIS scores was interesting in light of the frequent use of marihuana as a recreational drug among college students. There was clearly no indication of cognitive impairment associated with THC usage. Scores were consistent between test administration in both the verbal and performance areas. Because of the design no practice effect could be assumed nor was any guesswork necessary about the reliability of the measures. There was no change in the person's ability to abstract, conceptualize, determine part-whole relationship, use formulas, concentrate, attend to detail, understand antecedent consequent behavior, or recall previously learned material. No impairment was noted in perceptual or learning processes. Only one minor change was noted and that was an improvement in scores (during THC use) on Digit Span backwards, suggesting improved ability to attend.

There was a definite tendency to maintain weight in cancer patients treated with delta-9-THC. Weight gain was demonstrated in more than half the medicated group. This result in a randomized population of advanced patients who generally lose weight indicates that the results may take on different meaning, perhaps representing a combined effect of drug-induced psychological improvement, diminished pain and nausea, possibly even specific effects on the elusive mechanisms producing cachexia in cancer, and that the results may be interpreted as further evidence that THC has appetite-stimulating properties, as has been demonstrated by Hollister (1970) in normal volunteers.

Delta-9-THC has been proposed as a non-addicting analgesic in man. Marihuana smoking in man has also been reported to decrease the incidence of radiation sickness (Clarkson, n.d). The results obtained in this study did not provide definitive information. In this record, 7 out of 9 patients showed decreased pain on placebo. Three showed decreased nausea and vomiting on placebo but these patients had received active medication as the first treatment week and these results might well be interpreted as a carry-over effect from medication week into placebo week. This could be due to either a saturation effect or a persistent action of the drug well into the second week.

In general, the results of this study provide limited evidence that delta-9-THC has a beneficial effect on the symptoms of depression, pain, nausea, and vomiting, and show an attenuation of the cachexia in cancer patients.

REFERENCES

Abel, E.L. Marihuana and memory. <u>Nature</u>, 1970, <u>227</u>, 1151–1152.

Abel, E.L. Marihuana and memory: Acquisition or retrieval? <u>Science</u>, 1971, <u>173</u>, 1038–1040. (a)

Abel, E.L. Retrieval of information after the use of marihuana. <u>Nature</u>, 1971, <u>231</u>, 58. (b)

Allentuck, S., & Bowman, K.M. The psychiatric aspects of marihuana intoxication. <u>American Journal of Psychiatry</u>, 1942, <u>99</u>, 248–251.

Ames, F. A clinical and metabolic study of acute intoxication with cannabis sativa and its role in the model psychoses. <u>Journal of Mental Sciences</u>, 1958, <u>104</u>, 972–999.

Bialos, D. Adverse marihuana reactions: A critical examination of the literature with selected case material. <u>American Journal of Psychiatry</u>, 1970, <u>127</u>, 819–823.

Butler, J.R., Reid, B.E., & Peek, L.A. Life history antecedents in the college drug population. <u>Proceedings of the Annual Convention of the American Psychological Association</u>, 1973.

Carlini, E.A. Tolerance to chronic administration of cannabis sativa (marihuana) in rats. <u>Pharmacology</u>, 1968, <u>1</u>, 135–142.

Caswell, A., & Marks, D.F. Cannabis and temporal disintegration in experienced and naive subjects. <u>Science</u>, 1973, <u>179</u>, 803–805.

Clarkson, B. Personal communication. New York, Memorial Center for Cancer and Allied Diseases, n.d.

Department of Health Education and Welfare (DHEW). <u>Marihuana and health: A report to Congress</u>. Chevy Chase, Md.: Department of Health Education and Welfare, 1971.

Dornbush, R.L., Fink, M., & Freedman, A.M. Marihuana, memory and perception. <u>American Journal of Psychiatry</u>, 1971, <u>128</u>, 194.

Harms, E. The heroin-marihuana relationship: A basic aspect of drug management. <u>British Journal of Addiction</u>, 1972, <u>67</u>, 287–290.

Harris, R.E., & Lingoes, J.E. Subscales for the MMPI: An aid to profile interpretation. Mimeographed materials, Department of Psychiatry, University of California, Berkeley, 1955.

Heath, R. Marihuana. <u>Archives of General Psychiatry</u>, 1972, <u>26</u>, 577–584.

Hogan, R., Manaken, P., Conway, J., & Gillespie, H.K. Personality
    correlates of undergraduate marihuana use. Journal of Consulting and
    Clinical Psychology, 1970, 35, 58-63.

Hollister, L.E. Hunger and appetite after single doses of marihuana, ethanol,
    and dextroamphetamine. Clinical Pharmacology and Therapeutics, 1970.

Hollister, L.E., Richards, R.K., & Gillespie, H.K. Comparison of tetra-
    hydrocannabinol and synhexyl in man. Clinical Pharmacology and
    Therapeutics, 1968, 9, 783-791.

Isbell, H., Gorodetzsky, C., Jasenski, D., Claussen, U., Spulak, F., &
    Korte, R. Effects of delta 9 transhydrocannabinol in man.
    Psychopharmacologia, 1967, 11, 184-188.

Jones, R. Marihuana induced "high": Influence of expectation, setting and
    previous drug experience. Pharmacological Reviews, 1971, 23, 359-
    369.

Kotin, J., Post, R., & Goodwin, R. Delta 9-Tetrahydrocannabinol in
    depressed patients. Archives of General Psychiatry, 1973, 28,
    345-348.

Lemberger, L., Silberstein, S.D., Axelrod, J., & Kopin, I. J. Marihuana:
    Studies on the disposition and metabolism of delta 9-Tetrahydro-
    cannabinol in man. Science, 1970, 170, 1320-1322.

Mastrovito, R. Acute psychiatric problems and the use of psychotropic
    medications in the treatment of the cancer patient. Annals of the
    New York Academy of Sciences, 1966, 125, 1006-1010.

Manno, J.E., Kiplinger, G.F., Haine, S.E., Bennett, I.F., & Farney,
    R.B. Comparative effects of smoking marihuana or placebo on human
    motor and mental performance. Clinical Pharmacology and Therapy,
    1970, 11, 808-815.

Mayor's Committee on Marihuana. The marihuana problem in the City of
    New York. Lancaster, Pa.: Jacques Cattell Press, 1944.

McGlothlin, W.H., Arnold, D.O., & Rowan, P. K. Marihuana use among
    adults. Psychiatry, 1970, 33, 433-443.

Melges, P., Tinklenberg, J., Hollister, L., Gillespie, H. Temporal
    disintegration and depersonalization during marihuana intoxication.
    Archives of General Psychiatry, 1970, 23, 204-210.

Noyes, A.J. Cannabis analgesia. In press.

Pillard, R. Marihuana. New England Journal of Medicine, 1970, 283,
    294-303.

Schwarz, C.J. Toward a medical understanding of marihuana. Canadian Psychiatric Association Journal, 1969, 14, 591-600.

Siler, J.F., Sheep, W.L., Bates, L.B., Clark, G.F., Cook, G.W., & Smith, W.A. Marihuana smoking in Panama. The Military Surgeon, 1933, 269-280.

Stockings, G., & Tayleur, A. A new euphoriant for depressive mental states. British Medical Journal, 1947, 1, 918-922.

Task Force on Narcotics and Drug Abuse. Task Force Report: Narcotics and Drug Abuse. Washington: Government Printing Office, 1967.

Tinklenberg, J.R., Melges, F.T., Hollister, L.E., & Gillespie, H.K. Marihuana and immediate memory. Nature, 1970, 226, 1171-1172.

Waskow, I.E., Olsson, J.E., Solzmon, C., & Katz, M.M. Psychological effects of Tetrahydrocannabiol. Archives of General Psychiatry, 1970, 22, 97-107.

Weil, A.T., Zinberg, N.E., & Nelson, J.M. Clinical and psychological effects of marihuana in man. Science, 1968, 162, 1234-1242.

Williams, E.G., Hienmelsbach, C.K., Wikler, A., Reble, D.C., & Lloyd, B.J., Jr. Studies on marihuana and parahexyl compound. Public Health Reports, 1946, 61, 1059-1083.

CHAPTER 20

ANTIEMETIC EFFECT OF DELTA-9-TETRAHYDROCANNABINOL IN PATIENTS RECEIVING CANCER CHEMOTHERAPY

Stephen E. Sallan
Norman E. Zinberg
Emil Frei, III

Sidney Farber Cancer Center
Peter Bent Brigham Hospital
Harvard Medical School
Boston, Massachusetts

NOTE: This work was supported in part by a Cancer Center Support Grant Comprehensive (2PO2CA06516-12). It is here reprinted with permission from The New England Journal of Medicine, October 16, 1975, 293, 16, 795-797. We are indebted to Drs. Lester Grinspoon and Yvonne Bishop for assistance in this investigation.

ABSTRACT

Anecdotal accounts suggested that smoking marihuana decreases the nausea and vomiting associated with cancer chemotherapeutic agents. Oral delta-9-tetrahydrocannabinol was compared with placebo in a controlled, randomized, "double-blind" experiment. All patients were receiving chemotherapeutic drugs known to cause nausea and vomiting of central origin. Each patient was to serve as his own control to determine whether tetrahydrocannabinol had an antiemetic effect. Twenty-two patients entered the study, 20 of whom were evaluable. For all patients an antiemetic effect was observed in 14 of 20 tetrahydrocannabinol courses and in none of 22 placebo courses. For patients completing the study, response occurred in 12 of 15 courses of tetrahydrocannabinol and in none of 14 courses of placebo ($P < 0.001$). No patient vomited while experiencing a subjective "high." Oral tetrahydrocannabinol has antiemetic properties and is significantly better than a placebo in reducing vomiting caused by chemotherapeutic agents.

Nausea and vomiting of central origin occur after the administration of a variety of cancer chemotherapeutic agents and frequently constitute the major morbidity associated with such treatment. Control with classic anti-emetics is incomplete and variable.

Anecdotal accounts from patients suggested that smoking marihuana before receiving intravenous anti-tumor drugs resulted in diminution of nausea and vomiting, and, in contradistinction to the usual post-therapeutic anorexia, some were able to take food shortly after therapy. Effects of marihuana on nausea and vomiting in human beings deserve to be reported. It has been demonstrated that oral delta-9-tetrahydrocannabinol (THC) causes the same physiologic effects as smoking marihuana (Isbell, Gorodetzky and colleagues, 1967; Perez-Reyes, Lipton, Timmons and colleagues, 1973).

The purpose of this study was to determine the effects of orally administered THC on nausea and vomiting in patients receiving cancer chemotherapy.

PATIENTS, MATERIALS, AND METHODS

Twenty-two patients known to have a variety of neoplasms were enrolled in the study. Ten males and 12 females ranging in age from 18 to 76 years (median of 29.5) participated. Twenty patients had previously received cancer chemotherapeutic agents known to cause nausea and vomiting (adriamycin, 5-axacytidine, nitrogen mustard, imidazole carboxa-mide, procarbazine, high-dose cyclophosphamide or high-dose methotrexate, or combinations thereof). Twenty of the 22 were known to be refractory to conventional antiemetics. The other two patients had never been treated with chemotherapy before entering the study. Pregnant women and patients with a past history of emotional instability or untoward reactions to psycho-active drugs were not eligible.

The study was thoroughly explained to the patients. They were told that they would receive a placebo or a "marihuana-like drug for the purpose of controlling nausea and vomiting." Subjects agreed not to smoke marihuana during the course of the study.

THC was supplied by the National Institute on Drug Abuse. The drug was suspended in 0.12 ml of sesame oil and supplied in gelatin capsules. Identical-appearing placebo capsules contained only sesame oil. Initially, THC dosage was 15 mg given every four hours for three doses. Because of some variability in responses, the dose was changed to 10 mg per square meter body-surface area per dose. Nineteen patients received 15-mg doses, and three 20-mg doses.

A randomized, "double-blind," crossover experiment was employed, each patient being used as his own control. Optimally, patients received three one-day courses of drug (either THC or placebo). Each course consisted of three doses of drug, the first taken two hours before and the other two and six hours after chemotherapy. Patients were randomized to receive courses in one of four sequences: THC-placebo-THC; THC-placebo-placebo; placebo-THC-placebo; or placebo-THC-THC.

Nausea, vomiting, and food intake were assessed by the patient on the day after treatment through the use of self-administered questionnaires.* In addition, the patient, nurses, and other personnel in contact with the patient were interviewed by one of us (S.E.S), who also reviewed the questionnaires and nurses' notes.

RESULTS

Definitions of responses are based upon a comparison of THC and placebo courses.

Complete response to THC means that there was no vomiting in patients for whom the same antitumor drugs caused unequivocal moderate to severe vomiting after placebo. Conversely, a complete response to placebo theoretically is possible, but never occurred.

Partial response to THC means there was at least a 50% reduction in vomiting as compared to placebo after the same chemotherapy. Included in this group are the patients whose vomiting, which occurred shortly after chemotherapy during a placebo course, was delayed until escape from control of THC. These patients attained a "high" that wore off before the next dose, or after the last dose of THC, and during this time vomiting "broke through." A partial response to placebo is also a theoretical possibility but never occurred.

No response to the THC means that there was either no decrease or less than a 50% reduction in vomiting as compared with placebo after the same antitumor drugs. No response to placebo means that the patients vomited after chemotherapy as often or more often than after THC.

Absence of vomiting after both THC and placebo makes the response unevaluable because there was neither demonstrable emetic effect of chemo-therapy nor antiemetic effect of THC or placebo. One patient who had no prior chemotherapy before entering the study was excluded from analysis for this reason.

Eleven patients completed three courses of treatment, two completed two courses, and nine completed one course.

One of the 11 never vomited and was excluded from evaluation as noted above. The remaining 10 patients received 30 courses of drug, but a

---

* Questionnaire available on request.

single course was excluded from analysis because the dose of cancer chemotherapeutic agent was reduced by 50%. Therefore, 29 courses were
evaluated: 14 placebo and 15 THC. All courses of placebo resulted in no
response. Of the THC courses, there were five complete responses, seven
partial responses, and three no responses. The therapeutic response derived
from the THC was independent of the sequence of THC or placebo courses
administered. Accepting complete and partial responses as positive responses,
the difference between THC and placebo is highly significant (chi-square with
Yates's correction $P < 0.001$).

Of the two patients who completed two courses in the study, one died
of disease, and the other decided to smoke marihuana, thus becoming
ineligible to continue. Both these patients had no response after placebo;
after THC, both had partial responses.

Nine patients received one course of treatment. Six had placebo
only, and five of them vomited after chemotherapy. The patient who did not
vomit after placebo had no prior chemotherapy. His response to placebo,
therefore, is unevaluable because of the impossibility of differentiating an
antiemetic effect of placebo from the emetic effect of chemotherapy. Of the
six, two voluntarily withdrew from the study because they did not want to
risk another placebo course, one had chemotherapy discontinued, one died
of disease, and two are still in the study. Three had THC only. Of these,
two vomited and left the study, and the third went off study because of THC
toxicity.

In summary, 20 courses of THC were administered, resulting in five
complete responses, nine partial responses, three no responses, and three
unevaluable responses. Twenty-two courses of placebo resulted in no complete
responses, no partial responses, 16 no responses, and six unevaluable responses.

Side Effects

Of 16 patients receiving THC, 13 (81%) experienced a "high." This
effect was characterized by mood changes, which varied and consisted of one
or more of the following: easy laughing; elation; heightened awareness;
mild aberrations of fine motor co-ordination; and minimal distortion of their
activities and interactions with others. There were no hangovers or delayed
effects.

The next most common side effect was somnolence. For one third of
the patients, somnolence curtailed activities for two to six hours, but the
patients were easily aroused. Another third had somnolence which did not
curtail activities; the remainder experienced no somnolence.

Toxicity characterized by paranoid ideation, apprehension, fear,
panic, and frightening visual hallucinations has been reported after single
THC doses of 35 mg (Perez-Reyes, Lipton, Timmons and colleagues, 1973).
Only two of our patients (9%) experienced THC toxicity, both after three

doses of 20 mg. One had visual distortions lasting for a few seconds, and the other reported visual hallucinations of 10 minutes' duration and depression of several hours.

DISCUSSION

The results of this placebo-controlled "double-blind" study demonstrate that THC has antiemetic effects.

The study was designed to compare THC with placebo. It was not designed to evaluate placebo effect. No comparisons were made between placebo and absence of placebo, or between placebo and retrospective emesis control. If a placebo effect exists in this clinical and investigative setting, THC cannot be evaluated.

No patient vomited while experiencing a subjective "high." No "highs" were reported after placebo. In some patients, the "high" wore off before the next THC dose, and during this interval, nausea and vomiting frequently occurred. After this study, patients taking THC received their next dose as soon as the "high" began wearing off. Preliminary results indicate that this dose-scheduling adjustment sustains the antiemetic effect of THC.

Variability in gastrointestinal absorption of orally administered THC between, but not within, individual subjects has been reported (Perez-Reyes et al., 1973). Three of our patients (19%) reported the absence of a "high" after THC. The lack of THC effect ("high" and antiemesis) in at least some patients may be related to failure of absorption. Some patients who did not attain a "high" after the initial dose were able to do so with subsequent doses. This effect may be analogous to the experience of Weil, Zinberg, and Nelson (1968) with smoked marihuana: failure to respond to an initial dose of marihuana, and then response to subsequent doses. This phenomenon may also be related to induction of hepatic microsomal enzymes necessary for drug metabolism as suggested by Lemberger, Tamarkin, Axelrod and associates (1971).

Patients became "high" 20 to 60 minutes after ingestion of drug. The duration of the "high" varied from one to five hours, but was usually two to three hours, suggesting that the rigid four-hourly schedule between doses was probably too long for some patients, and possibly explaining some partial responses. When dosage was based on body-surface area, less variability in onset and duration of effects was noted.

Time of onset, duration of effect, and intensity of "high" were unrelated to previous marihuana use. Six patients admitted prior use of marihuana, but only one was considered more than an occasional user (defined here as smoking less than once a week).

It has been demonstrated that orally administered THC results in the same physiologic effects as inhaled marihuana (Isbell et al., 1967; Perez-Reyes et al., 1973). The previous studies showing inhaled marihuana to be more potent than oral THC (Isbell et al., 1967) were probably in error because the THC was delivered in poorly absorbed vehicles (Perez-Reyes et al., 1973). Inhalation appears to be more suitable for patients with suboptimal gastrointestinal absorption.

Hollister (1970) has shown that the effects of smoked THC clearly resemble those of marihuana. We have made preliminary observations comparing the antiemetic effect of smoked marihuana and oral THC. The marihuana belonged to individual patients and, therefore, was neither qualitatively nor quantitatively controlled. For most patients, both smoked and oral routes had identical effects. Theoretically, smoking might be the preferable route since it may result in less variability of absorption than the gastrointestinal route. Moreover, smoking provides greater opportunity for individual patient control by permitting the patient to regulate and maintain the "high."

THC has been reported to have a biphasic clinical effect, with initial stimulation and elation followed by sleepiness and tranquility (Hollister, 1974). With other antiemetics, such as the phenothiazine derivatives, sedative effect seems to parallel antiemetic effect (Moertel and Reitemeier, 1969). Although somnolence occurred in about two thirds of our patients, in the dosage used, THC prevented or reduced vomiting in most patients without appreciable curtailment of activities.

Appetite stimulation follows the smoking of marihuana (Hollister, 1971). Four of our patients reported food intake "more than usual" after chemotherapy when taking THC. No patient reported this effect after placebo.

These data demonstrate that THC is an effective antiemetic for patients receiving cancer chemotherapy. Failure of response in 19% of patients receiving THC perhaps is explicable on the basis of pharmacologic factors. THC can be used safely in the dosage of 10 mg per square meter per dose every four hours for at least three doses. Lack of effectiveness for some patients might be correctable by shortening the interval between doses to maintain a "high." The safety of such a dose-schedule adjustment is still to be determined.

REFERENCES

Hollister, L.E. Tetrahydrocannabinol isomers and homologues: contrasted effects of smoking. Nature, 1970, 227, 968-969.

Hollister, L.E. Structure-activity relationships in man of cannabis constituents, and homologs and metabolites of delta-9-tetrahydrocannabinol. Pharmacology, 1974, 11, 3-11.

Hollister, L.E. Hunger and appetite after single doses of marihuana, alcohol, and dextroamphetamine. Clin. Pharmacol. Ther., 1971, 12, 44-49.

Isbell, H., Gorodetzsky, C.W., Jasinski, D., et al. Effects of (-)delta-9-tetrahydrocannabinol in man. Psychopharmacologia, 1967, 11, 184-188.

Lemberger, L., Tamarkin, N.R., Axelrod, J., et al. Delta-9-tetrahydrocannabinol: metabolism and disposition in long-term marihuana smokers. Science, 1971, 173, 72-74.

Moertel, C.G., Reitemeier, R.J. Controlled clinical studies of orally administered antiemetic drugs. Gastroenterology, 1969, 57, 262-268.

Perez-Reyes, M., Lipton, M.A., Timmons, M.C., et al. Pharmacology of orally administered delta-9-tetrahydrocannabinol. Clin Pharmacol. Ther., 1973, 14, 48-55.

Weil, A.T., Zinberg, N.E., Nelsen, J.M. Clinical and psychological effects of marihuana in man. Science, 1968, 162, 1234-1242.

DISCUSSION

Lemberger: Dr. Sallan, you mentioned that the THC was given every 4 hours and you said they didn't have a high after the initial dose. Did you mean the initial series?

Sallan: There were some people who didn't have a high after their initial dose, actually after three doses on a given day, who were able to become high on their second day of treatment -- frequently a week to a month later.

Neu: I would like to ask Dr. Butler if you had a baseline check into side effects with patients before you administered the THC.

Butler: Yes, as a matter of fact, we observed all the inpatients for a period of a week prior to the beginning of the sedatives.

Burstein: I would like to ask Dr. Harris how he thinks THC might possibly interact with chemotherapy that Dr. Sallan's patients are receiving, in view of his results.

Harris: THC, at least in our hands, doesn't induce microsomal enzymes, but other cancer chemotherapy agents might be inducing the enzymes which alter the metabolism of THC. In addition to that, we have started, as you might expect, to put together combinations, which is exactly what is happening in the clinic these days. I don't think that anyone is getting a single antitumor agent any more. We do see some very strong interaction; in other words, we can get by with less of the standard cancer chemotherapy agent in the presence of THC. One thing about the analgesia. There were four attempts, to my knowledge, to do at least a reasonably con- trolled study of delta-9-THC in pain. The results are: one study reporting relatively good analgesic activity, two studies that you heard about during this conference -- the one in dental pain in North Carolina and the cancer pain from Richmond -- and a fourth study. The scores so far are one analgesia, one no effect, and two hyper-algesia. Putting that together, my guess is that delta-9-THC is not going to be an effective analgesic. I would say that people should be turning to something else in the marihuana field for that purpose, and I would discourage anyone from continuing along this line.

Sallan: I would like to ask a question of Dr. Harris in his antitumor work. I would like to ask about your experimental animals who in fact have a positive tumor response, and I ask that question because Dr. Golden a long time ago did a study with reserpine where he was able to get significant prolongation in the life of tumor-bearing animals. It was primarily based on decrease in their metabolic activities.

Harris: You can see that with reserpine very well, and if you noticed on the slides on increased life span, that the body weights changed in the animals. If you give reserpine in an antitumor regimen, the animals lose a great deal of body weight. The whole metabolic pattern is upset. With THC, after the first couple of administrations the rodents become rapidly tolerant to the effects, and by the third administration we see no behavioral effects at all. They continue to gain weight. Their activity is normal.

Cohen: In the same connection, hypothermia is supposed to reduce tumor growth, and we know that the cannabinoids are hypothermic in many species. What do you think about that?

Harris: We looked at that because it was one of the things we were interested in earlier when we first made our report. We looked at it two ways. First of all, the hypothermia of the animals again became rapidly tolerant, and so by the third administration they are not hypothermic anymore. Secondly, we ran chlorpromazine in really hypothermic doses, and that doesn't have any antitumor activity in the animal. So, from that point of view, I don't think you can explain it on hypothermia. You cannot slow down the growth just by putting the animals in the cold, and that's a general overall metabolic slowing of everything. As I say, when you do that, you get this marked decrease in body weight in the animals. I don't think this is what's happening with THC.

Burstein: Dr. Sallan mentioned that some of his patients are smoking marihuana and thereby getting a pretty good dose of cannabidiol. Perhaps these patients should be warned of the possible problem here.

Harris: Perhaps the problem should be further explored.

Sallan: If cannabidiol accelerates tumor growth, and we view it as anabolic to a certain extent, we know that presently anabolic steriors are not very good compounds. They have all sorts of side effects. I wonder whether anybody has looked into cannabidiol in anabolic situations.

Mechoulam: There again, a comment on the analgesia. Up to now, there has been no clear-cut separation of analgesia from any cannabis-like activity. The only clear-cut case, as I see it, is the Wilson and May paper in which they have found the opposite. 11-Nor-delta-8-THC has THC-like activity but no analgetic one, so I think that perhaps this only indicates that chances are that one can ultimately get separation -- pure analgesia without the THC effects. It is of interest that 9-beta-hydroxy-11-nor-hexahydro-THC is strongly analgesic.

Harris: I agree with what Dr. Mechoulam said. But until that compound gets into man, my bets about cannabis-like activity are off, because in all the test procedures we use for evaluating cannabinoid-like psychoactive effects, DMHP is very potent and very active, and yet in man, in any reasonable doses, doesn't produce this type of activity. I think we have to wait until we get it in man before we make statements.

Hill: I would like to comment on Dr. Sallan's data. We have observed at least two subjects who had severe vomiting in our laboratory. I think that they were probably naive users who wanted to taste marihuana in a legal setting. They were very sick. Do you know of any other incidences like that?

Sallan: I have had anecdotal evidence from people who tell me that the first thing that they feel when they smoke grass is nausea and vomiting. Yet when I got up at the cancer meetings and we presented our data, virtually everyone who stood up and asked a question prefaced it with, "We have heard the same story that marihuana decreases vomiting." I don't know.

Vachon: We have seen vomiting in our laboratory, but almost exclusively in people who were non-cigarette smokers, and it may have something related to that.

Smith: We have given it intravenously to a number of people breathing in mouthpieces, and I have been sitting in fear that they would vomit into my spirometer. About a third of the people we have had looked like they were about to vomit. A post-operative patient who is about to vomit gets a very pallid green look about him, and that's a fairly common observation. About half of those reported later that they did have nausea, but none of them vomited.

Lemberger: In all our studies giving it orally and intravenously, we have never seen any vomiting or nausea -- some dizziness at times, but no nausea or vomiting. That includes the synthetics as well.

Anticonvulsant Activity

CHAPTER 21

MARIHUANA AND EPILEPSY: ACTIVATION OF SYMPTOMS BY DELTA-9-THC

Dennis M. Feeney
Maura Spiker
Gerald K. Weiss

Departments of Psychology and Physiology
University of New Mexico
Albuquerque, New Mexico

NOTE: This work was supported by NINDS grant NS 10469-02
to Dennis M. Feeney and by funds from Abbott Laboratories.
We thank Toni Jelso, David Pitchford, and Bahadur Singh Longo
for their assistance on this project. Dr. Monique Braude of the
National Institute for Drug Abuse provided the delta-9-THC and
the cannabidiol. We wish to especially thank Dr. Hamilton
Redman and the Lovelace Foundation for donating the dogs for
study.

"There is not a substance in the materia medica, there is scarcely a
substance in the world, capable of passing through the gullet of man, that
has not at one time or another enjoyed a reputation of being an anti-epileptic."
This 100-year-old conclusion of Seivking (quoted by Meinardi and Magnus,
1974: 666) puts the issue of purported anticonvulsant effects of marihuana
into historical perspective. Considering the number of recent citations,
marihuana is developing a reputation of being an anticonvulsant even to the
degree that careful attention to details of existing evidence is sometimes
lacking. For example, citing an early study by Davis and Ramsey (1949),
the recent report on Marijuana and Health (1974: 135) states that "the THC-
like compounds worked as well or better than these drugs [diphenylhydantoin
and phenobarbital] in all children." The Davis and Ramsey study is often
cited as a demonstration of anticonvulsant effects in man but the report is
very brief and without a detailed description of methods or results and is
difficult to evaluate. Moreover, of the five patients studied one "had prompt
exacerbation of seizures" (1949: 285) under one of the THC homologs. The
early work of Lowe and Goodman (1947) on seizures induced in rats by
electroconvulsive shock (ECS) or Metrazol injection has also been misquoted.

Fried and McIntyre (1973) cite this study as showing that THC "was effective in attenuating Metrazol induced convulsions." Actually Lowe and Goodman (1949: 352) report that marihuana constituents and its synthetic homologs "were found ineffective and exhibited a marked lethal synergism with Metrazol," a result confirmed by Sofia, Solomon, and Barry (1971). These authors and others (Fujimoto, 1972; Chesher and Jackson, 1974; Consroe and Man, 1973; Karler, Cely and Turkanis, 1973; McCaughran, Corcoran and Wada, 1974) do report, however, that marihuana and cannabinoids block, shorten the duration, or raise the threshold for seizures elicited by ECS. Since this pattern of action is similar to the popular anticonvulsant diphenylhydantoin it seemed possible that cannabinoids might be useful in the treatment of epilepsy.

However, close examination of the effects of delta-9-THC on even these simple ECS or focal brain stimulation models of epilepsy indicates a variable effect on seizure duration. In previous work (Feeney, Wagner, McNamara and Weiss, 1973) we observed that delta-9-THC raised the threshold for evocation of seizures by electrical stimulation of the hippocampus in chronic cats (0.25-1.5 mg/kg, oral dosage). However, the delta-9-THC also produced an increase in the variability of seizure duration. Thus, under delta-9-THC seizure duration was less predictable and occasionally seizures of long duration were recorded. Inspection of our within-subject data indicated the increased variability was due to trial-to-trial fluctuations in responsiveness, an effect not easily attributed to uncontrolled variables. Additionally, there were no apparent differences in early and later drug effects which would account for the drug-induced increase in variability. Using very similar procedures Ishikawa, Yoshihisa, Katsuta, Ishiyama, and Tatsue (1966) reported a very similar increase in the variability of hippocampal seizure duration after administration of the anticholinergic drug scopolamine. Drew and Miller (1974) have proposed that marihuana has an anticholinergic action primarily affecting the hippocampus which has a rich cholinergic input (Lewis, Shute and Silver, 1956). Thus, there may not only be variability of response attributable to species differences or dosage, but with marihuana, also moment-to-moment fluctuations of responsiveness. This would suggest that marihuana may have more pronounced effects on measures of variability than measures of central tendency.

With regard to delta-9-THC and seizure duration, subsequently published work by Chesher and Jackson (1974) supports this interpretation. They measured effects on electroconvulsive seizures in mice at various times (1 to 4 hours) after administration of delta-9-THC and other cannabinoids. The highest dosages of delta-9-THC (200 mg/kg, oral) significantly reduced the duration of the tonic hind limb extensor phase of the seizure. Effects on the means were consistent, a 29% decrease at the one-hour test and a 12% reduction at the four-hour test by this high dose of delta-9-THC compared to a saline control group. These authors also report the standard errors for their data, and the effect of delta-9-THC on this measure of variability was quite dramatic. For the highest dose of delta-9-THC at the one-hour test there was an increase of 190% in the standard error compared to the saline control group. This effect of delta-9-THC on the standard error declined over time and at the four-hour test was 26% greater than the control group. In table 2 of Chesher and Jackson's comprehensive study they report 69 means and standard errors for electroconvulsive seizure duration at four one-hour time intervals after various dosages and combinations of cannabinoids. It is striking that the four largest standard errors in their table are from the four tests following the highest dosage of delta-9-THC. Dr. Chesher has kindly provided us with some of the raw data from that experiment, and the delta-9-THC induced increase in the variability of seizure duration is similar to our previously published data. This work suggests that the effects of marihuana, even on relatively simple models of epilepsy, may be complex and can exacerbate seizures.

There are very few studies of the effects of marihuana on natural models of epilepsy. Work on the epileptic baboon is inconclusive. Killam and Killam (1972) described a suppression of seizures by delta-9-THC; however, Meldrum, Fariello, Puil, Derouaux, and Naquet (1974) report a failure to replicate this result. Interestingly, these latter authors report a variable effect of delta-9-THC on seizures: a reduction in photomyoclonic responses on some trials and an enhancement on other trials.

To study further the effects of marihuana on epilepsy in a natural model we investigated the effects of relatively low dosages of delta-9-THC and cannabidiol in epileptic beagle dogs. These dogs display symptoms and drug responses similar to human epileptics (Redman, Hogan and Wilson, 1972). The seizures in these subjects are considered to be of temporal lobe origin (Wiederholt, 1974) and thus of particular interest because of our prior work with experimental hippocampal seizures. Clinical symptoms in these dogs are spontaneous and infrequent and so are a good population on which to test cannabinoids for a possible activation of epileptic symptoms.

Additionally, we studied the effects of delta-9-THC on alumina cream motor cortex foci in cats. This experimental model is considered a good approximation of human focal epilepsy (Ward, 1969).

METHODS

Seventeen male beagle dogs were selected from a colony established and bred for epilepsy at the Lovelace Foundation for Medical Education in Albuquerque. Dogs were selected that had a history of epileptic symptoms or were progeny of epileptic sires and had a high risk of developing epilepsy (Bielfelt, Redman and McClellan, 1971).

Briefly, three types of symptoms are observed in these subjects: (1) myoclonic jerks, brief shock-like contractions of a muscle group; (2) minor seizures, consisting of a loss of responsiveness, sometimes accompanied by chewing movements and/or myoclonic jerks and lasting approximately one minute; (3) generalized convulsions, which often begin with chewing movements and myoclonic jerks following by a tonic-clinic convulsion, salivation and urination, and a post-ictal depression, the entire episode usually lasting

a few minutes. These symptoms are not triggered by sensory stimuli although
one case of photic driving of myoclonic jerks has been reported (Redman et al.,
1972). The EEG has not been recorded during a spontaneous seizure in
these subjects, although interictal "spike" activity has been recorded from
the temporal lobe (Wiederholt, 1974). Epileptiform EEG activity and
seizures have been evoked in these subjects by several pharmacological
agents known to activate symptoms in human epileptics (Redman, Hogan and
Wilson, 1973; Wiederholt, 1974).

Experiment 1. Between subjects design: Behavioral observations

Fifteen of the debarked dogs were housed and observed in five out-
door runs. Three dogs were placed in each run which was 6 ft. by 12 ft. and
provided with a large doghouse and a 4 ft. wide sunshade. The subjects were
fed in the morning from 8:30 a.m. to 10:00 a.m. and allowed free access to
water. Caretakers spent at least two hours each day with the animals and
made daily reports of the subjects' behavior. They were alerted to watch for
epileptic symptoms.

Informal observations of the dogs' behavior began upon their arrival
to determine the most suitable time for systematic observations and to arrange
cage assignments to minimize fighting. The dogs were most active in the
evening and the last three hours of daylight were chosen for systematic
observations. Two observers scored the behavior of the dogs according to
rating scales and were given descriptions of the clinical symptoms of epilepsy
in the beagle.

The systematic observation sessions, carried out between 5:30 and
8:30 p.m., were divided into 10-minute periods for each dog run. A timing
device emitted an audible tone every 30 seconds and the observer noted the
behavior of the subjects in that run during that 30-second interval. Twenty
such intervals constituted a 10-minute observation period and the observer
then moved to the next run. There were three 10-minute observation periods
spaced one hour apart each evening for each run. These systematic observations, along with the informal observations of the caretakers, were conducted
on 44 consecutive days.

After 5 days of systematic observation, a daily dosing procedure was
begun. The dose was administered by the observer at approximately 5:00 p.m.,
30 minutes before the beginning of the observation period. The first 9 days
of dosing consisted of vehicle alone. A 5 cc syringe was filled by an
experimenter (not an observer) with 4 cc of beef bouillon and 1 cc of sesame
oil floated on top of the bouillon. Each syringe was tagged for a particular
dog and the mixture squirted down the throat of the subject.

Drug administration was begun after 9 days of vehicle treatment.
Because of hypothesized effects of delta-9-THC on sexual behavior (Kolodny,
Masters, Kolodner and Toro, 1974) the dogs in run No. 5 were assigned to
the high-THC dose condition as those subjects displayed some hypersexuality.

All of the other runs were randomly assigned to drug conditions. By chance, more subjects with a history of observed seizures were assigned to the cannabidiol treatment group. Details of the clinical history of these subjects have been published elsewhere (Bielfelt et al., 1971).

The design of the experiment is depicted below in Table 1. The dogs in two runs received delta-9-THC, in two other runs cannabidiol, and in one run the vehicle alone. Each drug group was divided into a low- and a high-dose condition but all of the dogs in a given run received the same dose. For the first 10 days, the dogs in the THC low-dose group received 0.5 mg/kg and concurrently the THC high-dose group received 3 mg/kg. For the second 10 days of drug administration, the low-dose group received 3 mg/kg and the high-dose group 5 mg/kg of delta-9-THC. The beagles in the cannabidiol low-dose group received 1 mg/kg and the cannabidiol high-dose group received 3 mg/kg for the first 10 days of the drug period. For the second 10-day drug period, the cannabidiol low-dose group was increased to 3 mg/kg and the high-dose group to 5 mg/kg. The vehicle was prepared as described above and the THC dissolved in a solution of 25% ethanol and 75% sesame oil and floated on top of the bouillon. The cannabidiol was dissolved in the sesame oil. For the final 10 days of the study, vehicle alone was administered to all of the subjects.

During the study, the observers and caretakers did not know when the drugging began, when the doses increased or were terminated. They did not know what dogs were receiving drugs. Classifications of all behaviors, including epileptic symptoms, were made by these observers. They did know we were studying the effects of marihuana on epilepsy.

Experiment 2. Within-subjects design: EEG and behavioral observations

Two epileptic beagles (357D & EP1D) not used in the above study were implanted with cortical and subcortical electrodes using sterile surgical procedure described previously (Feeney, 1971). Monopolar electrodes were placed bilaterally over the post cruciate gyri and bipolar electrodes bilaterally in the amygdala and dorsal hippocampus. For both dogs an initial two-hour baseline recording was taken two weeks after surgery. At weekly intervals thereafter, the first dog was dosed as described above once with 5 mg/kg of cannabidiol, then once with 0.5 mg/kg and three times with 5.0 mg/kg of delta-9-THC. The second dog was dosed initially with 0.5 mg/kg and then three times with 5.0 mg/kg of delta-9-THC and then once with 5.0 mg/kg of cannabidiol. Recordings were taken with the dog in an isolation chamber and observed continuously through one-way glass.

Table 1. Treatments and Observations

DOG	Observe 5 days	Vehicle Alone 9 days	Drug I 10 Days	Drug II 10 Days	Vehicle Alone 10 Days
Δ⁹-THC-Low			0.5 mg/kg Daily	3 mg/kg Daily	
EP3B	- - - - -	- - - - -	- - - - - - - - - -	M - - - - - M -	- - - - -
59D	- - - - -	- - - - -	- - - - - - - - - -	M - - - S	- - - - -
EP6A	- - - - -	- - - - -	- - - - - - - - - -	- - - - -	- - - - -
Δ⁹-THC-High			3 mg/kg Daily	5 mg/kg Daily	
163A	- - - - -	- - - - -	- - - - - - - S - -	- - - - M -	- - - - -
EP8D	- - - - -	- - - - -	- - - - - - - - - -	- - - - -	- - - - -
61A	- - - - -	- - - - -	- - - - - - - - - -	- - - - -	- - - - -
Cannabidiol-Low			1 mg/kg Daily	3 mg/kg Daily	
146D	- - - - -	- - - - -	- - - - - - - - - -	- - - - -	- - - - -
70A	- - - - -	- - - - -	- - - - - - - - - -	- - - - -	- - - - -
20D	- - - - -	- - - - -	- - - - - - - - - -	- - - - -	- - - - -
Cannabidiol-High			3 mg/kg Daily	5 mg/kg Daily	
145C	- - - - -	- - - - -	- - - - - - - - - -	- - - - -	- - - - -
EP2C	- - - - -	- - - - -	- - - - - - - - - -	- - - - -	- - - - -
58B	- - - - -	- - - - -	- - - - - - - - - -	- - - - -	- - - - -
Placebo					
EP1A	- - - - -	- - - - -	- - - - - - - - - -	- - - - -	- - - - -
EP8E	- - - - -	- - - - -	- - - - - - - - - -	- - - - -	- - - - -
20B	- - - - -	- - - - -	- - - - - - - - - -	- - - - -	- - - - -

Implanted* Subjects	Baseline Observation	5 mg/kg Cannabidiol	0.5 mg/kg Δ⁹-THC	5.0 mg/kg Δ⁹-THC	5.0 mg/kg Δ⁹-THC	5.0 mg/kg Δ⁹-THC
357C	-	-	-	M	M	M
EP1D	-	-	-	M	M	M & S

- = No epileptic symptoms
M = Spontaneous myoclonus
S = Seizure
* = The sequence of drug treatment was varied for these subjects – see text.

Since these initial electrophysiological results were promising, four of the dogs used in the behavioral study were implanted with electrodes approximately 3-4 months after completion of experiment 1. The three dogs from the vehicle control group were chosen for study since they had received no drugs and had shown no symptoms. Additionally, dog EP3B was implanted since he most often displayed myoclonus under delta-9-THC. These dogs were implanted as described above, but bipolar (transcortical) electrodes were used and a bipolar electrode placed in the mesencephalic reticular formation. These dogs received 3 doses of 5.0 mg/kg delta-9-THC, one dose of 5.0 mg/kg of cannabidiol, and a 20 mg/kg dose of delta-9-THC at weekly intervals in that order. A two-hour control analyzed for these subjects by a technician who was uninformed of the treatments. He scored the frequency of myoclonus over the two-hour session and duration of seizures in the records. Seizures were defined as persisting very high amplitude rhythmic discharges and the total seizure duration was measured in seconds. At the conclusion of the experiment the dogs were killed with an overdose of barbituate, perfused and the brain removed. The brain was fixed and imbedded in celloidin for histological examination.

Experiment 3. Effects of delta-9-THC on cortical epileptic foci in cats

Three cats were implanted with multiple cortical and subcortical electrodes using procedures described elsewhere (Feeney et al., 1973) and a canula implanted into the right anterior sigmoid gyrus. Baseline EEG recordings were taken weekly and appeared normal, and then 0.1 ml of alumina cream hydroxide was injected into the right anterior sigmoid gyrus via the canula. Within 3-8 weeks after this treatment all three cats displayed frequent epileptiform sharp waves which were most prominent at the focus. Two of the cats were observed having "grand mal" type seizures. These symptoms gradually subsided and by 5-8 months following alumina cream injection, the cats no longer had seizures and only rarely displayed epileptiform spikes. These subjects, now with quiescent motor cortex foci, were given 1.5 mg/kg of delta-9-THC orally (using the same procedure described above) on three successive days and the EEG was recorded for two hours following drug administration.

RESULTS

Experiment 1

The only epileptic symptoms observed during Experiment 1 were in three subjects from the delta-9-THC group during the period of drug administration.

The first symptoms were in dog 163A after 9 days of dosing with 3 mg/kg of delta-9-THC. Approximately 30 minutes after receiving the ninth dose, this dog was seen showing an uncharacteristic loss of responsiveness, ataxia, and the snout was covered with saliva. This syndrome is characteristic of post-ictal depression. While not directly observed it was evident a generalized seizure occurred sometime between dosing when the dog appeared normal and the beginning of the observation period 30 minutes later.

The second occurrence of epileptic symptoms was in dog EP3B on the eleventh day of THC administration, 30 minutes after the first dose of 3 mg/kg. The dog showed brief, intermittent, shock-like contractions of the muscles of the head, neck, and forequarters. These myoclonic jerks were spontaneous, not evoked by external stimuli. Fourteen myoclonic responses were noted in the first 10-minute observation period and they continued irregularly for two hours.

The third occurrence of epileptic symptoms was a generalized seizure in dog 59D on the morning after the twelfth dose of delta-9-THC (the second dose at 3 mg/kg). A caretaker noted tonic leg extension, profuse salivation, and a post-ictal coma. Because of the persisting coma and a leg wound sustained by a bite from a cagemate, this dog was isolated but continued on the drug regimen. Systematic behavioral observations were discontinued on this animal but he was frequently seen by caretakers and veterinarians. No further symptoms were observed.

The fourth and fifth observations of epileptic symptoms both occurred on the nineteenth day of drug administration again in dogs EP3B (after the ninth dose of delta-9-THC at 3 mg/kg) and in dog 163A (after the ninth dose at 5 mg/kg). These animals began showing myoclonic jerks 40 minutes after THC administration. For dog EP3B the myoclonus periodically occurred in rhythmic fashion about once per minute. These responses persisted intermittently for approximately two hours.

Experiment 2

Our electroencephalographic data from the six implanted dogs confirms the previous report (Wiederholt, 1974) of epileptiform sharp waves of relatively high amplitude in the amygdala and hippocampus of the epileptic beagle. Administration of 5 mg/kg of cannabidiol had no consistent effect on the EEG or behavior of these dogs. However, 30 to 60 minutes after each dosage of 5 mg/kg delta-9-THC the subjects began displaying myoclonic jerks identical to those described in the other subjects. The EEG following the high dosages of delta-9-THC showed a more synchronous pattern, displaying more sleep spindles than in the control records. Examination of the EEG record did not reveal any spike activity consistently preceding the myoclonic jerk. Spike activity in the limbic system was interspersed with, but apparently not causally related to, the clinical symptom (see Figure 1). The high incidence of delta-9-THC evoked myoclonus seen in these implanted dogs undoubtedly reflects the close and continuous individual observation of these subjects. The EEG and myoclonus data from the first two implanted dogs were not quantitatively analyzed and are presented in Table 1. The data from the remaining four implanted dogs was quantitatively analyzed and the EEG seizure activity and frequency of myoclonus was scored by an uninformed technician. For these subjects frequency of myoclonus observed before and for 2 hours after dosing at 5 mg/kg delta-9-THC is plotted in Figure 2. The mean number of myoclonic jerks observed over a two-hour and 15-minute period following 5 mg/kg of delta-9-THC was 19 and following 20 mg/kg was 20 myoclonic jerks.

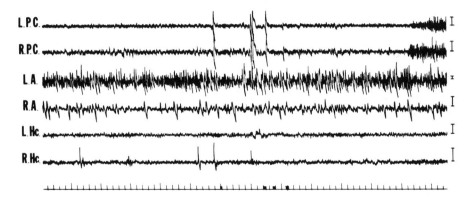

Figure 1.

      Electrophysiological recordings from an epileptic beagle (after administration of 5 mg/kg of delta-9-THC). Myoclonic jerks are indicated by the dark rectangles on the bottom trace which also indicates one-second intervals. The myoclonic jerks produced movement artifact in two monopolar cortical leads (upper two traces). The subcortical leads are bipolar, relatively free of movement artifact, and reveal prominent epileptiform spikes in the right hippocampus and some lower amplitude independent spiking in the right amygdala. Note that the spiking is poorly correlated with the myoclonic jerks. A sleep spindle appears in the far right of the cortical leads. Amplitude calibration, 100 μV; L.P.C., left post crucialis; R.P.C., right post crucialis; L.A., left amygdala; R.A., right amygdala; L.Hc., left hippocampus; R.Hc., right hippocampus.

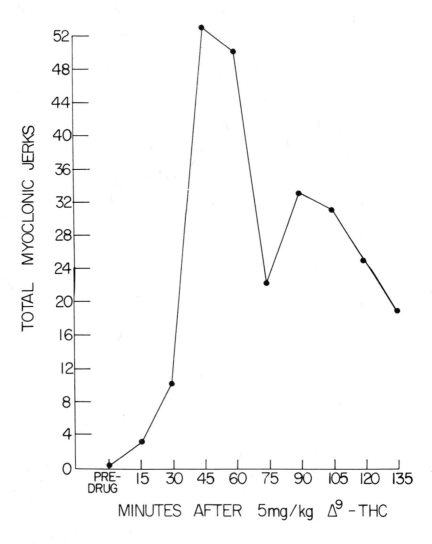

Figure 2.

Total number of myoclonic jerks observed in four epileptic dogs before and after three dosages of 5 mg/kg of delta-9-THC given at one-week intervals. All dogs displayed some myoclonus after every dose.

Seizures were also activated by delta-9-THC at both the 5 mg/kg and 20 mg/kg dosage. The persisting rhythmic, asymmetrical high voltage activity recorded unilaterally from temporal lobe and bilaterally from frontal cortex (often overdriving our amplifiers) was accompanied by a motionless "staring" and occasionally a slight trembling or twitching of a limb. The asymmetry of the drug-evoked EEG seizures is important as this would not be expected from a general drug effect and is likely a result of activation of a unilateral epileptic focus. The onset of a minor seizure is depicted in Figure 3. This typical seizure, recorded bilaterally from the cortex and in the left amygdala, was accompanied by a slight twitching of the right hind leg. Seizures occurred intermittently during the 2 hours following administration of delta-9-THC and were interspersed with epileptiform spikes and myoclonus.

In Figure 4 is plotted the mean amount of time (in seconds) of seizure activity during the two-hour recording sessions for each condition from the dogs used previously as control subjects. Dog EP3B did not complete all the sessions and his data are **not** included. It is clear that delta-9-THC evoked seizure activity in all three subjects. These "absence" type temporal lobe seizures would have gone unnoticed if not for the EEG recordings.

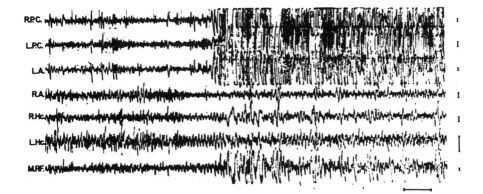

Figure 3.

Electrophysiological recordings of the onset of a minor seizure 30 minutes after receiving 5 mg/kg of delta-9-THC. This seizure was accompanied by an immobile staring and a slight twitching of the right hind leg. Calibrations are 50 μV and 2 seconds. The abbreviations are the same as in Figure 1 and MRF is the mesencephalic reticular formation. All recordings are bipolar, the cortical leads are transcortical.

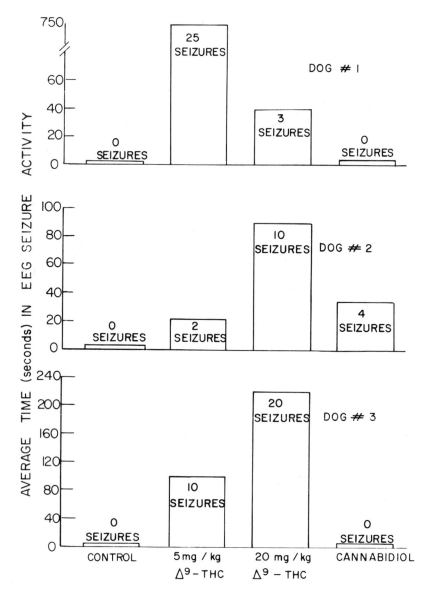

Figure 4.

The mean amount of time scored as seizure activity during
two-hour recording sessions for the three dogs initially used
as placebo controls and subsequently given drug treatments.
The 5 mg/kg delta-9-THC treatment was repeated three times,
the other conditions are the results from one session. The
mean number of clearly different seizures during the sessions
is also indicated.

The placement of the depth electrodes was verified histologically in the dogs. The electrodes were all accurately and symmetrically positioned.

Experiment 3

In the three cats with quiescent motor cortex foci a very clear increase in interictal spiking was observed along with increased sleep spindles and slow waves in the EEG compared to pre-drug control records. This was most dramatic in one cat that had displayed no spikes in four one-hour control records for the month prior to drug treatment. By 30 minutes after receiving delta-9-THC epileptiform spikes were frequently observed and occasionally clusters of focal spikes were recorded. This cat would often scratch the left side of its face during or immediately after the clusters of spikes in the right cortex. This observation gave the impression that this type of focal discharge was accompanied by localized somesthetic sensation. While not quantitatively analyzed, the delta-9-THC increased focal spiking appeared diminished by the third dose.

DISCUSSION

The data are clear: delta-9-THC, a psychoactive ingredient of marihuana, can activate myoclonus and seizures in the epileptic beagle. Cannabidiol, a relatively inactive ingredient, had no clear effects. With delta-9-THC, no effects were observed with the very low 0.5 mg/kg dose, but myoclonus and seizures were reliably elicited by 5 mg/kg. Additionally, delta-9-THC activated quiescent alumina cream foci in the motor cortex of cats.

The behavioral symptom most reliably elicited in the epileptic beagles was myoclonus, a brief shock-like contraction primarily of the muscles of the head, neck, and forequarters. This was most obvious for the six subjects implanted with electrodes for recording the EEG, probably detected because of the continuous individual observation of these subjects. All six of these dogs displayed myoclonus after every dose of 5 mg/kg of delta-9-THC. A close relationship between myoclonus and seizures is well documented in both human pathology and experimental models (Gastaut and Fisher-Williams, 1959). Convulsant drugs such as metraxol will elicit myoclonic jerks at dosages insufficient to produce a seizure. Also, spontaneous seizures in these dogs as well as in some human epileptics are occasionally preceded by myoclonus. Myoclonus has not been reported in normal subjects, including dogs (Dewey, Jenkins, O'Rourke and Harris, 1972; Joel, 1925) during marihuana or delta-9-THC intoxication, except at very high (12.8 mg/kg) intravenous dosages (Martinez, Stadnicke and Schaeppi, 1972).

Major convulsions of the "grand mal" type only occurred twice during this study, but it is striking that they both occurred in dogs receiving 3-5 mg/kg of delta-9-THC. Similarly, minor seizures were only reliably observed after dosages of 5-20 mg/kg of delta-9-THC. These minor seizures had minimal behavioral manifestations: an immobile staring and twitching or trembling of one leg or paw. The EEG displayed high voltage, rhythmic persistent discharge usually involving the amygdala on one side. The asymmetry of these epileptiform discharges is important because it distinguishes this drug effect from a nonspecific action of a neurotropic agent on normal brain. The asymmetrical epileptiform EEG activity evoked by delta-9-THC most likely indicates the drug interacted with an existing unilateral epileptic focus. This distinction is important in that it indicates that marihuana can activate or exacerbate existing epileptic pathology as opposed to causing epileptiform discharge de novo. Other investigators (Martinez et al., 1972) have reported "epileptiform" EEG activity in normal monkeys following intravenous administration of delta-9-THC. While the EEG effect they observed may have been abnormal -- a response to a powerful neurotropic drug -- it is not necessarily epileptic. Our subjects, on the other hand, had a history of seizures or were progeny of epileptic sires and under delta-9-THC displayed asymmetrical EEG seizures characteristic of temporal lobe epilepsy.

A general effect of the dosages of delta-9-THC used in this study was behavioral sedation and an increase in the spindle waves of slow wave sleep in the cortical EEG. For the cats with motor cortex foci the sedative effect was dramatic and the occurrence of cortical epileptiform spikes was correlated with the appearance of sleep spindles which has been noted previously (Wagner, Feeney, Gullotta and Cote, 1975). This sedative effect at low doses and activation of epileptic seizures at higher dosages is similar to a number of other drugs including chloropromazine (Schlichther, Bristow, Shultz and Henderson, 1956), antihistiminic agents (Rinaldi and Himwich, 1955), 5-hydroxytryptophan (Bogdanski, Weissback and Undenfriend, 1958), and steroids (Heuser, Ling and Buchwald, 1965). Additionally, previous work with the epileptic beagle has indicated that chloropromazine (Redman et al., 1973) and methohexital (Wiederholt, 1974) activate existing EEG symptoms in human temporal lobe epileptics (Mayr and Lechner, 1954; Musella, Wilder and Schmidt, 1971). It is well documented that natural sleep activates some types of epilepsies (Pompeiano, 1969; Janz, 1974). Also slow wave sleep and seizures share some common physiological mechanisms (Feeney and Gullotta, 1972; Wagner, Feeney, Gullotta and Cote, 1975). Thus the action of delta-9-THC on epilepsy in the beagle may be related to its sedative effects.

These conclusions regarding the activation of epileptic symptoms conflict with the numerous papers reporting anticonvulsant effects of cannabinoids. Those reports are largely based on the ability of cannabinoids to block seizures evoked by ECS or focal brain stimulation. In addition to the variability in the data outlined in the introduction, there are two other problems which seriously limit consideration of delta-9-THC for clinical use as an anticonvulsant: behavioral effects and tolerance. To obtain protection against ECS in 50% of the subjects, intraperitoneal doses of approximately 100 mg/kg of delta-9-THC, cannabidiol or cannabinol are required (Karler, Cely and Turkanis, 1973). Using oral dosages 160-200 mg/kg were required to reduce the duration of ECS seizures by Chesher and Jackson (1974). These dosages would produce severe behavioral impairments. Lower dosages of delta-9-THC are reported as effective in raising the threshold for seizures evoked by focal brain stimulation (Feeney et al., 1973) but this effect is dramatically reduced with repeated drug administration (Fried and McIntyre, 1973).

The conflicting conclusions may be partially semantic or reflect the particular approach of different investigators. Marihuana may not simply be either a convulsant or anticonvulsant, but rather be capable of blocking some types of seizures and exacerbating others. Admittedly our work may have been biased toward finding convulsant effects of the drugs since we selected subjects with histories or risk of developing epilepsy and our baseline and placebo controls showed no symptoms. We only recorded interictal spiking during our control periods. This is identical to what others have observed with the epileptic beagle (Wiederholt, 1974). This is also similar to what is observed with most human epileptics; seizures are rarely seen in the clinic without provocative treatments such as sleep deprivation, hyperventilation, photostimulation, or pharmacological treatment. Other investigators evaluating the effects of cannabinoids on epilepsy may bias their approach by utilizing maximal seizure responses before drug treatment and so be less likely to detect an exacerbation of seizures.

For therapeutic consideration as an anticonvulsant, a drug should: (1) block seizures at dosages having minimal toxic or behavioral effects; (2) sustain this property over repeated administration; and (3) have minimal risk of activating symptoms. From the data reviewed and the experiments conducted, delta-9-THC would fail on all of these criteria. Cannabidiol, on the other hand, does not reliably activate symptoms in the epileptic beagle and has been reported to block experimental seizures at dosages having behavioral effects similar to the popular anticonvulsant diphenylhydantoin (Izquierdo and Nasello, 1973; Izquierdo, Orsinger and Berardi, 1973). Cannabidiol should receive further study.

There is one final therapeutic aspect of marihuana use remaining to be discussed: the incidence of marihuana use by epileptics. Preliminary results of a survey we conducted of epileptic patients indicates that 29% of the sample in the 15-30 year-old age group smoked marihuana after being seen for treatment of epilepsy and this topic was almost never discussed with their physician. Given the findings of the present experiments, we would suggest that physicians discuss with their epileptic patients the possible activation of their symptoms by marihuana just as is routinely done for alcohol. Additionally phenobarbital, a popular anticonvulsant, interacts with delta-9-THC (Fujimoto, 1972) and thus smoking marihuana may alter the course of drug therapy. We do not know how well our animal models predict the reactions of the various human epilepsies to marihuana, but given the widespread popular use of this drug, its potential exacerbation of epileptic symptoms should receive further attention.

SUMMARY

To evaluate the effects of marihuana on epilepsy, fifteen naturally epileptic beagle dogs were given either placebo or various dosages of delta-9-THC or cannabidiol on twenty consecutive days. Myoclonic jerks and generalized seizures were observed only in those dogs receiving high dosages of delta-9-THC (3.0 or 5.0 mg/kg - oral). In six epileptic beagles implanted with cortical and subcortical electrodes delta-9-THC reliably evoked myoclonus and temporal lobe seizures. Additionally, low dosages of delta-9-THC (1.5 mg/kg - oral) activated epileptiform activity from quiescent alumina cream motor cortex foci in three chronic cats. These results indicate that delta-9-THC, a psychoactive component of marihuana, can activate existing epileptic pathology.

REFERENCES

Bielfelt, S. W., Redman, H. C., & McClellan, R. O. Sire- and sex-related differences in rates of epileptiform seizures in a purebred beagle dog colony. American Journal of Veterinary Research, 1971, 32, 2039-2048.

Bogdanski, D. F., Weissback, H., & Undenfriend, S. Pharmacological studies with the serotonin precursor 5-hydroxtryptophan. Journal of Pharmacology and Experimental Therapeutics, 1958, 122, 182-194.

Chesher, G. B., & Jackson, D. M. Anticonvulsant effects of cannabinoids in mice: Drug interactions within cannabinoids and cannabinoid interactions with phenytoin. Psychopharmacologia (Berl.), 1974, 37, 255-264.

Consroe, P. F., & Man, D. P. Effects of delta-8 and delta-9-tetrahydrocannabinol on experimentally induced seizures. Life Sciences, 1973, 13, 429-439.

Davis, J. P., & Ramsey, H. H. Antiepileptic action of marijuana-active substances. Federation Proceedings, 1949, 8, 284-285.

Dewey, W. L., Jenkins, J., O'Rourke, T., & Harris, L. S. The effects of chronic administration of trans-delta-9-tetrahydrocannabinol on behavior and the cardiovascular system of dogs. Archives internationales de Pharmacodynamie et de Therapie, 1972, 198, 118-131.

Drew, W. G., & Miller, L. L. Cannabis: Neural mechanisms and behavior -- a theoretical review. Pharmacology, 1974, 11, 3-11.

Feeney, D. M. Evoked responses and background unit activity during appetitive conditioning in dogs. Physiology & Behavior, 1971, 6, 9-15.

Feeney, D. M., & Gullotta, F. P. Suppression of seizure discharge and sleep spindles by lesions of the rostral thalamus. Brain Research, 1972, 45, 254-259.

Feeney, D. M., Wagner, H. R., McNamara, C., & Weiss, G. K. Effects of tetrahydrocannabinol on hippocampal evoked afterdischarges in cats. Experimental Neurology, 1973, 41, 357-365.

Fried, P. A., & McIntyre, D. C. Electrical and behavioral attenuation of the anti-convulsant properties of delta-9-THC following chronic administration. Psychopharmacologia, 1973, 31, 215-227.

Fujimoto, J. M. Modification of the effects of delta-9-tetrahydrocannabinol by phenobarbital pretreatment in mice. Toxicology & Applied Pharmacology, 1972, 23, 623-634.

Gastaut, H., & Fischer-Williams, M. The physiopathology of epileptic seizures. In J. Field, H. W. Magoun, & V. E. Hall (Eds.) Handbook of Physiology, Neurophysiology. Washington, D.C.: 1959, 1, 329-364.

Heuser, G., Ling, G.M., & Buchwald, N.A. Sedation or seizures as dose-dependent effects of steroids. Archives of Neurology, 1965, 13, 195-203.

Ishikawa, T.S., Yoshihisa, S., Katsuta, S., Ishiyama, S., & Tatsue, K. Hippocampal after discharge and the mode of action in psychotropic drugs. (Collected writings) In T. Tokizans & J. P. Shadi (Eds.) Correlative Neuroscience. Amsterdam: Elsevier Pub. Co., 1966, 577-602.

Izquierdo, I., & Nasello, A.G. Effects of cannabidiol and of diphenylhydantoin on the hippocampus and on learning. Psychopharmacologia (Berl.), 1973, 31, 167-175.

Izquierdo, I., Orsinger, O.A., & Berardi, A. C. Effect of cannabidiol and of other cannabis sativa compounds on hippocampal seizure discharges. Psychopharmacologia (Berl.), 1973, 28, 95-102.

Janz, D. Epilepsy and the sleep-waking cycle. In O. Magnus & A. M. Lorentz De Haas (Eds.) Handbook of Clinical Neurology, vol. 15, The Epilepsies. New York: American Elsevier Pub. Co., 1974, 457-490.

Joel, E. Beitrage zur pharmakologie der Korperstellung und der Labrinthreflexe. XIII: Haschisch. Pflugers Archives, 1925, 209, 526-536.

Karler, R., Cely, W., & Turkanis, S.A. The anticonvulsant activity of cannabidiol and cannabinol. Life Sciences, 1973, 13, 1527-1531.

Killam, K.F., & Killam, E.K. The action of tetrahydrocannabinol on EEG and photoclonic seizures in the baboon. Fifth International Congress on Pharmacology, 1972, 124. (Abstract)

Kolodny, R.C., Masters, W.H., Kolodner, R.M., & Toro, G. Depression of plasma testosterone levels after chronic intensive marijuana use. New England Journal of Medicine, 1974, 290, 872-874.

Lewis, P.R., Shute, G.C., & Silver, A. Confirmation from choline acetylase analysis of a massive cholinergic innervation to the rat hippocampus. Journal of Physiology, 1956, 191, 215-224.

Loewe, S. & Goodman, L. S. Anticonvulsant action of marijuana-active substances. Federation Proceedings, 1947, 6, 352.

Marijuana and Health, Fourth Annual Report to Congress from the Secretary of Health, Education and Welfare. Washington, D.C.: Government Printing Office, 1974.

Martinez, J.L., Stadnicke, S.W., & Schaeppi, U.N. Delta-9-tetrahydro-cannabinol: effects on EEG and behavior of rhesus monkeys. Life Sciences, 1972, 11, 643-651.

Mayr, R., & Lechner, H. Zur Frage der Provokation bei temporallappen-epilepsie im EEG. Wiener Klinische Wochenschrift, 1954, 66, 903-906.

Meinardi, H., & Magnus, O. Drug therapy. In O. Magnus & A. M. Lorentz De Haas (Eds.) Handbook of Clinical Neurology, vol. 15, The Epilepsies. New York: American Elsevier Pub. Co., 1974, 664-672.

McCaughran, J.A., Corcoran, M.E., & Wada, J.A. Anticonvulsant activity of delta-8- and delta-9-tetrahydrocannabinol in rats. Pharmacology Biochemistry & Behavior, 1974, 2, 227-233.

Meldrum, B.S., Fariello, R.G., Puil, E.A., Derouaux, M., & Naquet, R. Delta-9-tetrahydrocannabinol and epilepsy in the photosensitive baboon, Papio Papio Epilepsia, 1974, 15, 255-264.

Musella, L., Wilder, B.J., & Schmidt, R.P. Electroencephalographic activation with intravenous methohexital in psychomotor epilepsy. Neurology (Minneapolis), 1971, 21, 594-602.

Pompeiano, O. Sleep mechanisms. In H. H. Jasper, A. A. Ward, & A. Pope (Eds.) Basic Mechanisms in the Epilepsies. Boston: Little Brown, 1969, 453-473.

Redman, H.C., Wilson, G.L., & Hogan, J.E. Effect of chloropromazine combined with intermittent light stimulation on the electroencephalo-gram and clinical response of the beagle dog. American Journal of Veterinary Research, 1973, 34, 929-936.

Redman, H.C., Hogan, J.E., & Wilson, G.L. Effect of intermittent light stimulation singly and combined with pentylenetetrazol on the electroencephalogram and clinical response of the beagle dog. American Journal of Veterinary Research, 1972, 33, 677-685.

Rinaldi, F., & Himwich, W.E. Site of action of anti-Parkinson drugs. Confines of Neurology, 1955, 15, 209-224.

Schlichther, W., Bristow, M.E., Schultz, S., & Henderson, A.L. Seizures occurring during intensive chloropromazine therapy. Canadian Medical Association Journal, 1956, 74, 364-366.

Sofia, R.D., Solomon, T.A., & Barry, H., III. The anticonvulsant activity of delta-1-tetrahydrocannabinol in mice. The Pharmacologist, 1971, 13, 246.

Wagner, H.R., Feeney, D.M., Gullotta, F.P., & Cote, I.L. Suppression of cortical epileptiform activity by generalized and localized ECoG desynchronization. Electroencephalography and Clinical Neurophysiology, 1975, in press.

Ward, A.A. The epileptic neuron: Chronic foci in animals and man. In H. H. Jasper, A. A. Ward, and A. Pope (Eds.) Basic Mechanisms of the Epilepsies. Boston: Little Brown, 1969, 453-473.

Wiederholt, W.C. Electrophysiological analysis of epileptic beagles. Neurology, 1974, 24, 149-155.

CHAPTER 22

ANTICONVULSANT-CONVULSANT EFFECTS OF DELTA-9-TETRAHYDRO-CANNABINOL

Paul Consroe
Byron Jones
Hugh Laird II
Jeff Reinking

Department of Pharmacology and Toxicology
University of Arizona College of Pharmacy
Tucson, Arizona

NOTE: The present studies were supported, in part, by National Institute of Mental Health grant #MH23414 and National Institute on Drug Abuse grant #DA01448. We thank Dr. Monique Braude of the National Institute on Drug Abuse (ADAMHA) for the delta-9-THC and Ms. Lynne Rabe for her technical assistance.

It is fairly well established that delta-9-tetrahydrocannabinol (delta-9-THC), the major psychoactive constituent of marihuana, has anticonvulsant properties. A summary of the reported effects of delta-9-THC in laboratory animals for a variety of experimentally induced seizure paradigms is presented in Table 1. In general, behavioral seizures in rodents, frogs, and cats, and electrographic seizures in rats and cats produced by electrical stimulation are prevented by delta-9-THC. Additionally, auditory, tactile (reflex), and in some cases pentylenetetrazol (PTZ) induced seizures in rodents are also blocked by the cannabinoid.

Although delta-9-THC possesses anticonvulsant properties in many experimental seizure models, there is a paucity of information concerning the effects of the cannabinoid on chemical convulsants other than PTZ. Studies of such effects are important to obtain additional information on the spectrum of anticonvulsant activity and possible mechanisms of action of delta-9-THC. In the present anticonvulsant study, experiments were designed to obtain data on delta-9-THC's activity in rats against some well-known chemical convulsants and to further quantitate and compare its properties in electrical seizure models.

There is some evidence to indicate that, in addition to its anticonvulsant actions, delta-9-THC also possesses convulsant properties. A summary of the reported convulsant effects of delta-9-THC in laboratory animals is presented in Table 2. As shown, behavioral convulsions have occasionally been reported in rats, dogs, and monkeys after delta 9-THC administration, but generally these drastic effects only occur with lethal or near-lethal doses given acutely or with extremely high doses given chronically. In contradistinction to behavioral convulsions, EEG patterns interpreted as convulsant-like -- for example, "polyspikes," "epileptiform-like," "spikes and slow waves," and the like -- have frequently been shown to occur after delta-9-THC administration in the rat, dog, monkey, cat, and rabbit (Table 2). These EEG manifestations generally occur throughout a continuum of delta-9-THC dosage and importantly they occur without the corresponding appearance of behavioral convulsions.

Thus, it came as quite a surprise to us that 4 rabbits (all littermates) evinced clonic behavioral convulsions after acute administration of a low intravenous (i.v.) dose, that is, 0.5 milligrams per kilogram (mg/kg) of delta-9-THC (Consroe, Jones & Chin, 1975). We subsequently commissioned our local rabbit breeder/supplier to initiate inbreeding of these rabbits which resulted in producing offspring which convulse after i.v. delta-9-THC administration. These findings appeared quite significant in view of the well-known dose-response anticonvulsant properties of delta-9-THC (Table 1), and because of the extreme dosage and duration regimens of delta-9-THC administration apparently needed to produce behavioral convulsions (Table 2). Moreover, delta-9-THC induced behavioral convulsions had not previously been reported in rabbits despite the administration of a wide range of acute i.v. doses, that is 0.01-10 mg/kg (Table 2).

In the present convulsant study, experiments were designed to obtain basic pharmacological data on the convulsant effects of delta-9-THC in some of our specially bred New Zealand albino rabbits.

ANTICONVULSANT EXPERIMENTS

Methods

The effects of delta-9-THC were measured against electrically caused convulsions and chemically induced seizures and lethality in male Holtzman Sprague Dawley rats weighing 250-350 grams. Delta-9-THC was incorporated in a vehicle for oral (p.o.) administration containing 10% sesame oil, 1% polysorbate (Tween)-80, and 89% normal saline. Saline solutions of PTZ, picrotoxin, and strychnine were given subcutaneously (s.c.) and lidocaine was administered intraperitoneally (i.p.). Maximal (MEST) and minimal (EST) electroshock seizure thresholds were determined by delivering 0.2 second pulses via corneal electrodes from a standard 60-Hz electroshock

Table 1

Anticonvulsant Effects of Delta-9-THC in Laboratory Animals

Seizure Type	Species	Major Effects of Delta-9-THC on Seizure	Reference(s)
Maximal (Tonic) Electroshock Seizures (MES)	Rat	Dose-response protection, generally	Consroe & Man, 1973; Karler et al., 1974b; Loewe & Goodman, 1947; McCaughran et al., 1974
	Mouse	Protection (partial & dose-response); tolerance develops to anticonvulsant effect	Chesher & Jackson, 1974; Fujimoto, 1972; Garriott et al., 1968; Karler et al., 1973, 1974b, 1974c, 1974d; Sofia et al., 1971a, 1971b, 1974
		No protection reported	Dwivedi & Harbison, 1975
	Frog	Protection	Karler et al., 1974a
Electrically-induced Minimal (Clonic) Seizures	Rat	Protection against "kindled" seizures; tolerance develops to anticonvulsant effect	Corcoran et al., 1973; Fried & McIntyre, 1973
	Mouse	Elevation of 6-HZ- & not 60-HZ-electroshock seizure thresholds (EST)	Karler et al., 1974b
	Cat	Reduction of seizures induced by subcortical stimulation	Wada et al., 1973
Electrically-induced Electrographic (EEG) Seizures	Rat	Protection against cortical & subcortical EEG seizures, generally; tolerance develops to anticonvulsant effect	Corcoran et al., 1973; Fried & McIntyre, 1973; Izquierdo et al., 1973
	Cat	Reduction or enhancement of EEG seizures depending on stimulus strength	Feeney et al., 1973; Wada et al., 1973
Pentylenetetrazol (PTZ)-induced Seizures	Rat	No seizure protection & enhanced lethality	Loewe & Goodman, 1947
		Protection of maximal seizures & no effect on minimal seizures & lethality of PTZ	Consroe & Man, 1973
		Protection against minimal PTZ seizures only at toxic & lethal doses of delta-9-THC	McCaughran et al., 1974
	Mouse	Dose-response protection against minimal PTZ seizures	Dwivedi & Harbison, 1975
		Partial protection against maximal seizures; no protection or enhancement of minimal seizures & lethality of PTZ; strychnine seizures & lethality also enhanced	Chesher & Jackson, 1974; Karler et al., 1974b; Sofia et al., 1971b; Turkanis et al., 1974
Audiogenic (Clonic) &/or Tonic Seizures	Rat	Dose response protection	Consroe & Man, 1973; Consroe et al., 1973
	Mouse	Reduction in seizure susceptibility	Boggan et al., 1973
Photomyoclonic Seizures	Baboon	Protection	Killam & Killam, 1972
		No protection	Meldrum et al., 1974
Reflex ("spontaneous") Seizures	Gerbil	Protection; tolerance develops to anticonvulsant effect	Cox et al., 1975

Table 2

Convulsant effects of Delta-9-THC in Laboratory Animals

Species	Route & Duration of Delta-9-THC Administration	Dose(s) of Delta-9-THC (mg/kg)	Major Effects of Delta-9-THC	Reference(s)
Rat	intravenous; acute	10-20	Generalized body twitches ("popcorn" convulsions)	Braude, 1972
	oral; acute	225-3600	"popcorn" convulsions	Braude, 1972; Thompson et al., 1973b
	oral; 28-180 days	10-500	Clonic-type convulsions by day 50-75	Braude, 1972; Luthra & Rosenkrantz, 1974; Luthra et al., 1975; Rosenkrantz et al., 1975; Stadnicki et al., 1974; Thompson et al., 1973a
	inhalational, acute; 5 & 23 days	0.7-60	"Popcorn" convulsions with chronic administration	Rosenkrantz & Braude, 1974
	intravenous, intra-peritoneal, & oral; acute & chronic	0.5-30	Convulsant (?) cortical and subcortical EEG activity: "polyspikes," "high voltage sharp waves and/or "epileptiform-like" activity, with no behavioral convulsions	Lipparini et al., 1969; Moreton & Davis, 1973; Pirch et al., 1972; Stadnicki et al., 1974
	oral; chronic	10	Convulsant EEG activity & clonus in 1 of 6 rats on day 109 of treatment	Stadnicki et al., 1974
Dog	intravenous & oral; acute	3.9-210	Clonic-tonic convulsions with opisthotonos in 20-40% of prostrated animals with higher doses	Braude, 1972; Thompson et al., 1973b
	intravenous; acute	0.5-10	Convulsant (?) EEG activity with no behavioral convulsions	Domino, 1971
Monkey	intravenous; acute	3.9-256	Convulsions (behavioral) reported	Braude, 1972
	intravenous & inhalational; acute	0.05-12.8	Convulsant (?) EEG activity with no behavioral convulsions	Boyd et al., 1971, 1974; Heath, 1973; Martinez et al., 1972
Cat	intravenous & oral; acute & chronic	2-20	Convulsant (?) EEG activity with no behavioral convulsions	Barratt & Adams, 1972; Lipparini et al., 1969; Segal & Barak, 1972; Segal & Kenney, 1972
Rabbit	intravenous & intra-cerebral; acute	0.01-10	Convulsant (?) EEG activity with no behavioral convulsions	Consroe et al., 1975a; Fujimori & Himwich, 1973; Fujimori et al., 1973; Lipparini et al., 1969; Segal, 1974; Segal & Barak, 1972
	intravenous; acute	0.5	Clonic convulsions in 4 animals	Consroe, 1975a

apparatus (Woodbury and Davenport, 1952). Maximal (tonic extension of hindlimbs for 3 seconds) and minimal (forelimb clonus for 5 seconds) seizures were ascertained for electroshock and chemoshock in vehicle and delta-9-THC treated animals. Additionally, the effects of delta-9-THC on lethality of rats given the convulsant drugs were also determined. In a preliminary study 30 mg/kg delta-9-THC, given p.o. 1 1/2 hours earlier, was determined to be the ED80 -- that is, the dose effective in 80% of rats -- against maximal electroshock seizures (MES). Thus, in the present study a single p.o. dose of 30 mg/kg delta-9-THC was administered 1 1/2 hours prior to a convulsant challenge. All tests were carried out between 1000 and 1300 hours. Current-effect curves in electroshock tests and dose-effect curves in chemoshock and lethality studies, each having 3 to 6 points with data from 10 rats per point, were graphed according to the method of Litchfield and Wilcoxon (1949). From these curves, slopes and median values (CC50's, CD50's and LD50's) with corresponding 95% confidence limits (C.L.) were calculated wherever possible; tests for heterogenous data and parallelism were also carried out (Litchfield and Wilcoxon, 1949).

Results

In control animals, both maximal and minimal seizures were produced by electroshock and PTZ whereas only maximal seizures were observed with strychnine and only minimal seizures resulted from injection of lidocaine and picrotoxin. Table 3 illustrates the effects of delta-9-THC on maximal seizures. Delta-9-THC increased MEST 800% above control. An evaluation of the calculated slopes and CC50's (median convulsant currents) for delta-9-THC and vehicle treated animals indicated parallelism and hence a reliable (P<0.05) drug protective effect. In contrast, delta-9-THC did not alter strychnine-induced maximal seizures, as shown by the identical CD50's (median convulsant doses) for delta-9-THC and vehicle treated animals. Also, doses of PTZ in the lethal range (70-100 mg/kg) produced a high incidence of maximal seizures -- a CD50 of 88 mg/kg (with a 95% C.L. of 77.8-99.4 mg/kg)-- in vehicle treated rats. Although a CD50 could not be obtained in delta-9-THC-PTZ treated animals due to the almost complete lack of seizures obtained, the data clearly show that the cannabinoid significantly protects animals against maximal seizures over the full range of PTZ doses used.

The effects of delta-9-THC on minimal seizures are presented in Table 4. As indicated by the CC50's for EST and the CD50's for PTZ and lidocaine, delta-9-THC does not protect against these minimal seizures (P>0.95 for all delta-9-THC-vehicle comparisons). Although the range between 0 and 100% convulsant effect with picrotoxin was too narrow to obtain a CD50, delta-9-THC produced no sign of protection against minimal seizures at the 3 doses of picrotoxin used.

The effects of delta-9-THC on chemically induced lethality are presented in Table 5. Clearly, delta-9-THC did not alter the LD50's (median lethal doses) for the 4 convulsant drugs used (P>0.95 for all delta-9-THC-vehicle comparisons).

Table 3

Effects of Delta-9-THC and Delta-9-THC vehicle (V) pretreatment on electroshock (MEST), strychnine, and pentylenetetrazol (PTZ) induced maximal
seizures .

	MEST[a]	Strychnine[a]	PTZ[b]		
			70	80	100 (mg/kg)
V	70 mA	1.78 mg/kg	10%	40%	60%
	(51.8-94.5)	(1.5-2.12)			
Delta-9-THC	630 mA	1.78 mg/kg	0%	0%	10%
(30 mg/kg)	(352-1130)	(1.5-2.12)			

a. Numbers represent median convulsant currents (CC50's) for MEST and
median convulsant doses (CD50's) for strychnine; numbers in parentheses are
95% confidence limits. Each median value represents data obtained from
30-60 rats.

b. Percentages represent the percentage of animals exhibiting convulsions at
various doses of PTZ; data obtained from 10 rats per dose condition, i.e., a
total of 60 animals.

Table 4

Effects of Delta-9-THC and Delta-9-THC vehicle (V) pretreatment on Electroshock (EST), pentylenetetrazol (PTZ) , lidocaine, and picrotoxin induced
minimal seizures.

	EST[a]	PTZ[a]	Lidocaine[a]	Picrotoxin[b]		
				1.1	1.75	4.0 (mg/kg)
V	19 mA	47 mg/kg	70 mg/kg	20%	80%	100%
	(17.8-20.3)	(43.1-51.2)	(60.9-80.9)			
Delta-9-THC	18.8 mA	47 mg/kg	66 mg/kg	0%	80%	100%
(30 mg/kg)	(18.0-19.6)	(43.1-51.2)	(51.2-85.0)			

a. Numbers represent median convulsant currents (CC50's) for EST and median
convulsant doses (CD50's) for PTZ and lidocaine; numbers in parentheses are
95% confidence limits. Each median value represents data obtained from
30-60 rats.

b. Percentages represent the percent of animals exhibiting convulsions at
various doses of picrotoxin; data obtained from 10 rats per does condition,
i.e., a total of 60 animals.

Table 5

Median lethal doses (LD50's) of pentylenetetrazol (PTZ), lidocaine, strychnine, and picrotoxin following pretreatment with Delta-9-THC and Delta-9-THC vehicle (V).

	PTZ*	Lidocaine	Strychnine	Picrotoxin
V	79	116	1.78	3.0
	(70.0–89.8)	(98.3–136)	(1.50–2.12)	(2.6–3.4)
Delta-9-THC	79	115	1.78	3.4
(30 mg/kg)	(70.0–89.8)	(103–127)	(1.50–2.12)	(2.8–4.0)

* Numbers are mg/kg and numbers in parentheses represent 95% confidence limits. Each median value represents data obtained from 30–60 rats.

CONVULSANT EXPERIMENTS

Methods

As mentioned previously, our unexpected finding of delta-9-THC induced behavorial convulsions in 4 rabbit littermates prompted an attempt to breed these animals. Figure 1 illustrates the lineage of these 4 animals (Nos. 20, 21, 22, and 24) and of our present population of "delta-9-THC-seizure susceptible" New Zealand albino rabbits. The 7 experimental subjects (Ss) of the present report -- 5 females and 2 males -- consisted of 2 Ss (Nos. 22 and 24) from the F$_1$ generation, 3 Ss (Nos. 31, 33, and 34) from the F$_2$ generation, and 2 Ss (Nos. 40 and 42) from the F$_1$ backcross. After weaning at the local rabbitry, Ss were housed individually in our laboratory in a room maintained at constant temperature (25 $\pm$ 2°C) and under controlled lighting (12-hour light-dark). Ss were allowed access to food and water ad libitum and body weights ranged from 2.1 to 4.2 kg during this investigation.

Delta-9-THC was incorporated into a 4% polysorbate (Tween) 80-saline solution vehicle and doses of delta-9-THC and vehicle were injected into a marginal ear vein in the volume of 0.1 ml/kg. After injection, individual Ss were observed via a one-way vision window in a sound-attenuated chamber measuring 82 cm square by 70 cm high. Frequency and duration

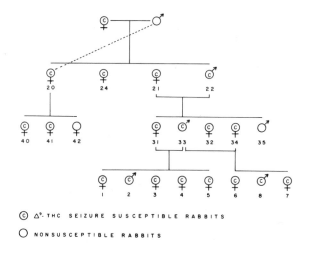

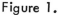

Figure 1.

of the following behaviors were measured by an experimenter-operated digital event recorder: limb clonus, front and/or hind limb extension, head tuck, body torsion, ears down, mydriasis, and nystagmus. Additionally, latency to convulsion (that is, first onset of clonus and/or tonus) was also measured. Each S received sequential injections of vehicle and subsequently delta-9-THC at various doses. Injections were given every other day to each S during 0800 to 1100 hours. Geometrically increasing doses of delta-9-THC were given to determine a threshold dose for eliciting convulsions. Once threshold was determined, a preliminary tolerance study was undertaken. A criterion for tolerance was adopted as the lack of spontaneous convulsion after administration of 2 consecutive treatments (at 2-day intervals) of the ex- perimentally derived threshold doses of delta-9-THC. Additionally, in 3 Ss showing tolerance, the threshold dose was doubled in an attempt to reinstate seizures. The criterion for lack of tolerance was defined as the continued occurrence of convulsion after 10 consecutive alternate-day treatments of delta-9-THC at one particular dose.

Results

Table 6 presents an overall behavioral characterization of the convul- sive activity observed in Ss responsive to delta-9-THC. The onset of seizure always occurred fairly rapidly after delta-9-THC administration where mean latencies to convulsion ranged from 116.8 to 158.8 seconds. A uniform seizure pattern developed in all Ss and consisted of front and/or hind limb clonus, mydriasis, nystagmus, and a positioning of both ears down and caudally (ears down). In addition, a flexure of the head ventrally (head tuck), body torsion, as well as front and/or hind limb extension were fre- quently observed. Convulsive activity generally persisted for about 5-15

Table 6. Characterization of Delta-9-THC Induced Convulsions in New Zealand Albino Rabbits

Subject No. & Sex	Convulsive Dose(s) (mg/kg) delta-9-THC	Total No. of Treatments Eliciting Convulsions	% of Treatments Eliciting:					Mean Latency (seconds) (± S.E.) to Convulsion
			Clonus, Mydriasis, Nystagmus, and Ears Down	Head Tuck	Body Torsion	Front Limb Extension	Hind Limb Extension	
22 M	0.2	6	100%	100%	83%	83%	50%	138.7 ± 10.5
24 F	0.1 & 0.2	12	100%	75%	58%	58%	50%	158.8 ± 5.2
31 F	0.1	10	100%	100%	100%	80%	90%	121.7 ± 6.3
33 M	0.4 & 0.8	11	100%	100%	64%	55%	64%	116.8 ± 4.7
34 F	0.4	10	100%	90%	40%	60%	50%	129.6 ± 8.8
40 F	0.4 & 0.8	14	100%	100%	57%	43%	57%	148.4 ± 6.1

minutes and was followed by postictal behavioral depression. Frequently, however, periodic episodes of seizure activity reoccurred during the subsequent 1 to 3 hours. Seizures did not result in death and Ss appeared completely normal within 8-12 hours after injection. In a correlative experiment, seizures were induced in a group of "normal" (non-convulsing) New Zealand albino rabbits with lidocaine (10 mg/kg, i.v.), PTZ (20 mg/kg, i.v.), picrotoxin (3 mg/kg, s.c.), strychnine (0.4 mg/kg, i.v.), or supramaximal electroshock (delivered via corneal electrodes) in an effort to qualitatively compare seizure endpoints. In general, picrotoxin induced seizures appeared to qualitatively resemble most closely those seizures elicited by delta-9-THC although picrotoxin (as well as PTZ and strychnine) produced a high frequency of subsequent lethality.

Table 7 presents data of threshold and tolerance determinations of delta-9-THC induced seizures. Despite some intersubject differences, convulsions were produced by a rather low and narrow dose range (0.1-0.4) mg/kg of delta-9-THC. Administration of vehicle (0 mg/kg delta-9-THC) did not elicit seizures and interestingly, delta-9-THC (up to 4 mg/kg) failed to induce convulsions in one S (No. 42). Additionally, in recent correlative experiments, we have repeatedly attempted to produce seizures in each of our Ss by various procedures other than with delta-9-THC administration. Thus far, subjecting Ss to stress (violent shaking), intermittent light stimulation (1-60 flashes/sec), and/or auditory stimulation (115 db relative to 2×10^{-4} dynes/cm^2) has failed to induce behavioral convulsions in non-drugged (delta-9-THC) rabbits.

Once a threshold dose of delta-9-THC was established, it was given every other day until the appearance of tolerance (that is, 2 consecutive treatments without seizures) or until a total of 10 treatments (each eliciting seizures) had been given. As shown in Table 7, tolerance to a threshold dose of delta-9-THC developed in 4 Ss (Nos. 22, 24, 33, and 40) and not in 2 others (Nos. 31 and 34). Additionally, the administration of a doubled threshold dose of delta-9-THC to 3 tolerant Ss (Nos. 24, 33 and 40) reinstated seizures. The other S (No. 22) which exhibited initial tolerance was found dead (of apparently natural causes) 2 days after its last injection of delta-9-THC and therefore could not be tested further. Nevertheless, only one S (No. 33) which developed tolerance to a threshold dose of delta-9-THC became tolerant to a suprathreshold dose of the cannabinoid. One might conclude from these data that tolerance to delta-9-THC induced convulsions is highly subject and dose dependent. Yet the variability observed in this preliminary investigation may be obviated by additional studies that utilize a larger number of Ss and a longer and perhaps more frequent treatment period of delta-9-THC administered.

DISCUSSION

The present data confirm and extend findings of both an anticonvulsant and convulsant effect of delta-9-THC, a truly unique drug. These divergent properties underscore the extremely complex pharmacological profile of this major psychoactive component of marihuana.

Table 7. Threshold and Tolerance Determinations of Delta-9-THC Induced Convulsions in New Zealand Albino Rabbits

Subject No. & Sex	Does of Delta-9-THC (mg/kg)							
	0	0.05	0.1	0.2	0.4	0.8	2.0	4.0
22 M	0/1	0/1	0/1	6/8*	--	--	--	--
24 F	0/1	0/1	2/4*	10/10	--	--	--	--
31 F	0/1	0/1	10/10	--	--	--	--	--
33 M	0/1	0/1	0/1	0/1	6/8*	5/7*	--	--
34 F	0/1	0/1	0/1	0/1	10/10	--	--	--
40 F	0/1	0/1	0/1	0/1	4/6*	10/10	--	--
42 F	0/1	0/1	0/1	0/1	0/1	0/1	0/1	0/1

Ratios refer to the number of treatments eliciting convulsions/total number of successive treatments at one particular dose.

* Criterion of tolerance met
-- Doses not tested

Concerning delta-9-THC's anticonvulsant properties, data of the present study appear consistent with data of most other studies showing protective effects in maximal electroshock and PTZ seizure paradigms. Except for one study in mice (Dwivedi and Harbison, 1975), protection against MES has been consistently demonstrated across species -- in rats (Consroe and Man, 1973; Karler, Cely and Turkanis, 1974b; Loewe and Goodman, 1947; McCaughran, Corcoran and Wada, 1974), in mice (Chesher and Jackson, 1974; Fujimoto, 1972; Garriott, Forney, Hughes and Richards, 1968; Karler, Cely and Turkanis, 1973, 1974b, 1974c, 1974d; Sofia, Kubena and Barry, 1971a, 1974; Sofia, Solomon and Barry, 1971b), and in frogs (Karler, Cely and Turkanis, 1974a). Similarly, protection against maximal PTZ seizures has been previously demonstrated in rats (Consroe and Man, 1973) and in mice (Turkanis, Cely, Olsen and Karler, 1974).

In the present study, a dose of delta-9-THC (30 mg/kg) which clearly blocked maximal electroshock and PTZ seizures, was ineffective in preventing minimal seizures produced by electroshock, PTZ, or picrotoxin and maximal seizures induced by strychnine. Similarly, chemically induced lethality was not altered by delta-9-THC pretreatment. These data suggest a differential selectivity of effect of the cannabinoid which appears to be congruent with many other reported findings. That is, doses of delta-9-THC in rodents which clearly afforded protection against MES were mostly ineffective against minimal seizures produced by electroshock, that is, 60 Hz-EST (Karler et al., 1974b) or PTZ (Chesher and Jackson, 1974; Consroe and Man, 1973; Karler et al., 1974b; McCaughran et al., 1974; Sofia et al., 1971b) or against PTZ induced lethality (Consroe and Man, 1973; Sofia et al., 1971b). However, one study in mice (Dwivedi and Harbison, 1975) indicated that PTZ induced minimal seizures and lethality are obtunded by delta-9-THC; the reasons for these discrepancies are not known.

Nevertheless, most of the presently available data describe a spectrum of activity qualitatively similar to that of phenytoin, that is, diphenylhydantoin (DPH), and by implication suggest a similar mechanism of action for delta-9-THC and DPH. In these regards, DPH protects against maximal electroshock and PTZ seizures (Woodbury, 1969) and fails to block minimal seizures produced by electroshock or PTZ (Turkanis et al., 1974; Woodbury, 1969) or lidocaine (deJong, 1970). Similarly, lethality caused by PTZ or strychnine (Sofia et al., 1971b; Woodbury, 1969) or lidocaine (deJong, 1970) is not prevented by DPH. Additionally, it has recently been reported (Turkanis and Karler, 1975) that the putative active metabolite of delta-9-THC, that is, 11-hydroxy-delta-9-THC (Lemberger, Martz, Rodda, Forney and Rowe, 1973), blocks post-tetanic potentiation, and this phenomenon is a well-known action of DPH (Woodbury, 1969). Moreover, cross-tolerance between delta-9-THC and DPH on MES (Karler et al., 1974c) and competition between delta-9-THC and DPH in blocking PTZ induced seizures (Dwivedi and Harbison, 1975) have been demonstrated; these findings suggest that both drugs may be acting at the same site of action.

Concerning the present convulsant experiments, the fact that delta-9-THC, in comparatively low i.v. doses, produced nonfatal behavioral seizures in our rabbits is significant for a number of reasons. The mere observation that behaviorial seizures resulted from delta-9-THC administration is salient since a major documented property of the cannabinoid is its ability to block experimentally induced convulsions in laboratory animals (Table 1). Moreover, even in the few studies which have reported behavioral convulsions with delta-9-THC, generally such effects only occur when extremely toxic acute and/or chronic doses of the cannabinoid are used (Table 2). EEG manifestations of delta-9-THC's activity, often described as "epileptic or convulsant-like," have been demonstrated in many species (Table 2) but their importance is obscure since corresponding behaviorial seizures in these animals have not been shown. In rabbits given delta-9-THC over a wide range of acute i.v. doses, that is, 0.01-10 mg/kg, reports of behavioral convulsions have been conspicuously absent despite corresponding observations of "convulsant-like" EEG patterns (Consroe et al., 1975a; Fujimori and Himwich, 1973; Fujimori, Trusty and Himwich, 1973; Lipparini, Scotti de Carolis and Longo, 1969). Additionally, implantation of delta-9-THC (30-60 micrograms) directly into the hippocampus of rabbits has been shown to cause epileptiform discharges without corresponding behavioral convulsions (Segal, 1974). Furthermore, behavioral convulsions were not reported in delta-9-THC treated rabbits given 3 mg/kg, i.v., daily for 6 days (Lipparini et al., 1969) or given up to 153.4 mg/kg, s.c., for 28 days (Thompson, Rosenkrantz, Fleischman and Braude, 1975). Therefore, it appears that the present finding of delta-9-THC induced behavioral convulsions in our rabbits is rather unique.

While controlled clinical data in humans are lacking, anecdotal accounts of anticonvulsant effects of marihuana in various seizure states, including some epilepsy conditions, have been published (O'Shaughnessy, 1842; Reynolds, 1890; Shaw, 1843). More recently, brief reports of a clinical study involving administration of some synthetic delta-3-THC derivatives (Davis and Ramsey, 1949) and a case history involving marihuana smoking (Consroe, Wood and Buchsbaum, 1975) also suggest that marihuana may be beneficial in some human epilepsies. These reports are interesting because of the documented anticonvulsant effects of delta-9-THC in laboratory animals and in view of the suggestion that these effects may resemble the actions of DPH, a well-known anticonvulsant drug.

In addition, brief reports of a clinical EEG study involving cannabidiol administration (Perez-Reyes and Wingfield, 1974) and a case history involving marihuana smoking (Keeler and Reifler, 1967) suggest that marihuana may also be detrimental in some human epilepsies. Likewise, these observations are interesting in view of the present and previous reports of delta-9-THC induced convulsions in laboratory animals. As previously mentioned, a majority of rabbits of common lineage have been found to exhibit behavioral convulsions after low i.v. doses of delta-9-THC administration (Figure 1). These findings appear to suggest the existence of a possible strain of New Zealand albino rabbit that is uniquely sensitive to the effects of delta-9-THC. Perhaps if seizures are a major sequela of delta-9-THC in a specialized rabbit strain, then similar effects might occur within a given population of other mammalian species, including man. Regardless of these hypotheses, the possible occurrence of a novel biological model to test the effects of marihuana and its congeners is an exciting avenue for further research.

REFERENCES

Barratt, E. S. , & Adams, P. The effects of chronic marijuana administration on brain functioning in cats. In J. M. Singh, L. Miller, & H. Lal (Eds.), Drug addiction: Experimental pharmacology. Mount Kisco, N.Y.: Futura Press, 1972.

Boggan, W. O. , Steele, R. A. , & Freedman, D. X. Delta-9-Tetrahydro-cannabinol effect on audiogenic seizure susceptibility. Psychopharm-acologia, 1973, 29, 101-106.

Boyd, E. S. , Boyd, E. H. , & Brown, L. E. The effects of some drugs on an evoked response senstitive to tetrahydrocannabinols. Journal of Pharmacology and Experimental Therapeutics, 1974, 189, 748-758.

Boyd, E. S. , Boyd, E. H., Muchmore, J. S. , & Brown, L. E. Effects of two tetrahydrocannabinols and of pentobarbital on cortico-cortical evoked responses in the squirrel monkey. Journal of Pharmacology and Experimental Therapeutics, 1971, 176, 480-488.

Braude, M. C. Toxicology of cannabinoids. In W. D. M. Paton and J. Crown (Eds.), Cannabis and its derivatives: Pharmacology and ex-perimental psychology. London: Oxford University Press, 1972.

Chesher, G. B. , & Jackson, D. M. Anticonvulsant effects of cannabinoids in mice: Drug interactions within cannabinoids and cannabinoid inter-actions with phenytoin. Psychopharmacologia, 1974, 37, 255-264.

Consroe, P. F. , Jones, B. C. , & Chin, L. Delta-9-Tetrahydrocannabinol, EEG and behavior: The importance of adaptation to the testing milieu. Pharmacology, Biochemistry and Behavior, 1975, 3, 173-177.

Consroe, P. F. , & Man, D. P. Effects of delta-8- and delta-9-tetrahydro-cannabinol on experimentally induced seizures. Life Sciences, 1973, 13, 429-439.

Consroe, P. F. , Man, D. P. , Chin, L. , & Picchioni, A. L. Reduction of audiogenic seizure by delta-8- and delta-9-tetrahydrocannabinols. Journal of Pharmacy and Pharmacology, 1973, 25, 764-765.

Consroe, P. F. , Wood, G. C. , & Buchsbaum, H. Anticonvulsant nature of marijuana smoking. Journal of the American Medical Association, 1975, 234, 306-307.

Corcoran, M. E. , McCaughran, J. A. , & Wada, J. A. Acute antiepileptic effects of delta-9-tetrahydrocannabinol in rats with kindled seizures. Experimental Neurology, 1973, 40, 471-483.

Cox, B. , Ham , M. T. , Loskota, W. J. , & Lomax, P. The anticonvulsant activity of cannabinoids in seizure sensitive gerbils. Proceedings of the Western Pharmacology Society, 1975, 18, 154-157.

Davis, J. P., & Ramsey, H. H. Antiepileptic actions of marijuana-active substances. Federation Proceedings, 1949, 8, 284. (Abstract)

deJong, R. H. Physiology and Pharmacology of Local Anaesthesia. Springfield, Ill. : Charles C. Thomas, 1970.

Domino, E. F. Neuropsychopharmacologic studies of marijuana: Some synthetic and natural THC derivatives in animals and man. Annals of the New York Academy of Sciences, 1971, 191, 166-191.

Dwivedi, C. , & Harbison, R. D. Anticonvulsant activities of delta-8 - and delta-9-tetrahydrocannabinol and uridine. Toxicology and Applied Pharmacology, 1975, 31, 452-458.

Feeney, D. M. , Wagner, H. R., McNamara, M. C. , & Weiss, G. Effects of tetrahydrocannabinol on hippocampal evoked afterdischarges in cats. Experimental Neurology, 1973, 41, 357-365.

Fried, P. A. , & McIntyre, D. C. Electrical and behavioral attenuation of the anti-convulsant properties of delta-9-THC following chronic administration. Psychopharmacologia, 1973, 31, 215-227.

Fujimori, M. , & Himwich, H. E. Delta-9-Tetrahydrocannabinol and the sleep-wakefulness cycle in rabbits. Physiology and Behavior, 1973, 11, 291-295.

Fujimori, M. , Trusty, D. M. , & Himwich, H. E. Delta-9-Tetrahydrocannabinol: Electroencephalographic changes and autonomic responses in the rabbit. Life Sciences, 1973, 12, 553-563.

Fujimoto, J. M. Modification of the effects of delta-9-tetrahydrocannabinol by phenobarbital pretreatment in mice. Toxicology and Applied Pharmacology, 1972, 23, 623-634.

Garriott, J. C. , Forney, R. B. , Hughes, F. W. , & Richards, A. B. Pharmacologic properties of some Cannabis related compounds. Archives Internationales de Pharmacodynamie et de Therapie, 1968, 171, 425-434.

Heath, R. G. Marijuana: Effects on deep and surface electroencephalograms of rhesus monkeys. Neuropharmacology, 1973, 12, 1-14.

Izquierdo, I., Orsingher, O. A. , & Berardi, A. C. Effect of cannabidiol and of other Cannabis sativa compounds on hippocampal seizure discharges. Psychopharmacologia, 1973, 28, 95-102.

Karler, R. , Cely, W. , & Turkanis, S. A. The anticonvulsant activity of cannabidiol and cannabinol. Life Sciences, 1973, 13, 1527-1531.

Karler, R. , Cely, W., & Turkanis, S. A. Anticonvulsant activity of delta-9-tetrahydrocannabinol and its 11-hydroxy and 8α, 11-dihydroxy-metabolites in the frog. Research Communications in Chemical Pathology and Pharmacology, 1974, 9, 441-452. (a)

Karler, R. , Cely, W., & Turkanis, S. A. Anticonvulsant properties of delta-9-tetrahydrocannabinol and other cannabinoids. Life Sciences, 1974, 15, 931-947. (b)

Karler, R. , Cely, W., & Turkanis, S. A. A study of the development of tolerance to an anticonvulsant effect of delta-9-tetrahydrocannabinol and cannabidiol. Research Communications in Chemical Pathology and Pharmacology, 1974, 9, 23-39. (c)

Karler, R. , Cely, W. , & Turkanis, S. A. A study of the relative anti-convulsant and toxic activities of delta-9-tetrahydrocannabinol and its congeners. Research Communications in Chemical Pathology and Pharmacology, 1974, 7, 353-358. (d)

Keeler, M. H. , & Reifler, C. F. Grand mal convulsions subsequent to marijuana use: Case report. Diseases of the Nervous System, 1967, 28, 474-475.

Killam, K. F., & Killam, E. K. The action of tetrahydrocannabinol on EEG and photomyoclonic seizures in the baboon. Fifth International Congress on Pharmacology, 1972, 124. (Abstract)

Lemberger, L., Martz, R., Rodda, B., Forney, R., & Rowe, H. Compara-tive pharmacology of delta-9-tetrahydrocannabinol and its metabolite, 11-OH delta-9-tetrahydrocannabinol. Journal of Clinical Investi-gation, 1973, 52, 2411-2417.

Lipparini, F. , Scotti de Carolis, A. , & Longo, V. G. A neuropharmacol-ogical investigation of some trans-tetrahydrocannabinol derivatives. Physiology and Behavior, 1969, 4, 527-532.

Litchfield, J. T. , & Wilcoxon, F. A. A simplified method of evaluating dose-effect experiments. Journal of Pharmacology and Experimental Therapeutics, 1949, 96, 99-133.

Loewe, S. , & Goodman, L. S. Anticonvulsant action of marihuana-active substances. Federation Proceedings, 1947, 6, 352. (Abstract)

Luthra, Y. K. , & Rosenkrantz, H. Cannabinoids: Neurochemical aspects after oral chronic administration to rats. Toxicology and Applied Pharmacology, 1974, 27, 158-168.

Luthra, Y. K. , Rosenkrantz, H. , Heyman, I. A. , & Braude, M. C.
Differential neurochemistry and temporal pattern in rats treated
orally with delta-9-tetrahydrocannabinol for periods up to six months.
Toxicology and Applied Pharmacology, 1975, 32, 418-431.

Martinez, J. L. , Stadnicki, S. W. , & Schaeppi, U. H. Delta-9-tetra-
hydrocannabinol: Effects on EEG and behavior of rhesus monkeys.
Life Sciences, 1972, 11, 643-651.

McCaughran, J. A. , Corcoran, M. E. , & Wada, J. A. Anticonvulsant
activity of delta-8- and delta-9-tetrahydrocannabinol in rats.
Pharmacology, Biochemistry and Behavior, 1974, 2, 227-233.

Meldrum, B. S. , Fariello, R. G., Puil, E. A. , Derouaux, M. , &
Naquet, R. Delta-9-Tetrahydrocannabinol and epilepsy in the
photosensitive baboon, Papio papio. Epilepsia, 1974, 15, 255-
264.

Moreton, J. E. , & Davis, W. M. Electroencephalographic study of the
effects of tetrahydrocannabinols on sleep in the rat. Neuropharmacology, 1973, 12, 897-907.

O'Shaughnessy, W. B. On the preparation of Indian hemp or gunjah.
Transactions of the Medical and Physical Society of Bombay, 1842,
8, 421-461.

Perez-Reyes, M. , & Wingfield, M. Cannabidiol and electroencephalographic epileptic activity. Journal of the American Medical
Association, 1974, 230, 1635.

Pirch, J. H., Cohn, R. A. , Barnes, P. R. , & Barratt, E. S. Effects of
acute and chronic administration of marijuana extract on the rat
electrocorticogram. Neuropharmacology, 1972, 11, 231-240.

Reynolds, J. R. Therapeutic uses and toxic effects of Cannabis indica.
Lancet, 1890, 1, 637-638.

Rosenkrantz, H., & Braude, M. C. Acute, subacute and 23-day chronic
marijuana inhalation toxicities in the rat. Toxicology and Applied
Pharmacology, 1974, 28, 428-441.

Rosenkrantz, H., Sprague, R. A. , Fleischman, R. W., & Braude, M. C.
Oral delta-9-tetrahydrocannabinol toxicity in rats treated for
periods up to six months. Toxicology and Applied Pharmacology,
1975, 32, 399-417.

Segal, M. Central implantation of cannabinoids: Induction of epileptiform
discharges. European Journal of Pharmacology, 1974, 27, 40-45.

Segal, M., & Barak, Y. Central excitatory effects of delta-1- and delta-6-
      tetrahydrocannabinol. Brain Research, 1972, 42, 547-548. (Abstract)

Segal, M., & Kenney, A. F. Delta-1- and delta-1(6)-tetrahydrocannabinol:
      Preliminary observations on similarities and differences in central
      pharmacological effects in the cat. Experientia, 1972, 28, 816-819.

Shaw, J. On the use of Cannabis indica in tetanus, hydrophobia, cholera
      with remarks on its effects. Madras Medical Journal, 1843, 5,
      74-80.

Sofia, R. D. , Kubena, R. K., & Barry, H. Comparison of four vehicles
      for intraperitoneal administration of delta-1-tetrahydrocannabinol.
      Journal of Pharmacy and Pharmacology, 1971, 23, 889-891. (a)

Sofia, R. D. , Solomon, T. A. , & Barry, H. The anticonvulsant activity in
      delta-1-tetrahydrocannabinol in mice. Pharmacologist, 1971, 13 (2),
      246. (Abstract) (b)

Sofia, R. D. , Kubena, R. K., & Barry H. Comparison among four vehicles
      and four routes for administering delta-9-tetrahydrocannabinol.
      Journal of Pharmaceutical Sciences, 1974, 63, 939-941.

Stadnicki, S. W., Schaeppi, U., Rosenkrantz, H., & Braude, M. C.
      Delta-9-Tetrahydrocannabinol: Subcortical spike bursts and motor
      manifestations in a Fischer rat treated orally for 109 days. Life
      Sciences, 1974, 14, 463-472.

Thompson, G. R., Mason, M. M. , Rosenkrantz, H. , & Braude, M. C.
      Chronic oral toxicity of cannabinoids in rats. Toxicology and Applied
      Pharmacology, 1973, 25, 373-390. (a)

Thompson, G. R., Rosenkrantz, H., Fleischman, R. W., & Braude, M. C.
      Effects of delta-9-tetrahydrocannabinol administered subcutaneously
      to rabbits for 28 days. Toxicology, 1975, 4, 41-51.

Thompson, G. R. , Rosenkrantz, H., Schaeppi, U. H., & Braude, M. C.
      Comparison of acute oral toxicity of cannabinoids in rats, dogs and
      monkeys. Toxicology and Applied Pharmacology, 1973, 25,
      363-372. (b)

Turkanis, S. A. , Cely, W., Olsen, D. M., & Karler, R. Anticonvulsant
      properties of cannabidiol. Research Communications in Chemical
      Pathology and Pharmacology, 1974, 8, 231-246.

Turkanis, S. A. , & Karler, R. Influence of cannabinoids on post-tetanic
      potentiation (PTP) at a bullfrog paravertebral ganglion. Federation
      Proceedings, 1975, 34 (3), 782. (Abstract)

Wada, J. A. , Sato, M. , & Corcoran, M. E. Antiepileptic properties of delta-9-tetrahydrocannabinol. Experimental Neurology, 1973, 39, 157-165.

Woodbury, D. M. Mechanisms of action of anticonvulsants. In H. Jasper, A. Ward, & A. Page (Eds.), Basic Mechanisms of the Epilepsies. Boston: Little, Brown, 1969.

Woodbury, L. A. , & Davenport, V. D. Design and use of a new electro-shock seizure apparatus, and analysis of factors altering seizure threshold and pattern. Archives Internationales de Pharmacodynamie et de Therapie, 1952, 92, 97-107.

CHAPTER 23

THE ANTIEPILEPTIC POTENTIAL OF THE CANNABINOIDS

Ralph Karler

Stuart A. Turkanis

Department of Pharmacology

University of Utah College of Medicine
Salt Lake City, Utah

NOTE: The authors are grateful to Dr. Monique C. Braude
for her continuous encouragement and support throughout this
work. The research was funded by the National Institute on
Drug Abuse research grant R01-DA-346, program project
grant 5P01-NS-4533, and pharmacology training grant GM-153.

INTRODUCTION

The anticonvulsant activity of marihuana and some of its surrogates
was first described by Loewe and Goodman in 1947; however, detailed studies
of the anticonvulsant activity of the cannabinoids were not undertaken until
recently when relatively pure cannabinoids became available.

There are numerous drugs that can block experimentally induced
seizures. Most of these agents remain laboratory curiosities because they
are either too toxic or they do not appear to offer any specific advantage
over the clinically established antiepileptics. Given the psychotoxicity of
marihuana, the cannabinoids would not appear to be therapeutically useful
as antiepileptics or, for that matter, for almost any other purpose. In addition,
the pharmacological properties of marihuana are legion and the drug's apparent lack of pharmacological selectivity bespeaks the poor clinical potential of marihuana itself (Paton, Pertwee and Tylden, 1973). There is, nevertheless, in the early literature evidence to suggest that some degree of anticonvulsant selectivity may be found within the individual cannabinoids.
First, Loewe and Goodman (1947) reported that the anticonvulsant activity
of some synthetic cannabinoids manifested itself in the absence of the motor

toxicity which is so characteristic of anticonvulsant doses of marihuana extract. Secondly, a limited clinical trial of some synthetic cannabinoids indicated that antiepileptic activity was not apparently associated with any psychic or motor toxicity (Davis and Ramsey, 1949); moreover, these cannabinoids checked seizures in patients who were inadequately controlled by conventional drug therapy. This complementary evidence prompted the initiation of our detailed investigation of the anticonvulsant activity of a number of cannabinoids.

The goal of this research is to determine the clinical potential of the cannabinoids as antiepileptics. The approach taken was to define the anticonvulsant properties of delta-9-tetrahydrocannabinol (delta-9-THC) so that it could be used as a reference standard for the evaluation of other cannabinoids, and to compare the cannabinoids with such established antiepileptics as diphenylhydantoin (DPH) and phenobarbital (PB).

ANTICONVULSANT PROPERTIES OF THE CANNABINOIDS

The data in Table 1 represent a summary of the effects of a single dose of the cannabinoids on a maximal electroshock (MES) test, which was used to assess anticonvulsant activity, and their effects on a bar-walk test, which was designed to measure neurotoxicity (Karler, Cely and Turkanis, 1974b). As can be seen, all four major naturally occurring agents -- delta-9-THC, delta-8-THC, cannabidiol (CBD), and cannabinol (CBN) -- are active anticonvulsants in this particular test. Furthermore, the principal, primary metabolite of delta-9-THC, the 11-hydroxy derivative, is also an anticonvulsant, as is the synthetic congener, dimethylheptylpyran (DMHP). Although the latter two substances are more potent than any of the naturally occurring cannabinoids, it is more significant to note here that both CBD and CBN are pharmacologically active. Hitherto, CBD and CBN were usually ignored in laboratory studies because of their purported pharmacological inactivity (Mechoulam, Shani, Edery and Grunfeld, 1970). Indeed, some of the early studies of these drugs did indicate a lack of psychoactivity, which in all likelihood accounts for the paucity of animal data on their other properties.

The data in Table 1 additionally illustrate that the anticonvulsant-dose 50 (ED50) for the 11-hydroxy metabolite is substantially lower than that for the parent compound, delta-9-THC. The relatively high potency of the metabolite raises the possibility that the anticonvulsant activity of delta-9-THC may be due, at least in part, to the metabolite, and this suggestion is further supported by the 11-hydroxy derivative's shorter time to peak effect. The results of a similar study in rats confirm both its potency and the more rapid onset of its peak effect compared with that of delta-9-THC. Furthermore, the mechanism of anticonvulsant action of 11-hydroxy-delta-9-THC appears to resemble that of DPH. Both drugs block post-tetanic potentiation in the isolated sympathetic ganglia (Turkanis and Karler, 1975); in contrast, delta-9-THC, even in massive doses, does not alter post-tetanic potentiation.

Table 1

Effects of a Single Dose of Cannabinoid in Mice in a
Maximal Electroshock and a Bar-walk Test*

Drug	Peak-effect Time (hr)**	ED50 (mg/kg)	TD50 (mg/kg)	Protective Index (TD50/ED50)
Delta-9-THC	2	101	84	0.8
Delta-8-THC	2	83	152	1.8
CBN	1	230	230	1.0
CBD	1	118	175	1.5
11-OH-delta-9-THC	1	14	22	1.6
DMHP	2	13	5.4	0.4

*   All experiments were performed at an ambient temperature of approxi-
    mately 22°C; ED50 and TD50 values were calculated by the method of
    Litchfield & Wilcoxon (1949) from conventional dose-response curves
    based on 3 to 6 doses with 15 to 20 animals for each dose; drugs were
    administered i.p.

** The peak-effect times for the anticonvulsant and toxic effects were
    similar.

Such an observation also suggests that the 11-hydroxy derivative accounts for
the anticonvulsant activity of delta-9-THC.

        The synthetic cannabinoid DMHP was included in this study because
it was one of the compounds subjected to the apparently successful but very
limited antiepileptic clinical trial referred to above. The ED50 for DMHP, as
shown in Table 1, indicates that it is more potent than delta-9-THC, but it
is not, as reported by Davis and Ramsey (1949) in their clinical trial, 150
times more potent in the MES test than is DPH. Although the data are not
given here, in our experiments these two drugs have similar potency. Hardman,
Domino and Seevers (1971) have suggested that such alleged differences in
the pharmacological activity of DMHP may emanate from its various isomers,
for the compound contains three asymmetric carbon atoms; therefore, eight
optical isomers are possible. In fact, the results of a study of the comparative activity of two isomers of DMHP do demonstrate different potencies. In

the mouse, the d, l, -threo form is several times more potent in the MES test than is the d, l, -erythro form (Karler et al., 1974b).

The protective indices in Table 1 illustrate that anticonvulsant activity is at least partially separable from motor or neurotoxicity; in other words, some degree of selectivity can be elicited from these drugs. The rationale for the calculation of the protective index is based on the clinical observation that the principal toxic limitation of antiepileptics is generally neurotoxicity. As can be seen, several of the cannabinoids have higher protective indices than does delta-9-THC. In this group CBD stands out for two reasons: First, its protective index of 1.5 is approximately the same as that of the very important antiepileptic PB (Swinyard, 1969); and secondly, unlike the others, CBD is devoid of both marihuana-like psychic and cardiac activity in humans, even in massive intravenous doses (Perez-Reyes, Timmons, Davis and Wall, 1973). The concurrence of relatively high anticonvulsant activity and low toxicity argues CBD's clinical potential as an antiepileptic agent, and a more detailed analysis of its pharmacological properties is, therefore, warranted. For this reason, we began to examine CBD's anticonvulsant properties relative to those of delta-9-THC.

The data in Table 2 represent, in three different species, the comparative activity of delta-9-THC and CBD in an MES test following acute treatment (Karler et al., 1974a, 1974b). From mouse to frog (Rana pipiens), there is a 1000-fold variation in potency for both delta-9-THC and CBD; this enormous difference in potency dramatically demonstrates the inherent dangers of extrapolating data from one species to another, including the human. The frog with its great sensitivity to the cannabinoids thus appears to constitute an ideal model for an anticonvulsant screening test, particularly

Table 2

Anticonvulsant Activity in an MES Test in Different
Species Acutely Treated with Delta-9-THC or CBD*

Species	ED50 (mg/kg)	
	delta-9-THC	CBD
Mouse	101	118
Rat	4.3	50
Frog (Rana pipiens)	0.1	0.1

* Drugs injected into peritoneum of mouse and rat and ventral lymph sac of frog.

when only small quantities of a drug are available. For example, the 8α, 11-dihydroxy metabolite was shown to be about as active an anticonvulsant as are delta-9-THC and the 11-hydroxy metabolite, at least in the frog (Karler et al., 1974a); but the extreme sensitivity of the frog in this test appears to be a unique response to the cannabinoids because the anticonvulsant potency of DPH and PB in the frog is approximately the same as that in the rat and mouse (Karler et al., 1974a). This uniqueness again underscores the potential complexity of any extrapolation of pharmacological effects from one species to another.

The frog as a routine test object, however, has its drawbacks, for its above-described sensitivity to the cannabinoids is seasonal, that is, limited to the summer. In the winter, Rana pipiens is responsive to neither delta-9-THC nor CBD, even in massive doses. The change in sensitivity, it should be noted, is not restricted to the cannabinoids, because winter frogs are not protected against seizures in the MES test by even relatively large doses of either DPH or PB; the seasonal change appears, therefore, to be a phenomenon involving anticonvulsants in general, rather than cannabinoids in particular.

The data in Table 3 summarize the activity of delta-9-THC, CBD, DPH, and PB in a variety of electrically and chemically (pentylenetetrazol, PTZ) induced seizure tests (Karler et al., 1974b; Turkanis, Cely, Olsen and Karler, 1974). These data show that, with one exception, all the drugs are capable of totally blocking hind-limb extension in maximal seizures induced either electrically or by PTZ; the exception is delta-9-THC, which has only limited effectiveness in blocking PTZ-caused maximal seizures. In this test the dose-response results indicate that only about 50% of the mice can be protected by delta-9-THC, even in doses as high as 400 mg/kg (Turkanis et al., 1974).

In the MES threshold test all the drugs can raise the current required to produce a maximal seizure, but in the 60-Hz-EST test only PB is an effective anticonvulsant (Table 3). In contrast, the threshold for minimal seizures is elevated by all the drugs in the 6-Hz-EST test. The effects of the drugs, however, in the PTZ minimal-seizure test are variable: Here, PB raises the threshold dose and delta-9-THC actually decreases the threshold dose for producing minimal seizures. The latter effect suggests that delta-9-THC can increase central-nervous-system (CNS) excitability; an increase in overt excitability has also been reported in animals chronically treated with delta-9-THC (Thompson, Fleischman, Rosenkrantz and Braude, 1974). In contrast to the delta-9-THC and PB results, both CBD and DPH appear to be inactive as anticonvulsants in the PTZ minimal-seizure threshold test; the latter two drugs produce similar effects in all six of the seizure tests. In some of the early reports, the anticonvulsant effects of delta-9-THC were considered comparable to those of DPH, but the results of the more detailed studies described in Table 3 indicate that there are differences between delta-9-THC and CBD, and that CBD more closely resembles DPH than does delta-9-THC.

Table 3

Comparison of the Anticonvulsant Properties of Delta-9-THC, CBD,
DPH and PB in Various Seizure Tests in Single Dose-treated Mice*

	Seizure Test**					
	Maximal		Threshold			
			Maximal Seizures	Minimal Seizures		
				60-Hz-	6-Hz-	
Drug	MES	PTZ	MES	EST	EST	PTZ
delta-9-THC (100 mg/kg)	+	+,0	+	0	+	-
CBD (120 mg/kg)	+	+	+	0	+	0
DPH (7 mg/kg)	+	+	+	0	+	0
PB (12 mg/kg)	+	+	+	+	+	+

*　　The dose of each drug represents the ED50 i.p. in the MES test, and all measurements of activity were made at the time of peak effect in the MES test: delta-9-THC, 2 hr; CBD, 1 hr; DPH, 2 hr; PB, 3 hr.

**　MES, maximal electroshock test; PTZ, pentylenetetrazol s.c.; 60- and 6-Hz-EST, 60- and 6-Hz-electroshock thresholds.

+,　effective in blocking hind-limb extension in maximal seizures or in elevating seizure threshold.

0,　not effective.

+,0, limited effectiveness.

-,　decreases seizure threshold.

THE RELATIONSHIP BETWEEN ANTICONVULSANT ACTIVITY
AND BRAIN CONCENTRATIONS OF DELTA-9-THC

The general theory that the 11-hydroxy metabolite is responsible for some of the pharmacological properties of delta-9-THC has been proposed by many investigators (see Lemberger, 1972). In the particular case of anti-convulsant activity both substances are active; and, as shown above, the metabolite is several times more potent than the parent drug. Thus, the possibility that the anticonvulsant activity is actually due to the formation of the 11-hydroxy derivative suggested another set of experiments: The time course of anticonvulsant activity and of the cannabinoid content of the brain was determined in order to correlate the brain concentration of delta-9-THC and its metabolite with the effect. Both rats and mice were used in these studies and the results are depicted in Figures 1 and 2. The relationship between cannabinoid-brain concentrations and anticonvulsant activity appears similar in both species; that is, neither delta-9-THC nor its 11-hydroxy metabolite correlates with the time course of activity. The lack of correlation is most striking at 4 hr in the rat and at 6 hr in the mouse. At these times there is no remaining anticonvulsant activity in the MES test, yet in both species substantial amounts of the parent compound and its metabolite are present in the brain. Several explanations for these results are possible. One explanation is that neither of these substances accounts for the anti-convulsant activity, but that a yet-unidentified metabolite is the active form

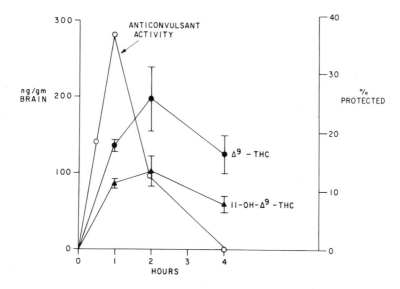

Figure 1. Time course of anticonvulsant activity and of brain concentrations of delta-9-THC and its 11-hydroxy metabolite in the rat. Anticonvulsant activity was measured as a percentage of the animals protected in an MES test; the cannabinoids were separated from brain extracts by thin-layer chromatography and quantitated with the use of 3H-delta-9-THC. The dose of delta-9-THC in these experiments was 5 mg/kg i.p.

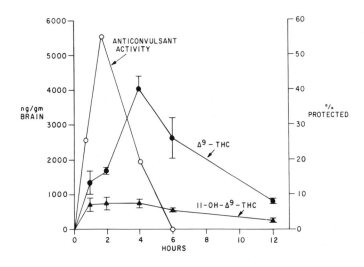

Figure 2. Time course of anticonvulsant activity and of brain concentrations of delta-9-THC and its 11-hydroxy metabolite in the mouse. Anticonvulsant activity was measured as a percentage of the animals protected in an MES test; the cannabinoids were separated from brain extracts by thin-layer chromatography and quantitated with the use of ^{3}H-delta-9-THC. The dose of delta-9-THC in these experiments was 80 mg/kg i.p.

of delta-9-THC. The "unidentified metabolite" interpretation is supported by the observations in the frog that the 8α, 11-dihydroxy metabolite of delta-9-THC is also a very active anticonvulsant (Karler et al., 1974a). Obviously, the possibility exists that still other metabolites are anticonvulsant.

Another explanation for the lack of correlation described above is the development of acute tolerance. While tolerance does develop to the protective effect of delta-9-THC in the MES test after repeated daily administration (Karler et al., 1974b, 1974c), it is not known whether tolerance develops acutely. The tolerance associated with repeated daily administration is characterized by the accumulation of cannabinoids in the brain; it appears, therefore, to be due to functional rather than dispositional changes (Karler and Turkanis, 1975).

INTERACTION OF CBD WITH OTHER ANTICONVULSANTS

Loewe (1944) first observed that CBD prolonged barbiturate sleep time; and Paton and Pertwee (1972), Fernandes, Warning, Christ and Hill (1973), and Siemans, Kalant, Khanna, Marshman and Ho (1974) confirmed this observation. On the basis of in-vitro studies they concluded that the prolongation of sleep time was probably the consequence of CBD's ability to inhibit barbiturate metabolism by the hepatic microsomal enzyme system. It has also been suggested that such inhibition of drug metabolism may be related to this cannabinoid's very high binding affinity for cytochrome P-450 (Bailey and Toft, 1973; Fernandes et al., 1973).

The fact that CBD can inhibit hepatic drug metabolism offers another potential use therapeutically. Drug combinations are frequently employed in the treatment of epilepsy, and conceivably CBD's ability to block drug metabolism could serve to prolong and enhance the anticonvulsant activity of drugs such as PB and DPH. There are published data which demonstrate that pretreatment of animals with CBD does in fact markedly enhance the anticonvulsant activity of these two drugs in the MES test (Turkanis et al., 1974). In these studies CBD was administered 20 hr prior to PB or DPH; there are other studies which describe a similar enhancement of activity by the concomitant administration of CBD with PB or DPH (Chesher and Jackson, 1974; Chesher, Jackson and Malor, 1975).

INFLUENCE OF REPEATED DAILY TREATMENT ON THE ANTICONVULSANT EFFECTS OF THE CANNABINOIDS

Tolerance of delta-9-THC has been generally reported to develop (see Paton, 1975), but there are some investigators who maintain that repeated treatment does not result in tolerance (Ham and Noordwijk, 1973; Ferraro and Grilly, 1973). Furthermore, still others claim that an increase, rather than a decrease, in sensitivity appears with chronic delta-9-THC treatment (Carlini, Mazur, Karniol and Leite, 1972). Presumably, the conflicting available data may be reconciled by the consideration that the response to chronic treatment depends in part upon the specific effect. Once again, in the particular instance of anticonvulsant activity, a marked tolerance rapidly develops in both rats and mice to the cannabinoids' protective effect in an MES test (Karler et al., 1974b, 1974c). A more detailed investigation of their anticonvulsant effects in mice in a variety of both maximal and minimal seizure tests indicates a very complex response to repeated treatment. A summary of these studies is shown in Table 4.

The animals were treated daily for the number of days noted with an intraperitoneal injection of an ED50 for the MES test (delta-9-THC, 100 mg/kg; CBD, 120 mg/kg; DPH, 7 mg/kg; and PB, 12 mg/kg). Anticonvulsant activity was measured at the time of peak effect following the final drug treatment and was expressed in terms of median-effective values, as determined from conventional dose-response curves. The resulting median-effective values from control (single-dose treated) and repeatedly drug-treated animals were compared for changes in sensitivity. A decrease in sensitivity (tolerance) in the MES test was observed for all the drugs; however, the responses in the other tests were variable. In the maximal EST test, the only change in sensitivity, tolerance, was seen with delta-9-THC; in this instance, CBD resembles DPH and PB because none of these drugs produced tolerance. Tolerance did not develop to either delta-9-THC or CBD in the 60-Hz-EST test, but it did to PB. The response to DPH in this test was strikingly different, because repeated treatment resulted in an increase in sensitivity

Table 4

Influence of Daily Anticonvulsant Treatment on the
Sensitivity of Mice in Four Electroshock Seizure Tests*

Drug	Days of Treatment	MES	Maximal EST	60-Hz-EST	6-Hz-EST
Delta-9-THC	3	↓**	↓**	0	↑**
CBD	4	↓**	0	0	↑**
DPH	4	↓**	0	↑**	0
PB	4	↓**	0	↓**	↓**

*   MES, a maximal electroshock test; maximal EST, maximal electroshock
     threshold; 60- and 6-Hz-EST, 60- and 6-Hz-electroshock threshold for
     minimal seizures.

**   Median-effective value after repeated daily treatment is significantly
     different from control (single dose-treated group), as indicated by a
     relative potency test ($P \leq 0.05$).

to the drug. A similar phenomenon appeared in the 6-Hz-EST test with
delta-9-THC and CBD, but in this case there was no quantitative change in
response by the DPH animals. Finally, tolerance also developed to PB in the
6-Hz-EST test.

The results in Table 4 clearly illustrate that tolerance does develop
to some of the anticonvulsant effects of the cannabinoids, but not to all of
them. In fact, the reverse situation obtains in the 6-Hz-EST test in which an
increase in sensitivity manifests itself with repeated treatment. A comparison
of the cannabinoids' results with those of DPH and PB indicates a general
similarity: Here, too, tolerance to the antiepileptics does not develop in all
the tests, for some tests are characterized by no change in sensitivity and
even, in one instance, an increase in sensitivity to DPH. Clinically, it
must be remembered, tolerance to the antiepileptic activity of either DPH or
PB does not develop (Buchthal and Lennox-Buchthal, 1972), despite the
indications in Table 4 of PB tolerance in three of the four tests. Only the
results from the maximal EST test correlate with clinical observations of
chronic DPH and PB use; and on the basis of this test, CBD more closely
resembles the well-established antiepileptics than does delta-9-THC.

EFFECTS OF THE CESSATION OF REPEATED, DAILY TREATMENT ON CNS EXCITABILITY

Upon withdrawal, CNS depressants characteristically produce a "rebound" hyperexcitability of the CNS. This phenomenon is dramatically demonstrated in some drug-dependent individuals by the seizure activity associated with the abstinence syndrome. Sudden termination of antiepileptic therapy may also precipitate seizures, presumably, in part, by a similar "rebound" mechanism. Although there is no evidence of the classical type of withdrawal effects associated with the use of marihuana, the following study of the effect of the cessation of treatment on CNS excitability was undertaken because the tests employed represent sensitive measures of excitability; therefore, changes smaller than those necessary for the onset of frank seizures can be detected. In our experiments CNS excitability was measured by determining the median-effective current or voltage necessary for the seizure threshold in three separate tests: the MES threshold, the 60-Hz- and the 6-Hz-EST. The threshold tests were administered 24 hr after the final drug treatment. The results in control (vehicle treated) and drug-treated groups were compared following withdrawal from delta-9-THC, CBD, DPH, and PB. The daily intraperitoneal dosages of these drugs were the same as those used to obtain the data shown in Table 4; the days of treatment prior to withdrawal were selected because they were previously shown to result in marked tolerance to the protective effect of these drugs (ED50) in a maximal electroshock test. The results are summarized in Table 5, and they indicate that drug treatment and subsequent withdrawal from delta-9-THC is coincident with an increased CNS excitability, as measured by a decrease in the electrical threshold for minimal seizures in both the 60-Hz- and 6-Hz-EST tests. The threshold for maximal seizures in the MES test, however, was unaffected by delta-9-THC. The results in the CBD-treated animals are strikingly different: Increased excitability upon withdrawal was not observed in any of the tests. On the contrary, in the 6-Hz-EST there is an actual decrease in CNS excitability. Withdrawal from DPH did not alter the threshold values in any of the tests; therefore, withdrawal from this drug is not associated with any changes in CNS excitability as measured under these experimental conditions. In contrast, the cessation of PB treatment produces hyperexcitability in the MES threshold and in the 60-Hz-EST tests. The results of threshold tests with PB are consonant with the clinical data on the abrupt withdrawal of PB from drug-abuse patients. Here, withdrawal is associated with symptoms of hyperexcitability, including seizures. The "rebound" hyperexcitability following delta-9-THC treatment may account for the report linking the use of marihuana with the precipitation of seizures in an epileptic (Keeler and Reifler, 1967).

CONCLUSIONS

The main goal of the work described above is to determine the clinical potential of the cannabinoids as antiepileptics. On the basis of laboratory data in animals and on clinical data, CBD appears to have a good potential for this purpose. In animals it has a relatively high protective

Table 5

Influence of Withdrawal from Daily Anticonvulsant Treatment
On the Thresholds for Electrically Induced Seizures

Drug	Days of Treatment	Change in Threshold After Withdrawal*		
		Maximal EST	60–Hz–EST	6–Hz–EST
Delta–9–THC	2	0	↓**	↓**
CBD	3	0	0	↑**
DPH	3	0	0	0
PB	3	↓**	↓**	0

* Threshold determined 24 hr after withdrawal.

** Change in threshold is significantly different from control (vehicle-treated), as indicated by a relative potency test (P ≤ 0.05); the median-effective values determined from conventional dose-response type curves (Litchfield & Wilcoxon, 1949).

index; that is, its anticonvulsant activity manifests itself at lower doses than does its neurotoxicity. The protective index for CBD is similar to that for the well-established antiepileptic PB. Furthermore, in humans CBD is devoid of the psychotoxicity and of the cardiac effects of delta-9-THC and its 11-hydroxy metabolite. The combination of these properties suggests that this cannabinoid may be an acceptable agent for human trial; however, any further assessment of the clinical potential of CBD must be deferred, because it has not been extensively studied and little is known about its general pharmacological and toxicological properties. Such data are necessary before any serious consideration can be given to the use of CBD or any other cannabinoid in humans.

REFERENCES

Bailey, K., & Toft, P. Difference spectra of rat hepatic microsomes induced by cannabinoids and related compounds. Biochemical Pharmacology, 1973, 22, 2780-2783.

Buchthal, F., & Lennox-Buchthal, M.A. Diphenylhydantoin: Relation of anticonvulsant effect to concentration in serum. In D. M. Woodbury, J. K. Penry, & R. P. Schmidt (Eds.), Antiepileptic Drugs. New York: Raven Press, 1972, 193-209.

Carlini, E. A., Mazur, J., Karniol, I. G., & Leite, R. Cannabis sativa: Is it possible to consider behavioural animal data as experimental models for some effects in humans? In W. D. M. Paton & J. Crown (Eds.), Cannabis and Its Derivatives. London: Oxford University Press, 1972, 154-175.

Chesher, G.B., & Jackson, D.M. Anticonvulsant effects of cannabinoids in mice: Drug interactions with cannabinoids and cannabinoid interactions with phenytoin. Psychopharmacologia, 1974, 37, 255-264.

Chesher, G.B., Jackson, D.M., & Malor, R.M. Interaction of delta-9-tetrahydrocannabinol and cannabinol with phenobarbitone in protecting mice from electrically induced convulsions. Journal of Pharmacy and Pharmacology, 1975, 27, 608-609.

Fernandes, M., Warning, N., Christ, W., & Hill, R. Interactions of several cannabinoids with the hepatic drug metabolizing system. Biochemical Pharmacology, 1973, 22, 2981-2987.

Ferraro, D.P., & Grilly, D.M. Lack of tolerance to delta-9-tetrahydrocannabinol in chimpanzees. Science, 1973, 179, 490-492.

Ham, M. ten, & Noordwijk, J. van. Lack of tolerance to the effect of two tetrahydrocannabinols on aggressiveness. Psychopharmacologia, 1973, 29, 171-176.

Hardman, H.F., Domino, E.F., & Seevers, M. H. General pharmacological actions of some synthetic tetrahydrocannabinol derivatives. Pharmacological Reviews, 1971, 23, 295-315.

Karler, R., Cely, W., & Turkanis, S.A. Anticonvulsant activity of delta-9-tetrahydrocannabinol and its 11-hydroxy and 8α, 11-dihydroxy metabolites in the frog. Research Communications in Chemical Pathology and Pharmacology, 1974, 9, 441-452. [a]

Karler, R., Cely, W., & Turkanis, S.A. Anticonvulsant properties of delta-9-tetrahydrocannabinol and other cannabinoids. Life Science, 1974, 15, 931-947. [b]

Karler, R., Cely, W., & Turkanis, S.A. A study of the development of tolerance to an anticonvulsant effect of delta-9-tetrahydrocannabinol and cannabidiol. Research Communications in Chemical Pathology and Pharmacology, 1974, 9, 23-29 [c].

Karler, R., & Turkanis, S.A. The development of tolerance and "reverse tolerance" to the anticonvulsant activity of delta-9-tetrahydrocannabinol and cannabidiol. In M. C. Braude & S. Szara (Eds.), Pharmacology of Marijuana. New York: Raven Press, 1975 (in press).

Keeler, M.H., & Reifler, C.B. Grand mal convulsions subsequent to marijuana use. Diseases of the Nervous System, 1967, 28, 474-475.

Litchfield, J.T. & Wilcoxon, F. A simplified method for evaluating dose-effect experiments. Journal of Pharmacology and Experimental Therapeutics, 1949, 96, 91-113.

Loewe, S. Studies on the pharmacology of marijuana. In The Mayor's Committee on Marijuana, The Marijuana Problem in the City of New York. Lancaster, Pa.: Jacques Cattell Press, 1944, 149-212.

Loewe, S., & Goodman, L.S. Anticonvulsant action of marihuana-active substances. Federation Proceedings, 1947, 6, 352.

Mechoulam, R., Shani, A., Edery, H., & Grunfeld, Y. Chemical basis of hashish activity. Science, 1970, 169, 611-612.

Paton, W.D.M. Pharmacology of marihuana. Annual Reviews of Pharmacology, 1975, 15, 191-220.

Paton, W.D.M., & Pertwee, R.G. Effect of cannabis and certain of its constituents on pentobarbitone sleeping time and phenazone metabolism. British Journal of Pharmacology, 1972, 44, 250-261.

Paton, W.D.M., Pertwee, R.G., & Tylden, E. Clinical aspects of cannabis action. In R. Mechoulam (Ed.), Marijuana. New York: Academic Press, 1973, 335-365.

Perez-Reyes, M., Timmons, M.D., Davis, K.H., & Wall, M.E. A comparison of the pharmacological activity in man of intravenously administered delta-9-tetrahydrocannabinol, cannabinol, and cannabidiol. Experientia, 1973, 29, 1368-1369.

Siemens, A.J., Kalant, H., Khanna, J.M., Marshman, J., & Ho, G. Effect of cannabis on pentobarbital-induced sleeping time and pentobarbital metabolism in the rat. Biochemical Pharmacology, 1974, 23, 477-488.

Swinyard, E.A. Laboratory evaluation of anticonvulsant drugs. Epilepsia, 1969, 10, 107-119.

Thompson, G.R., Fleischman, R.W., Rosenkrantz, H., & Braude, M.C. Oral and intravenous toxicity of delta-9-tetrahydrocannabinol in rhesus monkeys. Toxicology and Applied Pharmacology, 1974, 27, 648-665.

Turkanis, S.A., Cely, W., Olsen, D.M., & Karler, R. Anticonvulsant properties of cannabidiol. Research Communications in Chemical Pathology and Pharmacology, 1974, 8, 231-246.

Turkanis, S.A., & Karler, R. Influence of anticonvulsant cannabinoids on posttetanic potentiation of isolated bullfrog ganglia. Life Sciences, 1975, 17, 569-578.

DISCUSSION

Plotnikoff: In light of the presentations this morning, I am particularly struck by the psychic properties of delta-9, and I am curious if anyone has observed any interaction effects of anticonvulsants.

Feeney: I am unaware of any.

Turkanis: We have done some studies pretreating animals with cannabidiol, and even 24 hours after treatment with cannabidiol there is some enhancement of not only diphenylhydantoin activity, but also a similar enhancement of phenobarbital and a slight enhancement of delta-9 anticonvulsant activities. Whether this will be a problem clincally will be difficult to determine from our animal studies, but the potential for interaction is there.

Cohen: Dr. Consroe, what happened to your rabbits when you exposed them to the various convulsants -- metrazol, electric shock, and so on.

Consroe: Dr. Cohen, we haven't done that yet. We were limited by the number of rabbits that we had and we were very careful to choose what drugs we gave them. At this point, we are continuing some studies -- injecting other cannabinoids into these to see what happens. As far as I know right now, delta-8 causes the identical type convulsions that delta-9 does.

Vachon: Dr. Karler, in your studies on the last slide, you have administered treatment for two or three days; is that a sufficient length of time to ascertain the rebound effects?

Karler: Well, we chose that arbitrarily because at that time we had observed a marked tolerance in the electroshock test. We actually had done this with the single treatment; we never pursued that in the same detail, and I suppose like any other of the rebound phenomena, the longer we treat them and the higher the dose, we probably get more effect.

Harris: I am puzzled now. We have been talking about this for at least a decade. We have had animal data showing at least cannabidiol had relatively good anticonvulsant activity and a pretty good safety ratio, as good if not better than most of the drugs that are used in the marketplace. Is anyone carrying out any human studies to determine whether there is any anticonvulsant activity?

Mechoulam: Carlini is using something like 100 mg of cannabidiol. I hope that in a few months we will have some information.

Karler: I talked to Carlini and he is waiting for Mechoulam to give him drugs, but he had another problem, and he asked me the question, "How much do you give a human?" "How frequently do you dose him?" I told him I would give him some answers in about a year. We are about ready to give him some answers on how rapidly the human liver metabolizes cannabidiol, and maybe then we can get some idea of what dose we use, and how long will it hang around. I can say this, with the preliminary indications we have: cannabidiol is metabolized about as fast as delta-9-THC.

Lemberger: I agree with Lou Harris. It is somewhat disturbing since the National Institute of Health has a program and there is information that cannabidiol is an active anticonvulsant. The chronic toxicity should be done by NIH, and it should be tested. They are testing many other compounds. If this is an exciting anticonvulsant, I think they should test it.

Cohen: I don't know what the antiepileptic dose of cannabidiol is, but in a pilot study we have given a single dose, 1600 mgs. of cannabidiol orally without any effect whatsoever.

Braude: There is one question I think is important -- that is the question of repeated administration. Dr. Karler has shown you some data which, after two or three days, the effect turns into an entirely different picture. I would suggest that after a month of repeated administration, the picture might be completely different and the effect completely reversed.

Jones: I can think of at least one other not-so-exotic drug that at first produces depression and sedation, and things like that, but with continued administration at high doses, then one sees seizure, hallucination, delirium -- and that, of course, is alcohol. After a month or six weeks at high doses, even though the alcohol doses continue, the subject will go into d.t.'s. Almost the same thing is true of barbiturates, if you are talking about one gram a day. So it may not be so surprising that cannabis has this effect.

Karler: There may be changes occurring with chronic treatment, and I think they have to be looked at, and I have been telling you we are going to do it. There is another point here that comes up over and over again:

people tend to be disturbed by the fact that here we have a compound that
has both excitatory properties and anticonvulsant properties. I don't think
there is a single anticonvulsant that doesn't do this, including Dilantin. We
just have to get the right conditions.

Synthetic Cannabinoid-Like Compounds

CHAPTER 24

CLINICAL PHARMACOLOGY OF NATURAL AND SYNTHETIC
CANNABINOIDS

Louis Lemberger

Lilly Laboratory for Clinical Research
Lilly Research Laboratories

Departments of Pharmacology and Medicine
Indiana University School of Medicine
Indianapolis, Indiana

Cannabis sativa, the plant from which marihuana and hashish are derived, has been used for medicinal purposes for the past 5,000 years. About 3,000 B.C. the Chinese Emperor Shen Nung published a monograph in which cannabis was reportedly used for asthma, migraine, and certain gynecologic disorders. It was recognized as an official drug and was listed in the United States Pharmacopoeia until 1937, at which time the Narcotics and Marihuana Law came into effect.

Over the past few decades cannabis has been viewed differently by various groups in our society and it indeed has become a major social issue. However, for the purposes of this presentation, cannabis will be considered as a mixture of many cannabinoids with concern only for one of its constituents, delta-9-tetrahydrocannabinol (delta-9-THC). In 1964 Gaoni and Mechoulam (1964) isolated delta-9-THC (Figure 1) from cannabis, elucidated its structure, and demonstrated that it was the major psychoactive constituent of marihuana. It is essentially responsible for all of marihuana's effects. Delta-9-THC is especially of interest to scientists and clinicians because of its marked potency in producing its CNS effects, while possessing only a low incidence of toxicity (that is, it has a large therapeutic index).

The pharmacology of delta-9-THC has been extensively studied in man (Isbell, 1967; Hollister, Richards and Gillespie, 1968; Weiss, Watanabe, Lemberger, Tamarkin and Cardon, 1972; Galanter, Wyatt, Lemberger, Weingartner, Vaughan and Roth, 1972) (Table 1). After its inhalation, oral administration, or intravenous administration, delta-9-THC produces a marked tachycardia while having minimal effects on lying and standing blood pressure. It also causes a psychologic "high" or euphoria, psychomotor

405

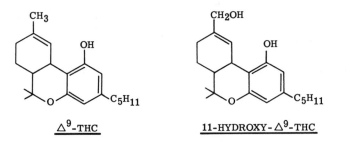

Figure 1. Chemical structure of delta–9–THC and its metabolite, 11–
hydroxy–delta–9–THC.

Table 1

CLINICAL PHARMACOLOGY OF $\triangle^9$-THC
AFTER SINGLE DOSES

1)   MARKED TACHYCARDIA

2)   MINIMAL EFFECT ON BLOOD PRESSURE
       (LYING OR STANDING)

3)   PSYCHOLOGIC "HIGH" (EUPHORIA)

4)   OTHER SYMPTOMS & SIGNS
       (DRY MOUTH, CONJUNCTIVAL INJECTION)

5)   PSYCHOMOTOR IMPAIRMENT

6)   RELAXATION AND SEDATION

impairment, and other symptomatology including dry mouth and conjunctival injection. After its initial stimulant phase, it produces relaxant and sedative effects. Thus, delta-9-THC appears to produce both stimulant and sedative type effects.

In animals and man, delta-9-THC is metabolized by liver microsomal enzymes to 11-OH-delta-9-THC, a monohydroxylated compound (Figure 1). This compound, although to date administered only by the intravenous route, appears to produce essentially the same pharmacologic effects as delta-9-THC (Lemberger, Crabtree and Rowe, 1972; Perez-Reyes, Timmons, Lipton, Davis and Wall, 1972; Hollister, 1974). It has been postulated that this metabolic product might be responsible for some of the psychologic effects of delta-9-THC.

Having earlier studied the pharmacologic effects of delta-9-THC and 11-OH-delta-9-THC, it became of interest to study the clinical pharmacology of DMHP (delta-6a, 10a-dimethylheptyl tetrahydrocannabinol) (Figure 2) a synthetic cannabinol which, from animal studies, appeared to be more potent than delta-9-THC. The clinical pharmacologic properties of DMHP are presented in Table 2 (Sidell, Pless, Neitlich, Sussman, Copelan and Sim, 1973; Lemberger, McMahon, Archer, Matsumoto and Rowe, 1974). After the intravenous administration of DMHP (total dose of 200 μg), subjects evidenced a marked tachycardia which occurred shortly after drug administration and peaked at 30-45 minutes. This was accompanied by the occurrence of a decrease in systolic blood pressure while the subjects were supine and a pronounced postural hypotension when the subjects stood (Figure 3).

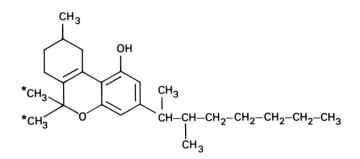

Figure 2. Chemical structure of DMHP.

Table 2

CLINICAL PHARMACOLOGY OF DMHP
AFTER SINGLE DOSES

1)   MARKED TACHYCARDIA

2)   MINIMAL BLOOD PRESSURE EFFECTS
     WHILE LYING
     PRONOUNCED POSTURAL HYPOTENSION

3)   ABSENCE OF PSYCHOLOGIC "HIGH"

4)   DRY MOUTH

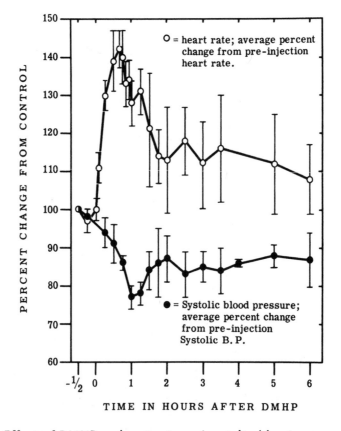

Figure 3. Effect of DMHP on heart rate and systolic blood pressure after
the intravenous administration of DMHP (200 μg intravenously).
Open circles indicate heart rate; closed circles indicate systolic
blood pressure.

In addition to the cardiovascular effects observed after DMHP administration, a major symptom was the production of dry mouth. In contrast to the studies conducted with delta-9-THC and the 11-OH compound, there was no evidence of any psychologic high in any of the three subjects to whom DMHP had been administered. The responses of one subject, who had previously been studied after delta-9-THC and 11-OH-delta-9-THC administration, are shown in Table 3. After delta-9-THC or 11-OH-delta-9-THC, this subject evidenced a "high," an increase in CMI score, and tachycardia. (This subject was the only one of nine subjects who exhibited an equal response to delta-9-THC and 11-OH-delta-9-THC, all other subjects reporting a much greater response to the 11-hydroxylated compound.) However, when this subject was given DMHP (200 μg intravenously), he had no psychologic "high" and no symptom signs; he did, however, have a marked tachycardia.

Thus, with this continuing interest in the structure-activity relation-ship of cannabinoids, my colleagues and I at the Lilly Research Laboratories were involved in the synthesis of analogs based upon the cannabinoid structure and the evaluation of their pharmacology. It appeared that these compounds might show promise as potential therapeutic agents due to their very high therapeutic index. The culmination of their research efforts was the development of a compound whose generic name is nabilone (Lilly Compound 109514, Figure 4). Pharmacologic studies conducted in animals revealed that this potent compound had certain properties in common with delta-9-THC. Toxicologic studies suggested that it should have a large therapeutic index.

Table 3

Comparative Pharmacology of

THC, 11-OH-THC, and DMHP

Treatment	Dose (mg) I.V.	"High" 0-10 Scale	Symptom Signs Score	Heart Rate (% of Control)
Vehicle	---	0	1	94
THC	1.0	9	40	112
11-OH-THC	1.0	9	35	131
DMHP	0.2	0	0	151

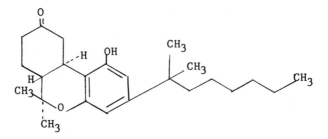

Figure 4. Chemical structure of nabilone (Compound 109514).

Nabilone resembles the cannabinols only with respect to the A and B rings; the C ring has a ketone instead of a methyl at position no. 9. Thus the compound is not a tetrahydrocannabinol. Preclinical pharmacologic studies revealed nabilone to possess interesting psychotropic properties in tests used to study potential new drugs in the CNS areas (Stark and Archer, 1975). It was thus of interest to study the clinical pharmacology of this synthetic cannabinol derivative (Lemberger and Rowe, 1976). Nabilone was administered to normal volunteers in single oral doses ranging from 0.1 to 5 mg. No clinically significant pharmacologic or psychologic effects were observed at single doses up to 2.5 mg; however, doses of 3 mg to 5 mg did produce minimal-to-moderate euphoria in all subjects. This euphoric effect was described by the subjects as resembling that previously experienced after alcohol or marihuana usage. In addition, subjects reported having dry mouth, drowsiness, and a feeling of fatigue. At times, dizziness occurred upon standing after the larger doses. All subjects reported being more relaxed and less anxious. There were no observable changes from baseline values with respect to routine blood chemistries, coagulation tests, or hematologic tests; and no effects were seen in routine chemistries, electrocardiogram, or lead II rhythm strips run at various times after drug administration. Even with larger doses which produced marked side effects, including pronounced postural hypotension, no electrocardiographic changes were observed, except for a slight increase in heart rate.

The dose-response relationship of nabilone on certain pharmacologic and psychologic effects was investigated in several normal volunteers. After the oral administration of 1 mg of nabilone, little effect was reported·on the response to a modified Cornell Medical Index Questionnaire (CMI) when compared to placebo. This dose did not produce any euphoria, although a dose of 2.5 mg produced a slightly greater effect on the CMI than the 1-mg dose; this did not appear to be of any clinical significance. In one of the subjects, this dose resulted in minimal euphoria. In contrast to these lower doses, the oral administration of 5 mg of nabilone produced a marked increase in the CMI score and a marihuana-like euphoria in all three subjects (Figure 5).

After the oral administration of 1 mg of nabilone, a slight decrease in heart rate occurred, whereas doses of 2.5 and 5 mg produced only an 8-10 beat/minute increase in heart rate when the subjects were recumbent (Figure 6). Although only a minimal tachycardia was seen when the subjects were in a lying position, a marked reflex tachycardia was evidenced upon standing secondary to the postural hypotension which occurs. Moreover, after the intravenous administration of 250 μg to 1 mg of this compound, only minimal increases in heart rate occurred, whereas the 1-mg dose of nabilone was accompanied by marked psychologic effects.

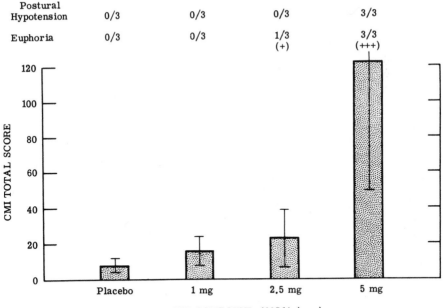

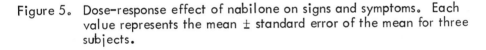

Figure 5. Dose-response effect of nabilone on signs and symptoms. Each value represents the mean ± standard error of the mean for three subjects.

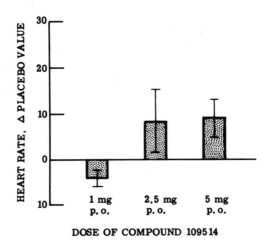

Figure 6.   Dose-response effect of nabilone on heart rate after the
            administration of single doses to normal volunteers. Each value
            represents the mean ± standard error of the mean for three
            subjects.

      Nabilone, at doses of 1 and 2.5 mg, produced only minimal effects
on lying and standing mean arterial blood pressure; in contrast, after the
administration of a 5-mg dose this compound produced a marked fall in
blood pressure upon standing (Figure 7). This dose, however, had no effect
on blood pressure when the subject was in a recumbent position.

      The effect of the repeated administration of nabilone on psychologic
and cardiovascular function has also been investigated. After the repeated
administration of nabilone (1 mg b.i.d.) to one subject, symptoms, as determined by the CMI questionnaire, were evidenced following the second dose.
These symptoms peaked on the second day and disappeared by the fourth day
(Figure 8), suggesting that tolerance developed. This subject experienced
similar effects after the repeated administration of 2 mg of nabilone twice
daily (Figure 8). In both cases the subject was more relaxed and less anxious
during the week on drug when compared to placebo. The results of the
repeated administration of 2 mg b.i.d. in three subjects are shown in
Figure 9. Again, an increase in symptoms occurred after day 1, peaked on
the second day, and was followed by a gradual decrease in symptoms.

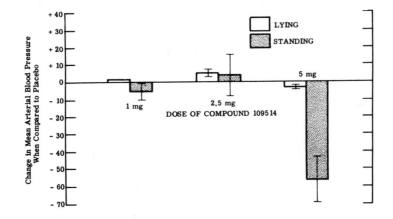

Figure 7. Dose-response effect of nabilone on mean arterial blood pressure after the administration of single doses to normal volunteers. Values represent the change in mean arterial blood pressure when compared to placebo while subjects were lying or standing. Each value represents the mean ± standard error of the mean for three subjects.

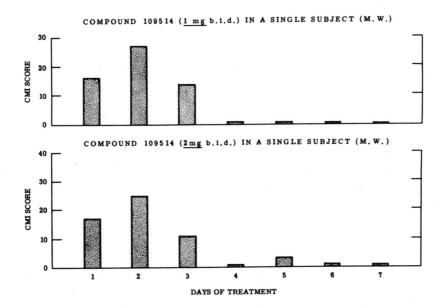

Figure 8. The effect of nabilone (1 mg b.i.d. or 2 mg b.i.d.) on signs and symptoms after its repeated administration to a single subject.

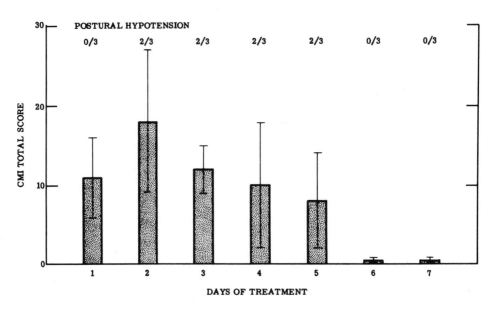

Figure 9. The effects of nabilone (2 mg b.i.d.) on signs and symptoms after
its repeated administration. Each value represents the mean ±
standard error of the mean for three subjects.

Similarly, postural hypotension occurred in two of the three subjects after
day 2 (the third dose), then disappeared in all subjects by the sixth day
(Figure 9). Although euphoria was reported in one of the subjects,
tolerance rapidly developed to this effect. In an attempt to determine if
tolerance had in fact developed to certain of the effects of nabilone, a
challenge dose of 5 mg nabilone was administered on the eighth day after
repeated administration of the compound. After the administration of this
single 5-mg dose, subjects reported only a minimal increase in CMI score.
Only one of the subjects evidenced a mild euphoria and postural hypotension
(Figure 10). After one week's duration, during which time the subjects
received no medication, they were again challenged with a single 5-mg dose
of nabilone. These subjects now manifested a marked increase in symptoms
and signs as evidenced by increase in the CMI score. In addition, all three
subjects had euphoria and two of the three evidenced postural hypotension
(Figure 10).

In summarizing the effects of various natural and synthetic cannabinoids
on a variety of clinical parameters, it is clear (Table 4) that it is possible
to separate certain of the adverse effects of delta-9-THC from what might
perhaps be its more desirable effects, for example, the relaxant effects.
Since delta-9-THC has been implicated as a potential therapeutic agent

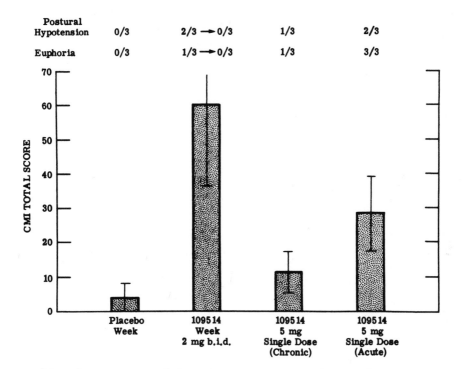

Figure 10. The effect of nabilone administration on the development of signs and symptoms, euphoria, and postural hypotension. The drug was administered as described in the text. Each value represents the mean ± standard error of the mean for three subjects.

with multiple uses such as an antidepressant in patients with terminal cancer (Regelson, Butler, Schulz, Kirk, Peek and Green, 1975), in the treatment of glaucoma (Hepler and Frank, 1971), as a bronchodilator in asthmatics (Vachon, Fitzgerald, Solliday, Gould and Gaensler, 1973; Tashkin, Shapiro and Frank, 1973), and as an antiemetic in patients receiving cancer chemotherapy (Sallan, Zinberg and Frei, 1975), if there is to be any useful therapeutic use resulting from the extensive research that is being carried out with marihuana, it is likely that synthetic cannabinoids will have to be discovered and developed which produce similar beneficial effects. It is unlikely that delta-9-THC itself could ever be a useful drug since this compound occurs as a resin and therefore lacks the suitability of being prepared in pharmaceutical preparations for widespread use. In addition, it has multiple pharmacologic effects such as producing tachycardia, an effect which would limit its use in elderly people.

Table 4

CLINICAL PHARMACOLOGY
OF SEVERAL CANNABINOIDS
AFTER ORAL OR INTRAVENOUS ADMINISTRATION

EFFECT	Δ^9THC 1 mg	11-OH Δ^9THC 1 mg	DMHP .25 mg	109514 .5 mg i.v.	109514 2 mg oral
TACHYCARDIA	+++	+++	+++	+	0
BLOOD PRESSURE					
lying	±	±	0	0	0
standing	±	±	+++	++	0
PSYCHOLOGIC HIGH	++	+++	0	+	±
DRY MOUTH	+++	+++	+++	+++	+
SEDATIVE, RELAXANT	+++	+++	±	+++	+++

The clinical studies reported here clearly demonstrate that by molecular manipulation one can separate many of the adverse effects of delta-9-THC or other cannabinoids to achieve potentially useful therapeutic agents. The development of nabilone, a crystalline cannabinoid which retains many of the advantageous effects of delta-9-THC, and whose absorption and pharmacologic effects are reproducible, may be of benefit in evaluating the role of cannabinoids in the treatment of several disease states in which delta-9-THC has previously been reported to be of therapeutic value. In addition, unlike many of the other cannabinoids, nabilone, which exists as a crystalline material rather than in the form of a resin, should be more acceptable for producing stable pharmaceutical formulations. Although there was a rapid development of tolerance to several of the effects of nabilone, these studies suggest that tolerance can develop to several effects while not developing to other effects.

REFERENCES

Galanter, M., Wyatt, R.J., Lemberger, L., Weingartner, H., Vaughan, T.B., & Roth, W.T. Effects on humans of delta-9-tetrahydrocannabinol administered by smoking. Science, 1972, 176, 934-936.

Gaoni, Y. & Mechoulam, R. Isolation, structure and partial synthesis of active constituent of hashish. Journal of the American Chemical Society, 1964, 86, 1646-1647.

Hepler, R.S. & Frank, I.R. Marihuana smoking and intraocular pressure. American Journal of Ophthalmology, 1972, 74, 1185-1190.

Hollister, L.E. Structure-activity relationships of cannabis constituents in man. Clinical Pharmacology & Therapeutics, 1974, 15, 208-209.

Hollister, L.E., Richards, R.K., & Gillespie, H.K. Comparison of tetrahydrocannabinol and synhexyl in man. Clinical Pharmacology and Therapeutics, 1968, 9, 783-791.

Isbell, H. Effects of (-)delta-9-trans-tetrahydrocannabinol in man. Psychopharmacologia (Berl.), 1967, 11, 184-188.

Lemberger, L., Crabtree, R.E., & Rowe, H.M. 11-hydroxy-delta-9-tetrahydrocannabinol. Pharmacology, disposition, and metabolism of a major metabolite of marihuana in man. Science, 1972, 177, 62-64.

Lemberger, L., McMahon, R., Archer, R., Matsumoto, K., & Rowe, H. Pharmacologic effects and physiologic disposition of delta-6a, 10a-dimethylheptyl tetrahydrocannabinol (DMHP) in man. Clinical Pharmacology and Therapeutics, 1974, 15, 380-386.

Lemberger, L., & Rowe, H. The clinical pharmacology of nabilone (Lilly compound 109514), a modified cannabinol derivative. Clinical Pharmacology and Therapeutics, 1976 (in press).

Perez-Reyes, M., Timmons, M.C., Lipton, M.A., Davis, K.H., & Wall, M.E. Intravenous injection in man of delta-9-tetrahydrocannabinol and 11-OH-delta-9-tetrahydrocannabinol. Science, 1972, 177, 633-634.

Regelson, W., Butler, J.R., Schulz, J., Kirk, T., Peek, L., Green, M.L., and Zakio, O. Delta-9-THC as an effective antidepressant and appetite stimulating agent in advanced cancer patients. In S. Szara and M. C. Braude (Eds.), International Conference on the Pharmacology of Cannabis. Savannah: Raven Press, 1975.

Sallan, S., Zinberg, N., & Frei, E., III. Oral delta-9-tetrahydrocanna-
    binol (THC) in the prevention of vomiting associated with cancer
    chemotherapy. Proceedings of the American Association for Cancer
    Research, 1975, 16, 144.

Sidell, F.R., Pless, J.E., Neitlich, H., Sussman, P., Copelan, H.W.,
    & Sim, V.M. Dimethylheptyl-delta-6a, 10a-tetrahydrocannabinol:
    Effects after parenteral administration to man. Proceedings of the
    Society for Experimental Biology and Medicine, 1973, 142, 867-873.

Stark, P., & Archer, R.A. Preclinical pharmacologic profile of a psycho-
    active cannabinoid. Pharmacologist, 1975, 17, 210.

Tashkin, D.P., Shapiro, B.J., & Frank, I.M. Acute pulmonary physio-
    logical effects of smoked marijuana and oral delta-9-tetrahydro-
    cannabinol in healthy young men. New England Journal of
    Medicine, 1973, 289, 336-341.

Vachon, L., Fitzgerald, M.X., Solliday, N.H., Gould, I.A., &
    Gaensler, E.A. Single-dose effect of marihuana smoke. New
    England Journal of Medicine, 1973, 288, 985-989.

Weiss, J.L., Watanabe, A.M., Lemberger, L., Tamarkin, N.R., &
    Cardon, P.V. Cardiovascular effects of delta-9-tetrahydrocanna-
    binol in man. Clinical Pharmacology & Therapeutics, 1972, 13,
    671-684.

CHAPTER 25

HETEROCYCLIC ANALOGS OF THE CANNABINOIDS

Harry G. Pars
Raj K. Razdan

SISA Incorporated
Cambridge, Massachusetts

NOTE: This presentation is based on subject matter which
has been accepted for publication by the Journal of Medicinal
Chemistry (see Pars and associates, 1976; Razdan and associates,
1976).

This paper presents chemical and pharmacological data on a series of
nitrogen- and sulfur-containing benzopyrans structurally and historically
related to the cannabinoids. These new classes of compounds are benzopyranopyridines, thiopyranobenzopyrans, thienobenzopyrans, and their water-
soluble ester derivatives. Representatives of these agents are currently under
investigation in animals and man to determine their therapeutic potential.

INTRODUCTION

Interest in developing and pursuing these and other analogs of the
cannabinoids as new drugs was stimulated by the following general observations:

(1)   Cannabinoids themselves have pharmacological profiles
        of action which made them unique among known thera-
        peutic agents.

(2)   There is no known physical dependence liability
        associated with cannabis.

419

(3)   Cannabinoids show extraordinarily low-toxicity
        in laboratory animals, including low-lethality
        and little or no respiratory depression.

(4)   Centuries of folklore use suggests the potential
        for pain relief, sedation, and other therapeutic
        indications for cannabis-like drugs.

It has been stated (Bergel, 1965) that ". . .it is regrettable that
neither hashish nor one of its major constituents has an honest nitrogen from
which one could make a soluble salt. . . ." In 1946 Anker and Cook succeeded
in synthesizing a nitrogen-containing cannabinoid, which they reported to be
inactive as an analgesic agent. Following this work, Pars, Granchelli,
Keller and Razdan (1966) reported the synthesis of a pharmacologically active
series of nitrogen analogs. Although the initial nitrogen-containing substances were not water-soluble, soluble ester-salts of delta-9-THC were
subsequently synthesized and investigated (Zitko and associates, 1972).

Interest in preparing the nitrogen analogs was originally stimulated by
the observation that THC is one of very few potent drugs which act on the
central nervous system, yet has no nitrogen in its structure. In designing these
compounds, Pars and Razdan (1971) considered the following factors: (a)
phenethylamine orientation as found in the large majority of alkaloids (for
example, phenethylamines, morphine, indoles, indolylethylamines); (b) aryl
tetrahydropyridine moiety, which is found in particular in psychotomimetic
agents (for example, LSD, yohimbine); and (c) aryl piperidine moiety, which
is present in many CNS active agents. Additional points of similarity were
observed in the structures of morphine, THC, and LSD) (Figure 1). All have
a planar ring (benzene in the case of morphine and delta-9-THC, and indole
in LSD) joined to a β-hydrogen atom two carbon atoms away. With nitrogen
in the C-ring of THC, other points of striking structural similarity become
evident between the nitrogen analog I and LSD, and between the nitrogen
analog II and morphine (Razdan and Pars, 1970) (Figure 2).

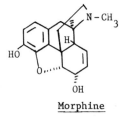

Morphine

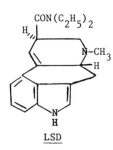

LSD

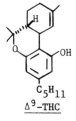

Δ^9-THC

Figure 1.

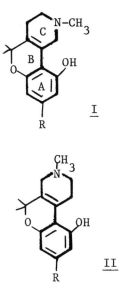

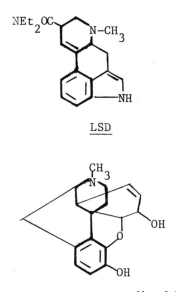

Figure 2.

In addition to the nitrogen analogs I and II, the heterocyclic analogs shown in Figure 3 have been prepared to date. All of these compounds bear the common structural feature of the benzopyran ring system.

All the pyrans (I to XII) except X were prepared according to the general Scheme I. The appropriate resorcinol and the keto ester were allowed to react under Pechmann conditions to give the pyrones as shown. The pyrones were then reacted with methyl magnesium iodide or bromide and followed up by an acid work-up to produce the pyrans. To prepare the various N-substituted pyrans of Table 1, the N-benzyl pyran was prepared and then debenzylated catalytically over Pd/C to give the nor-base which was alkylated to the final compound. The sulfur analog X was prepared from VIII by dehydrogenation.

NITROGEN ANALOGS

Table 1 lists a series of N-substituted benzopyranopyridines and the results of general screening in mice. The list includes the levo and dextro forms of threo and erythro isomers of compound 26 (SP-1). The latter is the most potent of the series, and is comparable to the diastereoisomeric, synthetic cannabinoid DMHP and its stereoisomers (Aaron and Ferguson, 1968). Also included are derivatives of compound II, with the nitrogen in the phenylpropylamine orientation.

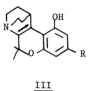
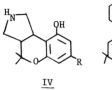
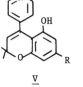
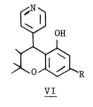

III IV V VI

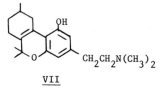
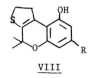
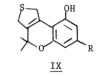

VII VIII IX

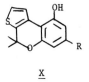
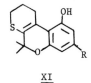
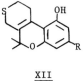

X XI XII

Figure 3.

Scheme I

  +  Pechmann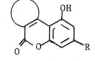

keto ester   Resorcinol   Pyrone

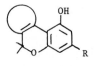

1) CH₃MgX

2) H⁺

Pyran

Figure 4.

Table 1

Comparative Activity of Various Nitrogen Analogs in Mice

A. Derivatives of Compound I

Compd. Number	R	R'	R"	Mouse Data mg/kg iv. MED$_{50}$	LD$_{50}$
1	CH$_3$	CH$_3$	H	5.6	>32
2	CH$_3$	n-C$_5$H$_{11}$	H	18	>32
3	CH$_3$	CH(CH$_3$)C$_5$H$_{11}$	H	>10	>10
4	CH$_3$	CH(CH$_3$)-(S)	H	>10	>10
5	CH$_3$	CH(CH$_3$)C$_{12}$H$_{25}$	H	>10	>10
6	CH$_3$	CH(CH$_3$)CH(CH$_3$)C$_5$H$_{11}$	H	1	22.4
7	CH$_3$	"	COCH$_3$	3.2	32
8	CH$_2$C$_6$H$_5$	"	H	10	>32
9	H	"	H	1.8	18
10	COCH$_3$	"	H	5.6	>32
11	COCH$_3$	"	COCH$_3$	1.8	>32
12	C$_2$H$_5$	"	H	5.6	>10
13	n-C$_3$H$_7$	CH(CH$_3$)CH(CH$_3$)C$_5$H$_{11}$	H	.42	>3.2
14	CO-◁	"	H	10	>32
15	CH$_2$-◁	"	H	1.8	>10
16	n-C$_5$H$_{11}$	"	H	1.8	>10
17	CH$_2$-□	"	H	.56	25
18	CH$_2$CH$_2$C$_6$H$_5$	"	H	3.2	>10
19	CH$_2$CH=CH$_2$	"	H	.75	>10
20	CH$_2$CH=CH$_2$	"	COCH$_3$	.42	32
21	n-CH$_2$CH=CHCl	"	H	.42	>32
22	CH$_2$CH=CHCl(cis)	"	H	.42	>10
23	CH$_2$CH=CHCl(trans)	"	H	.24	>10

Table 1, continued.

Compd. Number	R	R'	R"	Mouse Data mg/kg iv. MED$_{50}$	LD$_{50}$
24	$CH_2CH=CHC_6H_5$	$CH(CH_3)CH(CH_3)C_5H_{11}$	H	>10	>10
25	$CH_2CH=C(CH_3)_2$	"	H	3.2	>10
26 (SP-1)	$CH_2C\equiv CH$	"	H	.042	40
27	$CH_2C\equiv CH$	"	$COCH_3$	.18	>100
28	$CH_2C\equiv C-CH_3$	"	H	1.0	32
29	$CH_2C\equiv CH$	$n-C_7H_{15}$	H	.13	>32
30	$CH_2C\equiv CH$	$n-C_9H_{19}$	H	.32	>20

B.   Isomers of Compound 26

Compound Number	Isomer	Mouse Data mg/kg iv. MED$_{50}$	LD$_{50}$
26a	(+)Erythro	0.013	>10
26b	(-)Erythro	0.056	>10
26c	(+)Threo	0.13	>10
26d	(-)Threo	0.13	>10

C.   Derivatives of Compound II

Compound Number	R	R'	Mouse Data mg/kg iv. MED$_{50}$	LD$_{50}$
31	$CH_2C_6H_5$	CH_3	18	>32
32	CH_3	C_9H_{19}	1.8	>32
33	CH_3	"	10	>32
34	H	"	>10	>10
35	$CH_2CH=CH_2$	"	>32	>32
36	$(trans)-CH_2CH=CHCl$	"	>32	>32
37	$CH_2C\equiv CH$	"	18	>32

All of these compounds were evaluated in a general pharmacology screen in mice (Pars and associates, 1976). The procedure used was a modification of the Irwin mouse screen (see Irwin, 1964). Minimum effective doses (MED50's) and lethal doses (LD50's) were determined. These nitrogen analogs were, like the cannabinoids, insoluble in aqueous media. They were solubilized in polyethylene glycol 200 and administered intravenously. The overt drug effects seen were qualitatively similar for all compounds tested. Most prominent effects were decreased locomotor activity, increased sensitivity to stimuli, depression, and, at high doses, static and dynamic ataxia. Adams' most potent carbocyclic compound DMHP (Adams, Harfenst and Loewe, 1949) (Figure 5) has an MED50 of 0.075 mg/kg in this test. Compound 6, the nitrogen analog of DMHP, was less potent with an MED50 of 1 mg/kg. Altering the side chain (R') of compound 6 further reduced potency (compounds 1 to 5). Acetylation of the phenolic OH of compound 6 had little effect on its potency (compound 7). Shifting the ring-position of the nitrogen of compound 6 had no effect on potency (compound 32). Changing the substituent on the nitrogen of compound 6 sometimes increased potency slightly and sometimes reduced potency (see for example compounds 8, 10, 12, 13-19, 21-23, and 28). A propargyl substituent (compound 26 or SP-1) substantially increased potency as do other three-carbon substituents (19, 21-23). N-Propargyl compounds with long n-alkyl side chains were also potent in this test (29 and 30). Compound 26 was equipotent with DMHP. A detailed comparison is discussed later in this paper. Resolution of compound 26 into its four stereoisomers showed the erythro isomers (26a, 26b) to be more potent than the threo isomers (26c, 26d). Compound 26 and its erythro isomers were the most potent nitrogen analogs tested. Alteration of the structure of compound 26 in the side chain (R'), by acetylation of the phenolic OH, slightly reduced potency (compound 27). Shifting the ring-position of the nitrogen (that is, 26 to 37) significantly reduced its potency.

BASIC ESTERS OF A NITROGEN ANALOG

A comparison of the various basic esters, "water-soluble derivatives," of compound 26 and related compounds in selected pharmacological tests is given in Table 2 (Razdan and associates, 1976a). The structure-activity (SAR) picture that emerges from these tests is as follows:

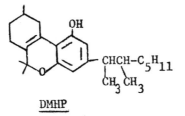

DMHP

Figure 5.

Table 2

Basic Esters of Compound 26 and Related Compounds--
Comparative Profiles(a)

Compd. Number	R	R'	DOPA 5 mg/kg	Mouse Fighting mg/kg	Motor Activity 10 mg/kg	Analgesia ED_{50}, mg/kg	Dog Ataxia mg/kg	Sedative-Hypnotic mg/kg(TST)
26(SP-1)	H	C_9H_{19}	+ + +	1(+ +) 5(+ +)	1(+ + +)	W(4.3) RTF(13.8) HP(7.7)	1(+ +)	0.1(+100) 0.25(+56) 0.5(+44)
38(SP-106)	$\overset{O}{\overset{\|}{C}}CH_2CH_2CH_2N$⬡ ·HCl	"	+	1(+) 5(+ +)	1(+ +)	W(12.0) RFT(12.5) HP(4.2)	1(+ +)	0.1(+38) 0.25(+33) 0.5(+48)
39	$\overset{O}{\overset{\|}{C}}\underset{CH_3}{C}HCH_2CH_2N$⬡ ·2HCl	"	+	10(IA)	+ +	W(12.21) RFT(9.8)	1(+)	0.25(+58) 0.5(+45)
40	$\overset{O}{\overset{\|}{C}}-\underset{CH_3}{\overset{CH_3}{C}}-CH_2CH_2N$⬡ ·2HCl	"	+	10(IA)	+ +	W(17.5) RFT(>20)		0.5(+15)
41	$\overset{O}{\overset{\|}{C}}CH_2CH_2CH_2N$⬠$CH_3$ ·2HCl	"	+	10(+)	+ +	IA	1(+)	
42	$\overset{O}{\overset{\|}{C}}CH_2CH_2CH_2N$⬡ ·HCl	"	+	10(+)	+	W(26.8)	1(+ +)	0.5(+92)

No.	Structure	R	DOPA	Mouse fighting	Motor activity	Dog ataxia		
43	$\overset{O}{\overset{\|}{C}}$CHCH$_2CH_2$N(CH$_3$)$_2$ ·2HCl (with CH$_3$)		+	10(IA)	+	W(7.3) RFT(10.7)		0.5(+38) 1.0(+104)
44	$\overset{O}{\overset{\|}{C}}CH_2CH_2$N⟨⟩ ·2HCl		+	10(++)	+	W(12.3) HP(22.3)		0.5(+69)
45	$\overset{O}{\overset{\|}{C}}CH_2CH_2CH_2$N⟨⟩ ·HCl	C$_5$H$_{11}$	+	10(++)	++	W(>10)	1(+)	
46	$\overset{O}{\overset{\|}{C}}CH_2CH_2CH_2$N⟨⟩ ·HCl	C$_5$H$_{11}$	+	5(+)	+	IA		
47	$\overset{O}{\overset{\|}{C}}CH_2CH_2CH_2$N⟨O⟩ ·2HCl	C$_9$H$_{19}$	+	5(++)	+	W(9.5) RTF(14.4)	1(++)	1.0(+30)
48	$\overset{O}{\overset{\|}{C}}$CHCH$_2CH_2$N⟨O⟩ ·2HCl (with CH$_3$)	C$_9$H$_{19}$	+	10(+)	++	W(>10)		0.5(+36)
49	$\overset{O}{\overset{\|}{C}}CH_2CH_2$N(C$_2H_5$)$_2$ ·HCl		+	10(++)	+	W(>40)	10(++)	
50	Diquarternary Salt(2CH$_3$I) of 45		+	10(++)	+	IA	10(+)	

(a) All doses are in mg/kg (po); in the DOPA potentiation test, results have been graded as + (slight), + + (moderate) and + + + (marked) increases. In the mouse fighting and motor activity tests, + corresponds to 1–33%, + + (33–66%) and + + + (66–100%) reduction. In the dog ataxia test, + corresponds to decreased activity only and + + to decreased activity and ataxia; W = writhing; RFT = rat tail flick; TST = change in total sleep time; IA = inactive.

In general, formation of the basic esters of 26 reduces its activity in the DOPA test and in the rat motor activity procedure. A similar effect is also observed in tranquilizing activity (mouse fighting), with the reduction being more pronounced in the case of hindered esters like α-methyl or α, α-dimethyl derivatives (compare 39 or 40 with 38; 43 with 42; 48 with 47). The effect on analgesia varies with the nature of the substituent R. Thus, ω-piperidine and morpholine groups retain analgetic activity; α-methyl substitution in both cases has little or no effect; α, α-dimethyl substitution decreases activity. Methyl substitution in the 2-position of the piperidine ring (42 and 43) retains activity and varying the length of the chain also has little effect. Replacement of piperidine or morpholine by pyrrolidine (41) eliminates and diethylamine (49) reduces analgetic activity. Similarly, quarternization of the basic nitrogen (50) or replacement of the aromatic side chain alkyl group C_9H_{19} by n-C_5H_{11} (48) eliminates activity. The limited sedative-hypnotic studies in cats show that this activity can be retained but is somewhat decreased by making a very hindered (α, α-dimethyl) ester. An interesting fact which emerges from these studies is the selectivity of action (analgesia and sedative-hypnotic) in the ester derivatives compared to the parent phenol (compare 26 with 38, 39 and 43).

SULFUR ANALOGS AND THEIR BASIC ESTERS

Sulfur analogs including their basic esters are listed in Table 3 (Razdan and associates, 1976b). The SAR in this series of analogs is as follows: Only the 5-membered-ring compounds (51 and 54) gave significant activity in the DOPA test, and the activity was reduced when the five-membered-ring was aromatized (compound 59). Basic esters (52 and 53) of the parent phenol (51) showed reduced activity in this test. A similar SAR was observed in the nitrogen analogs of Table 2. In the mouse fighting and rat motor-activity tests, no SAR trends were obvious. Interesting analgetic activity was found only in the parent phenol 55, and this activity was reduced in the ester derivatives 56 and 57. This is in contrast to the nitrogen analogs where esterification with the piperidino and morpholino acids retained analgetic activity. In sedative-hypnotic activity tests in cats (see Table 4), compound 51 showed marginal activity whereas the esters 55 and 57 were inactive. These results also differ from those found with the nitrogen (Table 2) and carbocyclic analogs (Table 4) some of which showed potent sedative-hypnotic activity.

For activity with sulfur analogs, it appears that (1) the heterocyclic atom should be adjacent to the double bond in order to elicit interesting activity, for example, 51 and 55, (2) ring size has no influence, and (3) a planar ring, as in compound 59, eliminates activity.

Table 3

Sulfur Analogs and Their Basic Esters—Comparative Profiles[a]

Compd. Number	Structure	DOPA 5 mg/kg	Mouse Fighting mg/kg	Motor Activity 5 mg/kg	Analgesia ED_{50}, mg/kg	Dog Ataxia mg/kg
51	(R = H)	+ + +	5(+) 10(+ +)	+	W(71.8) HP(12.1)	0.1(+)
52	R=CO(CH$_2$)$_3$N· ·HCl	+	10(+ +)	+	W(24)	1 (IA)
53	R=CO(CH$_2$)$_3$N· ·HCl	+ +	5(+) 10(+ +)	+	HP(>50)	1 (IA) 10(+ +)
54	OH	+ + +	10(+ +)	+	W(51.7) HP(>120)	
55	(R = H)	+	10(+)	+	W(8.6) HP(5.7) RTF(2.7)	1(+ +)
56	R=CO(CH$_2$)$_2$N· ·HCl	+	5(+)	+ + +	W(14.7)	
57	R=COCH(CH$_3$)CH$_2$CH$_2$N· ·HCl	+	10(+ + +)	+	W(22.6)	
58	OH	+ +	5(+)	10(+)	W(>40) HP(>40)	10(+ +)
59	OH	+	10(+)	+	W(>10)	

(a) All doses are in mg/kg (po); in the DOPA potentiation test, results have been graded as + (slight), + + (moderate) and + + + (marked) increases. In the mouse fighting and motor activity tests, + corresponds to 1-33%, + + (33-66%) and + + + (66-100%) reduction. In the dog ataxia test, + corresponds to decreased activity only and + + to decreased activity and ataxia; W = writhing; RTF = rat tail flick; HP = hot plate; and IA = inactive.

Table 4

Alkyl Substituted Analogs--Comparative Profiles(a)

Compd. Number	Ring A	DOPA 5 mg/kg	Audiogenic Seizure 10 mg/kg	Mouse Fighting 10 mg/kg	Analgesia ED50, mg/kg	Sedative-Hypnotic mg/kg	TST	Dog Ataxia mg/kg
51		+++	++	++	W(71.8) HP(12.1)	1 / 2	+30 / +31	0.1(+) / 10(++)
60		++	++	++	W(4.7) HP(1.4)	0.1 / 0.25	+21 / +50	0.1(++) / 1(++)
61		+	+	++	W(34)			10(++)
62		+	+	+	W(>40)			10(++)
63		++	+	++	W(25.3) HP(45.1)	0.5 / 1.0	+59 / +65	1(+) / 10(++)
64		+	+++	+++	W(13.3) HP(13.2)	0.5	+58	1(++) / 10(++)
65		+	IA	+	W(22.6)			1(++) / 10(++)
66		++	IA	++	W(>40) RTF(>40)			10(++)
DMHP		+	+++	+++	W(19.6) HP(12.4)	0.5	+62	1(+) / 10(++)
67		+ (@ 30 mg/kg)	++ (@ 30 mg/kg)	++	W(10.5) HP(25.0)	0.5	+54	1(+) / 10(++)

(a)All doses are in mg/kg(po); in the DOPA potentiation test, results have been graded as + (slight), ++ (moderate), +++ (marked) increases; in the audiogenic seizure test, + corresponds to 1-33%, ++ (33-66%) and +++ (66-100%) protection after 1 hr; in the mouse fighting test, + corresponds to 1-33%, ++ (33-66%), +++ (66-100%) reduction; in the dog ataxia test, + corresponds to decreased activity only and ++ to decreased activity and ataxia; W=writhing; RTF=rat tail flick; HP=hot plate; TST=change in total sleep time; IA=inactive.

THE EFFECT OF ALKYL SUBSTITUENTS

The effect of alkyl substitution in the alicyclic ring of selected sulfur and carbocyclic analogs were also studied. These results are summarized in Table 4 (Razdan and associates, 1976c).

Substitution at the C-1 position in the five-membered sulfur and carbocyclic series (compounds 60 and 64) produced the most pronounced changes in the pharmacological activity. Thus a dramatic increase in potency in the analgesic and sedative-hypnotic tests was noted in the sulfur series (compare 60 with 51). On the other hand, in the five-membered carbocyclic analogs, the potency in the audiogenic seizure test (anticonvulsant activity) increased the most, but the change in analgesic activity was moderate and there was no change in the sedative-hypnotic activity (compare 64 with 63). In both series, however, the potency was increased in the dog ataxia test, as compounds 60 and 64 were more active than 51 and 63.

In contrast to the marked pharmacological changes caused in the five-membered series, moving the methyl group to the C-10 position in the six-membered carbocyclic series, compound 67 affected the activity only slightly, similar to the findings of Adams (1949) and Todd (1943). Our results for compound 67 compared to DMHP (methyl at C-9) show that the anticonvulsant activity was decreased only slightly, the analgesic activity was increased (slightly), and the dog ataxia test results were unchanged.

It appears then that methyl substitution in the close proximity of the phenolic hydroxyl group is important in influencing activity of certain cannabinoids, particularly those which have a planar five-membered alicyclic ring rather than a six-membered ring.

PHARMACOLOGICAL PROFILE OF 26 COMPARED TO DMHP

Adams' most potent carboxycyclic compound, DMHP, a stereoisomeric mixture, has been studied extensively in laboratory animals (Adams et al., 1949; Dagirmanjian and Boyd, 1962; Hardman, Domino and Seevers, 1971; Loev and associates, 1973); and in man (Sidell and associates, 1973; Lemberger, McMahon, Archer, Matsumoto and Rowe, 1974). The most potent nitrogen analog, compound 26, also a stereoisomeric mixture, was compared to DMHP in a variety of tests in different animal species (Pars et al., 1976). The results are summarized in Table 5.

In the mouse screen, the MED_{50}'s and LD_{50}'s for 26 and DMHP were not statistically different. Effects produced were similar, the most prominent of which were general depression and, at high doses, static and dynamic ataxia. Both compounds also showed similar overt behavior effects in the cat, dog, and rhesus monkeys: depression, static ataxia, and ataxia. In addition, ptosis was observed in the monkey and relaxation of the nictitating membrane was seen in the cat. Depression in the dog did not resemble that

Table 5

Comparison of the Pharmacological Profiles of 26 and DMHP

26 (SP-1)   DMHP

	26 (mg/kg)	DMHP (mg/kg)
Primary screen, mouse, iv MED_{50}	0.042 (0.018–0.10)[a]	0.075 (0.031–0.18)[a]
LD_{50}	40 (32–50)[a]	63 (50–79)[a]
Overt behavior, cat, iv MED	0.006	0.05
monkey, iv MED	0.012	0.05
dog, iv MED	0.006	0.05
Synaptic reflexes, cat, iv MED		
intact	↓ ; 0.006–0.012	↓ ; 0.0004
Cardiovascular, iv MED		
anesthetized cat, BP and respir.	↓0.025	↓0.025
unanesthetized dog, BP only	↓0.100	↓0.400
Conditioned avoidance, gerbil, sc, ED_{50}	>1	>1
Hexobarbital potentiation, mouse, iv, ED_{50}	3.0 ± 1.4	0.72 ± 0.31
Inclined screen, mouse, iv, ED_{50}	0.92 ± 0.22	2.2 ± 0.99

(a) 95% confidence limits.

produced by the classical sedative-hypnotics or tranquilizers. Although the dog was clearly sedated, it was hyperactive to stimuli. In these three species, 26 was more potent than DMHP.

It was shown that β-adrenergic stimulation could account in part for the overt behavior effects seen with these compounds. Thus, in the cat, 5 mg/kg i.v. of the β blocking agent, dichloroisoproterenol (DCI), both prevented and reversed many of the depressant effects of DMHP and 26. This dose of DCI had minimal or no effect on ataxia or on the relaxation of the nictitating membrane which is produced by both compounds.

Compound 26 and DMHP were also active in other tests for CNS depression (polysynaptic reflex and hexobarbital potentiation) and in a test for neuromuscular effects (inclined screen). These results were consistent with the overt behavior test findings. Both compounds depressed the cat's polysynaptic reflex, with 26 less potent than DMHP. Both compounds potentiated hexobarbital activity and caused animals to fall from the inclined screen but their potencies were not statistically different in these tests. Neither compound affected conditioned avoidance performance at doses up to 1 mg/kg s.c.

In cardiovascular studies in the anesthetized cat, both compounds lowered mean arterial pressure without significantly altering pulse pressure. They were equipotent in their hypotensive activity, with similar minimum effective doses causing comparable decreases in mean blood pressure (26 - 19 mmHg, DMHP - 15 mmHg). Both compounds decreased heart rate and respiratory rate. Cardiovascular responses to acetylcholine were not affected by either compound at doses up to 0.1 mg/kg i.v. Cardiovascular activity was also tested in the unanesthetized dog. Both compounds decreased mean blood pressure and at their respective MED's, 26 was more potent than DMHP. Each compound was less potent in the unanesthetized dog than in the anesthetized cat. Decreases in heart rate were also noted in the dog but were attributable to the administration vehicle (PEG 200) and were not drug-related. No consistent effect on respiration was found. It should be noted that in the dog both compounds had overt behavior effects at doses below those which affected blood pressure. This contrasts with results reported in man, where DMHP and its diastereoisomers have been shown to lower blood pressure at doses where no overt CNS effects are observed (Lemberger et al., 1974).

In summary, the pharmacological profiles of 26 and DMHP were similar. Both compounds exhibited significant CNS depressant activity and hypotensive activity. In overt behavior studies in the mouse, cat, monkey, and dog, general depression (of spontaneous activity, awareness, and, except in the mouse and dog, responses to stimuli) and static and dynamic ataxia were observed. Polysynaptic reflex depression, hexobarbital poten-tiation, and inclined screen activity were consistent with the observed overt behavior effects. Part of the overt behavior effects of both compounds appeared to be mediated through β-adrenergic systems since they could be blocked by DCI. 26 was more potent than DMHP for overt behavior effects

Table 6

Comparison of 26 with Morphine and Pentazocine

	Compound 26	Morphine	Pentazocine
Hot Plate,[a] ED_{50}	3.6(3.0–4.3) mg/kg s.c.	1.2(0.9–1.2) mg/kg s.c.	>200 mg/kg s.c.
Tail-flick, ED_{50} (D'Amour Smith)	>20 mg/kg i.v. Some non-dose related activity between 2.5 and 20 mg/kg i.v.	4.8 ± 0.6 mg/kg s.c.	Inactive up to 120 mg/kg s.c.
Phenylquinone Writhing, ED_{50}	0.021(0.010–0.046) mg/kg i.v.	0.54(0.42–0.70) mg/kg s.c.	2.3(1.2–4.6) mg/kg s.c.
Anti-diarrheal % Inhibition of[b] gastrointestinal propulsion	50% at 10 mg/kg p.o. 67% at 100 mg/kg p.o.	52% at 10 mg/kg p.o.	5% at 10 mg/kg p.o. 29% at 100 mg/kg p.o.
Morphine Dependent Monkey:[a] A. Single dose suppression in withdrawn monkey.	Exacerbates abstinence at 1 and 2 mg/kg s.c., but also produced signs of CNS depression.	Suppresses abstinence	No suppression of abstinence.
B. Non-withdrawn Monkey.	Produces reaction resembling precipitated abstinence at 2, 4 and 8 mg/kg s.c., but mixed with sedation and accompanied by mydriasis.	Produces morphine sedation.	Precipitates abstinence.

[a]NAS/NRC Data, Committee on Problems of Drug Dependence (E. L. May, Private Communication).

[b]Diphenoxylate (Lomotil) shows 53% inhibition at 20 mg/kg p.o.

in the cat, dog, and monkey, and hypotensive activity in the unanesthetized dog, less potent for polysynaptic reflex depression and equipotent with DMHP in other tests performed.

COMPARISON OF 26 WITH NARCOTIC AND NARCOTIC-ANTAGONIST ANALGESICS

The design considerations previously described for introducing nitrogen into the carbocyclic nucleus of tetrahydrocannabinols also led us to compare the pharmacology of these nitrogen analogs with that of narcotic and narcotic-antagonist analgesics. Table 6 summarizes and compares the activities of 26, morphine, and pentazocine in various tests for narcotic-agonist properties.

Like both morphine and pentazocine, 26 exhibited antiwrithing activity in the phenylquinone test. Compound 26 was active in the Eddy hot plate test and was also equiactive with morphine for inhibition of gastro-intestinal propulsion; but differed from morphine and was similar to penta-zocine in the tail-flick test where it was without significant activity. In the morphine-dependent monkey (Villarreal, Seevers and Swain, 1974), both withdrawn and non-withdrawn, 26 presented a mixed picture of narcotic antagonist-like activity combined with depressant activity, which is unlike that of morphine or pentazocine.

Based on the finding that 26 precipitated abstinence in the morphine dependent monkey, Harris and Dewey (1974) reexamined these compounds for narcotic-antagonist activity using the mouse tail-flick test. Compound 26 and other nitrogen analogs in the series were found to have narcotic-antagonist properties characterized by a long onset and duration of activity. Thus 26 showed an onset at 4 hr, a peak activity about 24 hr and a duration of nearly 4 days.

In summary, the pharmacological profiles of these compounds are unique and distinct compared to other CNS drugs. Two of these, compound 26 (SP-1) and its water-soluble derivative, 38 (SP-106) are being studied further in animals and in man.

REFERENCES

Aaron, M.S., & Ferguson, C.P. J. Organic Chem., 1968, 33, 684.

Adams, R., Harfenst, M., & Loewe, S. J. Amer. Chem. Soc., 1949, 71, 1624, and earlier papers cited therein.

Anker, R.M., & Cook, A.H. J. Chem. Soc., 1946, 58.

Bergel, F. In G.E.W. Wolstenholme (Ed.), "Hashish: Its chemistry and pharmacology," CIBA Foundation Study Group No. 21. London: J. & H. Churchill Ltd., 1965, 81.

Bergel, F., Morrison, A.L., Rinderknecht, H., Todd, A.R., MacDonald, A.D., & Woolfe, G. Journal of the Chemical Society, 1943, 286, and earlier papers cited therein.

Dagirmanjian, R., & Boyd, E.S. J. Pharmac. and Exp. Therap., 1962, 135, 25.

Dewey, W.L., Harris, L.S., Howes, J.F., Kennedy, J.S., Granchelli, F.E., Pars, H.G., & Razdan, R.K. Nature, 1970, 226, 1265.

Dren, A.T. Symposium on "Approaches to centrally acting drugs derived from the cannabinoid nucleus." Presented at the 68th American Chemical Society Meeting, Atlantic City, N. J., 1974 (Abstract).

Hardman, H.F., Domino, E.F., & Seevers, M.M. Pharmacological Reviews, 1971, 23, 295.

Harris, L.S., & Dewey, W.L. Symposium on "Approaches to centrally acting drugs derived from the cannabinoid nucleus." Presented at the 68th American Chemical Society Meeting, Atlantic City, N. J., 1974 (Abstract).

Irwin, S. In J. A. Nodine & P. E. Siegler (Eds.), "Animal and clinical pharmacologic technique in drug evaluation." Chicago: Year Book Publishers, 1964, 36-54.

Lemberger, L., McMahon, R., Archer, R., Matsumoto, K., & Rowe, H. Clinical Pharmacology and Therapeutics, 1974, 15, 380.

Loev, B., Bender, P.E., Dowalo, F., Macko, D.E., & Fowler, P.J. Journal of Medicinal Chemistry, 1973, 16, 1200.

May, E.L. Private communication.

Pars, H.G., Granchelli, F.E., Keller, J.K., & Razdan, R.K. Communication to the Editor, Journal of the American Chemical Society, 1966, 88, 3664.

Pars, H.G., & Razdan, R.K. Annals of the New York Academy of Sciences, 1971, 191, 15.

Pars, H.G., Granchelli, F.E., Razdan, R.K., Rosenberg, F., Teiger, D., & Harris, L.S. Journal of Medicinal Chemistry, 1976, in press.

Razdan, R.K., & Pars, H.G. In C.R.B. Joyce & S.H. Curry (Eds.), The Botany and Chemistry of Cannabis. London: J. & H. Churchill, 1970, 137.

Razdan, R.K., Zitko-Terris, B., Pars, H.G., Plotnikoff, N.P., Dodge, P.W., Dren, A.T., Kyncl, J., & Somani, P. Journal of Medicinal Chemistry, 1976, in press (a).

Razdan, R.K., Zitko-Terris, B., Handrick, G.R., Dalzell, H.C., Pars, H.G., Howes, J.F., Plotnikoff, N., Dodge, P., Dren, A.T., Kyncl, J., Shoer, L., & Thompson, W.R. Journal of Medicinal Chemistry, 1976, in press (b).

Razdan, R.K., Handrick, G.R., Dalzell, H.C., Howes, J.F., Winn, M., Plotnikoff, N., Dodge, P.W., & Dren, A.T. Journal of Medicinal Chemistry, 1976, in press (c).

Sidell, F.R., Pless, J.E., Neitlich, H., Sussman, P., Copeland, W.W., & Sim, V.M. Proceedings of the Society of Experimental Biology and Medicine, 1973, 142, 867.

Villarreal, J.E., Seevers, M.H., & Swain, H.M. Symposium on "Approaches to Centrally Acting Drugs Derived From the Cannabinoid Nucleus." Presented at the 68th American Chemical Society Meeting, Atlantic City, N. J., 1974 (Abstract).

Zitko, B.A., Dalzell, B.C., Dalzell, H.C., Dewey, W.L., Harris, L.S., Pars, H.G., Razdan, R.K., & Sheehan, J.C. Science, 1972, 177, 442.

CHAPTER 26

PRECLINICAL NEUROPHARMACOLOGY OF THREE NITROGEN-

CONTAINING HETEROCYCLIC BENZOPYRANS DERIVED FROM THE

CANNABINOID NUCLEUS

Anthony T. Dren

Department of Pharmacology and Medicinal Chemistry
Abbott Laboratories
North Chicago, Illinois

The centuries of folklore ascribing medicinal properties to cannabis in
the areas of pain relief, sedation, digestive problems, and mood elevation
(Snyder, 1971; Li, 1974) have culminated in the recent surge of scientific
interest to provide documented proof of the therapeutic efficacy thought to
reside in the cannabinoid class of compounds. Delta-1-trans-tetrahydrocan-
nabinol (delta-1-THC), one of the principal cannabinoids of interest in Cannabis sativa, lends itself well to chemical modification. The chemical structure of delta-1-THC is shown in Figure 1. Our modifications of the molecule
have been carried out in a collaborative effort with Sharps Associates (Cambridge, Massachusetts) and are outlined by dashed lines. These alterations
include: (1) modification of the carbocyclic C-ring to form nitrogen-containing heterocyclic derivatives; (2) esterification of the phenolic hydroxy
to form basic esters; and (3) alternate substituents in place of the n-pentanyl
side chain.

Three compounds which have had extensive preclinical evaluation
and are currently undergoing clinical investigation are shown in Figure 2.

The first compound, Abbott-40174, which also has the designation
SP-1, is the prototype of this nitrogen-containing heterocyclic series and is
characterized by an N-propargyl substitution on the C-ring and a dimethyl-
heptyl branched alkyl side chain which Adams, Harfenst, and Loewe (1949)
found to be the most potent homolog in a carbocyclic cannabinoid series.
These structural changes improve the physical properties of Abbott-40174,
making it a white, crystalline solid as compared to the water-insoluble
delta-1-THC resinous material (Pars and associates, 1976).

C-RING MODIFICATIONS:

    (1) HETERO-ATOMS IN RING
    (2) POSITION OF DOUBLE BOND
    (3) DEGREE OF UNSATURATION
    (4) POSITION AND NUMBER OF SUBSTITUENTS

HYDROXY MODIFICATIONS:

    (1) ESTERIFICATION
    (2) ETHER DERIVATIVES

SIDE CHAIN MODIFICATION:

    (1) BRANCHED C_9 DERIVATIVES
    (2) p-FLUOROPHENYL DERIVATIVES

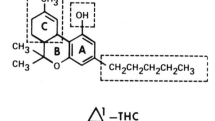

Figure 1. Alterations of the Delta-1-THC molecule used to prepare hetero-cyclic benzopyrans.

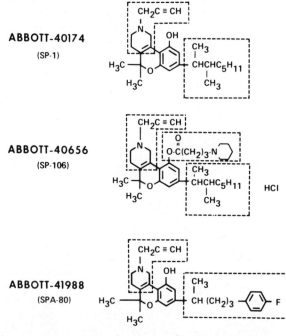

Figure 2. Nitrogen-containing heterocyclic benzopyrans derived from the cannabinoid nucleus.

The second compound, Abbott-40656 or SP-106, differs from Abbott-40174 by the presence of an ester group on the phenolic hydroxy (Razdan and associates, 1976). The formation of this basic ester conveys water solubility to the otherwise insoluble Abbott-40174.

The third compound, Abbott-41988 or SPA-80, differs from Abbott-40174 in that the side chain has been changed to a para-flurophenyl derivative (Winn and associates, 1976). This compound is also a water-insoluble, crystalline solid.

The preclinical studies presented here revealed that the pharmacological spectra of these compounds include tranquilizer, analgetic, sedative-hypnotic, and intraocular pressure lowering properties. However, their activity profiles are unlike the relatively large number of psychotherapeutic agents having utility in these areas. Since the pharmacological spectra of many psychotherapeutic agents also include the capacity to reinforce intravenous self-administration behavior in animals, the dependency producing characteristics of the water soluble analog, Abbott-40656, were evaluated by determining its reinforcing properties in rhesus monkeys under experimental conditions in which other psychoactive agents are self-administered.

These three compounds are either in Phase I or early Phase II clinical trials. At this time, there are no clinical data to support or reject our projections as to therapeutic efficacy or to the predictability of our animal models.

TRANQUILIZER PROPERTIES

Potential tranquilizer activity was demonstrated in several test procedures. These included: (1) reduction of footshock-induced fighting behavior in mice; (2) reduction of spontaneous motor activity and methamphetamine-induced hyperactivity in mice and rats; and (3) blockade of provoked aggressive behavior in rhesus monkeys. All three derivatives showed activity in these test procedures at oral doses of approximately 0.5 to 5 mg/kg. The footshock-induced fighting test can be used to illustrate this activity. In this test, male albino mice were paired on an equal weight basis and each pair was trained to fight in response to footshock. The mice responded to the footshock with distinct and clearly recognized aggressive responses which were counted during a control period prior to drug administration and at various time intervals after drug was given. Test sessions were of one-minute duration. The number of attacks in each test session after drug administration was converted to a percentage of the predrug control value.

The effects of the heterocyclic benzopyrans on mouse fighting behavior are compared to delta-1-THC, diazepam, and chlorpromazine in Table 1. In this test procedure, the heterocyclic benzopyrans, as well as delta-1-THC, were nearly as effective as either diazepam or chlorpromazine in blocking footshock-induced aggression in mice.

Table 1

Drug Effects on Footshock-Induced Fighting Behavior in Mice

Compound	MG/KG	% Change in Fighting at 90 Minutes
Placebo	--	-6
Abbott-40174 (SP-1)	0.5	-10
	1.0	-42*
	5.0	-50*
	10.0	-62*
Abbott-40656 (SP-106)	1	-24
	5	-58*
	10	-64*
Abbott-41988 (SPA-80)	10	-47*
Delta-1-THC	1	-19
	5	-36*
	10	-68*
Diazepam	0.5	-10
	1.0	-28
	5.0	-85*
Chlorpromazine	1.0	-45
	5.0	-75*

* $P < 0.05$, student t test, paired comparison.
N = Three or four pairs of mice/dose.

ANALGETIC ACTIVITY

The antinociceptive properties of the benzopyran derivatives were evaluated in three test procedures: (1) the mouse hot-plate test; (2) the acetic acid writing test in mice; and (3) the rat tail-flick test. Comparisons were made to delta-1-THC and to three analgesic reference standards: codeine phosphate, d-propoxyphene, and anileridine HCl. Portions of these data have been reported previously by Young, Dodge, Dren, and Plotnikoff (1975).

The procedure used in the acetic acid writing test was modified from that of Whittle (1964). Groups of 5 female I. C. R. mice were gavaged with test compound one hour prior to the intraperitoneal injection of 0.4 ml of 0.5% acetic acid. The number of acid-induced writhes were counted over a 20-minute period. Graded activity was calculated as the percent difference in the average number of writhes between test groups and controls.

For the hot-plate test, the method of Woolfe and MacDonald (1944) was used. Groups of 10 female, Swiss-Webster mice, which responded to a hot-plate temperature of $56°C$ by licking their hind paws within 5-15 seconds, were selected after the determination of two control pain thresholds at least 30 minutes apart. Response times were determined at various time intervals after oral drug administration. Graded activity was determined as the percent increase in response time over control with the ED_{50} representing the dose producing a 50% increase in average response time.

For the rat tail-flick test, a modification of the D'Amour and Smith method (1941) was employed. Groups of 10 male Sprague-Dawley rats, their tails blackened with India ink, were exposed to heat from a light source focused on the tail from a power rheostat adjusted so that normal escape responses occurred in about 6-12 seconds. This adjustment in the intensity of the stimulus was made in order to measure "moderately potent" analgesics as reported by Gray, Osterberg, and Scuto (1970). Two trials were run to establish the normal reaction times prior to the oral administration of test compound. Measurements of the responses after drug were made at various time intervals and graded activity was calculated as the percent increase in reaction times.

The ED_{50} values determined in these studies are summarized in Table 2. The three heterocyclic benzopyrans were considerably more potent than either delta-1-THC, cocaine, or d-propoxyphene, with Abbott-41988 being the most potent in all three test procedures. The potency of Abbott-41988 was comparable to that of anileridine HCl.

SEDATIVE-HYPNOTIC ACTIVITY

The sedative-hypnotic activity of these compounds was evaluated on the basis of EEG sleep pattern analysis in cats. Adult male cats were prepared surgically with chronic indwelling electrodes implanted to monitor brain EEG potentials, eye movements, and neck muscle potentials. The animals were acclimated to dimly lit, sound-attenuated chambers which were constructed with plexiglass doors to allow observation of gross motor behavior on closed circuit television. All experimental sessions began at approximately 5:00 p.m. and polygraph recordings were made continuously thereafter throughout the night.

These recordings were evaluated visually with an established set of criteria to quantify changes in sleep-waking patterns. Each one-minute segment of the polygraph tracing was classified as one of four possible categories: (1) awake; (2) spindle sleep; (3) slow wave sleep; and (4) rapid eye movement (REM) sleep, according to criteria established by Lanoir and Killam (1965).

Table 2

Comparison of the Antinociceptive Activity*
of Heterocyclic Benzopyrans to Reference Standards

Compound	Mouse Writing Test	Mouse Hot Plate Test	Rat Tail Flick Test
Abbott-40174 (SP-1)	4.3 (3.2-5.9)	7.7 (4.1-12.7)	13.8 (4.5-23.9)
Abbott-40656 (SP-106)	13.7 (7.8-22.1)	4.2 (2.0-6.8)	12.5 (9.4-15.7)
Abbott-41988 (SPA-80)	5.3 (4.2-6.8)	5.7 (2.1-10.4)	5.9 (2.7-10.5)
Delta-1-THC	52.5 (38-63)	9.6 (2-17)	27.2 (1.4-123)
Codeine Phosphate	15.2 (11.2-17.5)	38 (25-55)	112 (25-398)
d-Propoxyphene HCl	52.8 (39-65)	57.7 (17-87)	52.7 (17-97)
Anileridine HCl	6.0 (2.4-10.8)	10.9 (8.6-13.6)	5.6 (2.8-8.6)

* Values represent graded oral ED_{50}'s (mg/kg) with 95% confidence limits.

All compounds were administered orally by mixing them in a small amount of cat food which was presented to the cat just prior to each experimental session. The drugged food was generally consumed within one to five minutes and the cats were then left undisturbed for the remainder of the experimental session. A three-day protocol was followed: Day 1, adaptation; Day 2, vehicle control (placebo); Day 3, one dose of the test compound. Each animal served as its own control, and drug data are expressed as differences from the paired placebo control experiment.

The changes in total sleep time and in the various stages of sleep produced by Abbott-40656 in cats are shown in Figure 3. The height of the bars on this graph represents the average change in minutes produced by Abbott-40656 as compared to placebo control experiments.

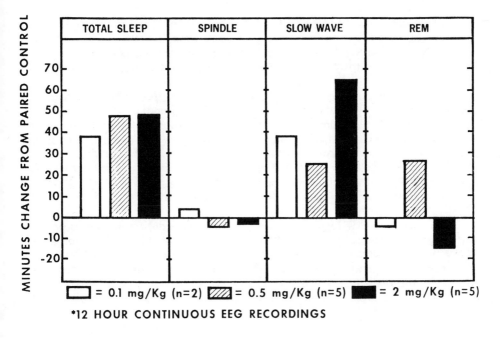

Figure 3. Effects of oral Abbott-40656 on EEG sleep patterns in cats.

Abbott-40656 produced a consistent increase in total sleep time but exhibited a rather flat dose-response curve. Its principal effect on the various sleep stages to account for the increase in total sleep time was an increase in the slow wave stage of sleep. There was only a minimal change in spindle sleep, and REM sleep did not change consistently. The effects of Abbott-40174 and Abbott-41988 in cats were very similar to these illustrated for Abbott-40656.

In cats, the activity of these benzopyrans was markedly different from that of the reference standards, pentobarbital sodium, or flurazepam HCl While the benzopyrans produced a marked increase in sleep time in this species in the dose range of 0.1 to 2.0 mg/kg, p.o., pentobarbital began to exhibit a slight sedation at 10 mg/kg and flurazepam was essentially inactive in this dose range.

The effects of a single dose of Abbott-40656 on all-night EEG sleep patterns in cats are shown in Figure 4. The panels illustrate 12 hours of continuous minute-to-minute changes in EEG sleep stages occurring on a placebo control night and on a night when the same animal received a 1.0 mg/kg oral dose of Abbott-40656. The four levels on each panel represent the four EEG sleep stages: (1) the top level indicating an awake period; (2) the next, spindle sleep; (3) the third, slow wave sleep; and (4) the fourth, REM sleep.

On the placebo control panel, the cyclic changes in EEG sleep patterns are clearly evident. On the Abbott-40656 panel, there is an obvious decrease in the amount of wakefulness and consequently an increase in the total amount of sleep time. The increase in slow wave sleep is difficult to distinguish when the data are presented in this format. However, it is quite obvious that Abbott-40656 did not markedly suppress the REM stage of sleep which is a phenomenon that we and many others have observed as an effect of several well-known sedative-hypnotic agents.

To illustrate this latter point, the effects of sedative-hypnotic pentobarbital sodium (Nembutal®) are illustrated in Figure 5. Notice that while pentobarbital also decreased the amount of awake time, there was also a marked suppression of the REM phase of sleep during the first six hours of the session. In this regard, there is a marked distinction between the effects of the benzopyran derivatives and the barbiturate-like sedative-hypnotic agents.

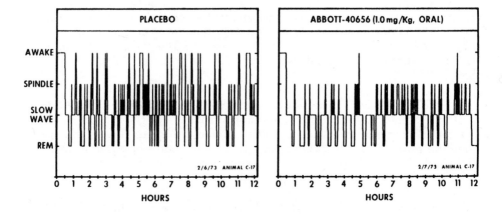

Figure 4. Effects of Abbott-40656 on cat EEG sleep patterns over 12 continuous hours compared to placebo.

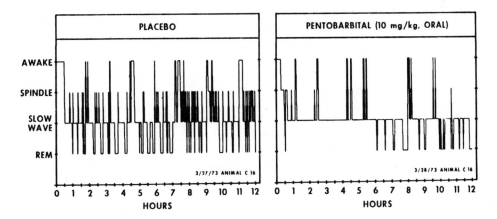

Figure 5. Effects of Pentobarbital on cat EEG sleep patterns over 12 continuous hours compared to placebo.

INTRAOCULAR PRESSURE LOWERING ACTIVITY

The intraocular pressure lowering properties reported for delta-1-THC in animals and man prompted us to evaluate the heterocyclic benzopyrans for this activity (Green and Podos, 1974; Green, 1975; Hepler and Frank, 1971). Dren, Bopp, and Ebert (1975) have reported that Abbott-40656 and Abbott-40174 lower normal and elevated intraocular pressures in rabbit eyes.

In their studies, unanesthetized male albino rabbits weighing 2-4 kg were placed in plastic restrainers and both eyes were anesthetized by topically applied lidocaine hydrochloride (0.1 ml of 0.1%) prior to determining intraocular pressure. Either a Schiotz tonometer loaded with a 5.5 g weight or a Bausch and Lomb Applamatic tonometer was used to measure intraocular pressures.

The effect of Abbott-40656 on the intraocular pressure of normal rabbits was determined initially. Following two control determinations taken 30 minutes apart, test compounds were applied topically and readings made at 30, 60, 90, and 180 minutes afterward. Abbott-40656 was tested topically (0.1 ml) in concentrations of 0.01, 0.1, and 1%. Control animals received physiological saline. Abbott-40656 effectively decreased the intraocular pressure of normal rabbit eyes. Multifactor analysis of variance of the intraocular pressure determinations made over the four-hour period indicated that the overall effect of Abbott-40656 was significant at the 0.1 and 1% concentrations. In these same studies, Abbott-40174 was found to be equivalent in potency to Abbott-40656.

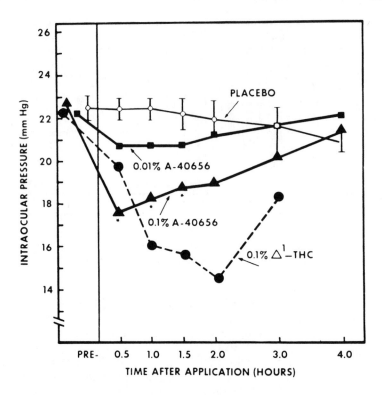

Figure 6. Topically applied Abbott-40656 and delta-1-THC
              lower intraocular pressure in normal rabbit eyes.

In Figure 6, the intraocular pressure-lowering properties of 0.1%
delta-1-THC are compared to Abbott-40656. The delta-1-THC was dissolved
in olive oil and then suspended in 0.5% carboxymethylcellulose (1:9 mixture)
for topical application.

The average ocular pressure of the eyes treated topically with the
higher concentration of Abbott-40656 (0.1%) was significantly lower than
that of the control group at 0.5 through 1.5 hours after drug administration.
There were no significant differences in the pressures of the placebo controls
and lowest dose (0.01%) group at any of the time intervals. A gradual but
slight reduction in the intraocular pressure of the placebo control group was
observed during the 4-hour period. There were no significant differences between the control and the 0.1% Abbott-40656 test group at 3 and 4 hours.

In a separate but similar study, the intraocular pressure lowering properties of delta-1-THC were also demonstrated as shown in Figure 6. Delta-1-
THC at 0.1% concentration produced a slightly greater and more prolonged
lowering of intraocular pressure than did Abbott-40656.

ACUTE TOXICITY

The acute oral LD_{50} of the heterocyclic benzopyrans in mice and rats are compared to the LD_{50}'s of various reference standards in Table 3. Abbott–40174 and Abbott–41988 were considerably less toxic than Abbott–40656. This differentiation in acute toxicity may in part be explained by the water-solubility of Abbott–40656. The LD_{50} of Abbott–40656, however, was considerably greater than that of pentobarbital sodium in mice but somewhat lower than that of codeine phosphate.

SELF–ADMINISTRATION STUDIES

The pharmacological spectra of many psychoactive agents having sedative–hypnotic, tranquilizer and/or analgetic properties include the capacity to reinforce self–administration behavior in animals. This test procedure has been used to indicate the abuse potential of compounds in man. Therefore, we have evaluated the dependency–producing characteristics of the water–soluble derivative Abbott–40656 (SP–106) by determining its reinforcing properties in rhesus monkeys under experimental conditions in which other psychoactive agents are positive reinforcers of self–administration behavior. These data have been reported previously by Jochimsen and Dren (1974).

Table 3
Acute Oral Toxicity in Mice and Rats

Compound	Mouse LD_{50}*	Rat LD_{50}*
Abbott–40174 (SP–1)	2500 (1670–3750)	900 (650–1240)
Abbott–40656 (SP–106)	570 (500–650)	130 (107–159)
Abbott–41988 (SPA–80)	3000 (2600–3500)	>1000
Codeine Phosphate	693 (601–820)	NOT TESTED
Pentobarbital Sodium	240 (222–259)	NOT TESTED

*Mg/kg, orally. Values in parentheses represent 95% confidence limits.

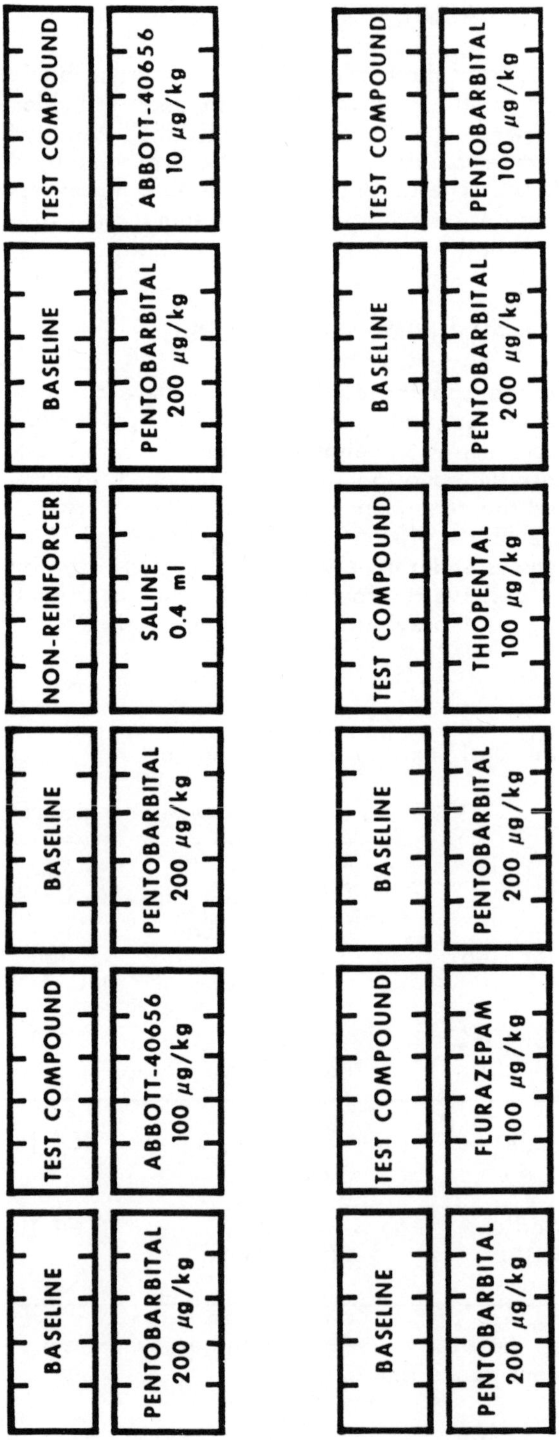

Figure 7. Pentobarbital substitution protocol followed over 12 consecutive weeks to compare i.v. self-administration of CNS depressants in rhesus monkeys.

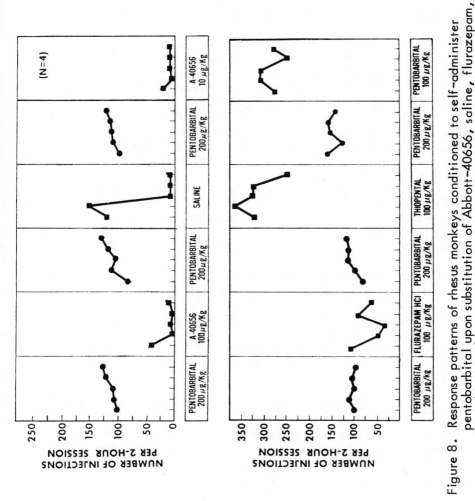

Figure 8. Response patterns of rhesus monkeys conditioned to self-administer pentobarbital upon substitution of Abbott-40656, saline, flurazepam, and thiopental.

In our procedure, male rhesus monkeys are surgically prepared with chronic indwelling silastic catheters implanted in the jugular vein. After surgery, the animals were housed in primate restraining chairs and were transported from our animal quarters to experimental chambers for each test session. In the chambers, the animals were able to self-administer drug solutions by pressing a lever switch to activate an automatic infusion pump connected to the intravenous catheter. Each lever press resulted in a single injection. The animals were allowed access to drug solutions for 2 hours each day for 5 consecutive weekdays. These were followed by a 2-day rest period.

The general protocol that we followed was based on a substitution procedure as shown in Figure 7. The animals were initially conditioned to respond for pentobarbital, at a dose of $200 \mu g/kg$ injection as the reference standard. When the animals began to respond regularly for pentobarbital, which required a period of several weeks, a one-week period was designated as a baseline. The animals were then given access to a non-reinforcing substance such as physiological saline for one week or to some test compound such as Abbott-40656 at a specific dose level on alternate weeks. In between, the animals were always returned to a pentobarbital baseline.

When either Abbott-40656, at doses of 100 and 10 $\mu g/kg$ injection, or saline was substituted for pentobarbital, as shown in the upper row of panels of Figure 8, the animals extinguished their lever-pressing behavior, indicating that Abbott-40656, like saline, was not reinforcing in barbiturate-dependent monkeys.

In the lower row of panels shown in Figure 8, reference standards known to be positive reinforcers of self-administration behavior were substituted for pentobarbital in the same animals that did not respond for either Abbott-40656 or saline. Both flurazepam and thiopental maintained self-administration behavior in these animals, and in the last panel we illustrate that the mean rate of responding is dose-dependent. When the dose of pentobarbital was lowered to 100 $\mu g/kg$ per injection, the rate was approximately doubled.

We also investigated the reinforcing properties of Abbott-40656 in monkeys previously conditioned to self-administer cocaine HCl, our psychostimulant reference standard, and morphine sulfate, our narcotic analgesic reference standard. As we found in the barbiturate model, Abbott-40656 did not maintain self-administration behavior in either the cocaine- or morphine-dependent animals.

SUMMARY

In summary, the preclinical neuropharmacological evaluation of three nitrogen-containing heterocyclic benzopyrans derived from the cannabinoid nucleus indicates that in a number of animal species the pharmacological spectra of these compounds include tranquilizer, analgetic, sedative-hypnotic, and intraocular pressure lowering properties. Unlike a variety of psychoactive agents having therapeutic utility in these areas, the water-soluble analog Abbott-40656 did not maintain intravenous self-administration behavior in rhesus monkeys previously made dependent on either pentobarbital, cocaine, or morphine sulfate.

Phase I clinical trial studies in normal human volunteers were recently initiated with these derivatives and are still in progress. Therefore, the potential therapeutic efficacy of these compounds in man is as yet unknown.

REFERENCES

Adams, R., Harfenst, M., & Loewe, S. New analogs of tetrahydrocannabi-
    nol. XIX. J. Med. Chem. Soc., 1949, 71, 1624-1628.

D'Amour, F. E. and Smith, D. L. A method for determining the loss of pain
    sensation. J. Pharmacol. Exp. Therap., 1941, 72, 74-79.

Dren, A.T., Bopp, B. A., & Ebert, D. M. Nitrogen-containing benzopyran
    analogs: Reduction of intraocular pressure in rabbits. Pharmacologist,
    1975, 17, 267.

Gray, W. E., Osterberg, A. C., & Scuto, T. J. Measurement of the anal-
    gesic efficacy and potency of pentazocine by the D'Amour and Smith
    method. J. Pharmacol. Exp. Therap., 1970, 172, 154-162.

Green, K. & Podos, S. M. Antagonism of arachidonic acid-induced ocular
    effects by delta-1-tetrahydrocannabinol. Investigative Ophthalmology,
    1974, 13, 422-429.

Green, K. Marihuana and the eye. Investigative Ophthalmology, 1975,
    14, 261-263.

Hepler, R. S., & Frank, I. M. Marihuana smoking and intraocular pressure.
    Journal of the American Medical Association, 1971, 217, 1392.

Jochimsen, W. G., & Dren, A. T. Abbott-40656 (SP-106), a water soluble
    benzopyran: Evaluation of its reinforcing properties in the rhesus
    monkey. Fed. Proc., 1974, 33, 527.

Lanoir, J. & Killan, E. K. Alteration in the sleep-wakefulness patterns by
    benzodiazepines in the cat. Electroenceph. Clin. Neurophysiol.,
    1968, 25, 530-542.

Li, H. C. An archeological and historical account of Cannabis in China.
    Journal of Economic Botany, 1974, 28, 437-448.

Litchfield, J. T. & Wilcoxon, F. A simplified method of evaluating dose-
    effect experiments. J. Pharmacol. Exp. Therap., 1949, 95, 99-113.

Pars, H. G., Granchelli, F. F., Razdan, R. K., Rosenberg, F., Teiger, D.,
    & Harris, L. S. Drugs derived from cannabinoids, Part I. Nitrogen
    analogs: Benzopyranopyridines and benzopyranopyrroles. Journal of
    Medicinal Chemistry, 1976 (accepted for publication).

Razdan, R. K., Terris, B. Zitko, Pars, H. G., Plotnikoff, N. P., Dodge,
    P. W., Dren, A. T., Kyncl, J., & Somani, P. Drugs derived from
    cannabinoids, Part II. Basic esters of nitrogen and carbocyclic analogs
    of cannabinoids. Journal of Medicinal Chemistry, 1976 (accepted for
    publication).

Snyder, S. H. Uses of marijuana. New York: Oxford University Press,
    1971.

Whittle, B. A. The change in capillary permeability in mice to distinguish
    between narcotic and non-narcotic analgesics. Brit. J. Pharmacol.,
    1964, 22, 246-253.

Winn, M., Arendsen, D., Dodge, P., Dren, A., Dunnigan, D., Hallas, R.,
    Hwang, K., Kyncl, J., Lee, Y., Plotnikoff, N., Young, P., Zaugg,
    H., & Dalzall, H. Drugs derived from cannabinoids, Part V. Delta^{6a},
    ^{10a}-tetrahydrocannabinol and heterocyclic analogs containing aro-
    matic side chains. Journal of Medicinal Chemistry, 1976 (accepted
    for publication).

Woolfe, G. & MacDonald, A. D. Evaluation of analgesic action of pethi-
    dine hydrochloride (Demerol Ⓡ). J. Pharmacol. Exp. Therap., 1944,
    80, 300-307.

Young, P. R., Dodge, P. W., Dren, A. T., & Plotnikoff, N. P. Analgetic
    activity studies with Abbott-41988, a benzopyranopyridine compound.
    Pharmacologist, 1975, 17, 188.

CHAPTER 27

COMPARATIVE TOXICITIES OF TETRAHYDROPYRIDOBENZOPYRANS

George R. Thompson
Christine L. Yang

Abbott Laboratories
North Chicago, Illinois

Various forms of marihuana preparations have been used and abused for nearly 5,000 years (Rossi, 1970). However, precise systematic delineation of toxicologic and pharmacologic effects has only been possible since the recent isolation and identification of delta-9-tetrahydrocannabinol (delta-9-THC) as the major active component (Gaoni and Mechoulam, 1964), and delta-8-THC as a minor active constituent in cannabis (Hively, Mosher and Hoffman, 1966). The signs of acute toxicity produced by these cannabinoids in rats, dogs, and monkeys included severe hypothermia, bradypnea, rapid weight loss, ataxia, muscle tremors, prostration, and hyperreactivity to stimuli (Thompson, Rosenkrantz, Schaeppi and Braude, 1973). In addition, dogs and monkeys exhibited salivation, emesis, and drowsiness. Rats treated chronically with cannabinoids developed tolerance to most signs of depression and, ultimately, exhibited increased activity and convulsions (Thompson, Mason, Rosenkrantz and Braude, 1974). These cannabinoids, therefore, produced similar signs of toxicity in various species, but some species differences were apparent.

Abbott-40174, Abbott-40656, and Abbott-41988 are tetrahydropyridobenzopyrans that are chemically and generically distinct from tetrahydrocannabinols (Figure 1). These three compounds are benzopyran derivatives with a nitrogen inserted into the "C" ring and modifications in the attached side-chains. These congeners demonstrated pharmacological activity as analgesics, sedative-hypnotics, tranquilizers and/or antihypertensives. Alteration of the chemical structures in Abbott-40174, Abbott-40656, and Abbott-41988 produced quantitative differences in their pharmacological activities (for example, the analgetic activity of Abbott-41988 was greater than that of Abbott-40174 and Abbott-40656, while the tranquilizing activity was reduced). Consequently, potential toxicological differences needed to be evaluated prior to commencement of efficacy studies in man.

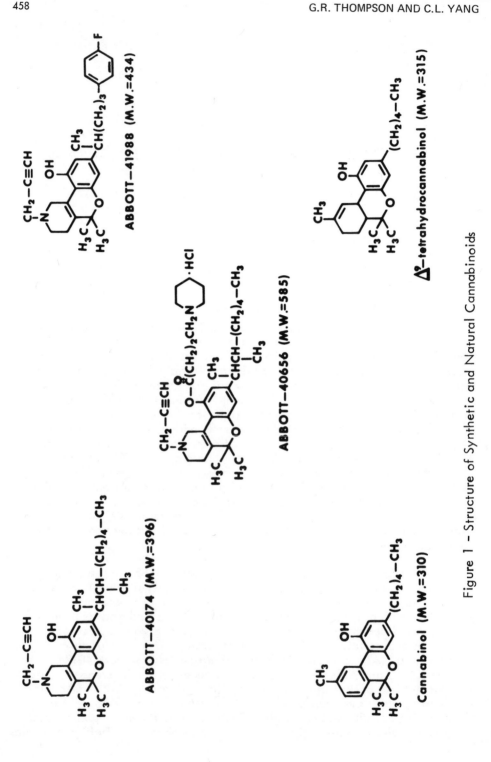

Figure 1 - Structure of Synthetic and Natural Cannabinoids

LD50 values for ABBOTT-40174, ABBOTT-40656, and ABBOTT-41988 were determined in male Sprague-Dawley rats and in female Swiss-Webster mice (Table 1). ABBOTT-40656 was the most acutely toxic compound in both rats and mice. ABBOTT-40174 was substantially less toxic than ABBOTT-40656 while ABBOTT-41988 was even slightly less toxic than ABBOTT-40174 in both species. All three compounds were more potent in male rats than in female mice. The differences in chemical structure, therefore, resulted in different potencies for acute toxicity.

The subacute toxicities of these three compounds have been determined in three animal species (Table 2). The duration of compound administration varied from 3 to 35 consecutive daily treatments. All three compounds were administered per os to each species, and ABBOTT-40174 and ABBOTT-40656 were also administered intravenously. Only ABBOTT-40656 was evaluated for subacute toxicity after intramuscular treatments.

The subacute toxicities of ABBOTT-40174, ABBOTT-40656, and ABBOTT-41988 in rats were characterized by sedation, body weight loss, hypothermia, and bradypnea. Long-Evans rats treated orally with ABBOTT-40174, ABBOTT-40656, or ABBOTT-41988 at 2-50 mg/kg/day for one month exhibited drug- and dose-related decreased body weights (Figure 2). Rapid body weight loss occurred for the first 3 days of treatment and was similar in magnitude for all three congeners. Tolerance was evident by day 7. The duration of body weight loss corresponded to the duration of inactivity and sedation, and body weight recovery occurred as tolerance developed to signs of behavior depression. Rates of weight gain in treated groups during

Table 1

LD Values for A-40174, A-40656, and A-41988
in Female Mice and Male Rats[a]

Route of Administration	Test Species	Observation Time (Day)	Test Compound[b]		
			A-40174	A-40656	A-41988
oral	mouse	7	$2.5(1.7-3.8)^c$	0.57(0.50-0.65)	3.0(2.6-3.5)
oral	rat	7	0.9(0.7-1.2)	0.13(0.11-0.16)	>1.0

[a] Values were determined according to the method of Litchfield and Wilcoxon (1949).

[b] All compounds were suspended or dissolved in 0.5% methocel.

[c] Values in parentheses indicate 95% confidence limits (in gm/kg).

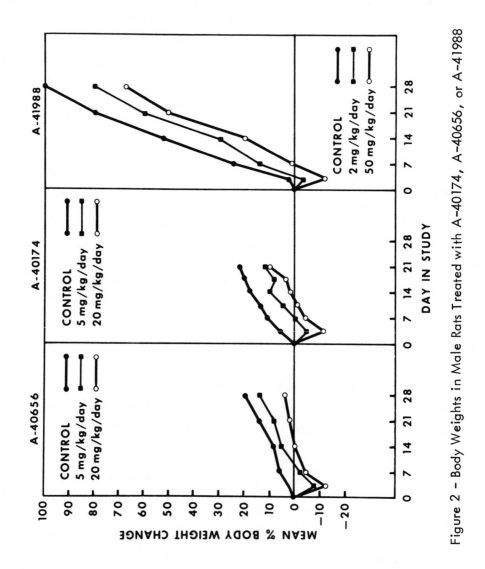

Figure 2 – Body Weights in Male Rats Treated with A–40174, A–40656, or A–41988

Table 2

Subacute Toxicity Studies for A-40174, A-40656, and A-41988

Test Species	Route of Administration	Test Compound		
		A-40174	A-40656	A-41988
Rat	P.O.	21[a]	30	30
	I.V.	15, 19	30	--
Dog	P.O.	3	3, 35	3, 30
	I.V.	5, 14, 32	30	--
Rhesus Monkey	P.O.	23	30	30, 35
	I.V.	14, 28	--	--
	I.M.	--	14, 30	--

[a] Treatment duration (in days).

the last three weeks of treatment were similar to controls. However, body weights for treated rats never recovered to control levels. The apparent differences in growth rates for control and treated rats in the Abbott-41988 experiment resulted from the substantially smaller initial body weights (60% less) of these younger animals.

Hypothermia and bradypnea in these rats occurred within 15 minutes and 4 hours after the first treatment in rats treated i.v. and p.o., respectively (Figures 3 and 4). Tolerance to bradypnea was evident by day 3. Decreased rectal temperatures in rats treated intravenously with Abbott-40656 did not recover until day 14 in a 28-day study, and rectal temperatures in rats treated with Abbott-40174 never recovered to control levels in a 14-day study. Tolerance to hypothermia in rats treated p.o. with Abbott-41988 occurred by day 3. These data indicated that body weight decrements, hypothermia, and bradypnea occurred in rats treated with all three congeners. Hypothermia was more persistent than body weight loss and bradypnea in rats treated i.v. with Abbott-40656 or Abbott-40174.

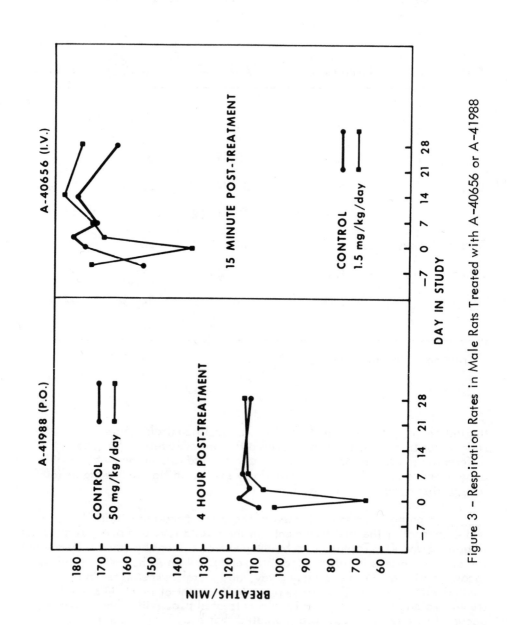

Figure 3 – Respiration Rates in Male Rats Treated with A-40656 or A-41988

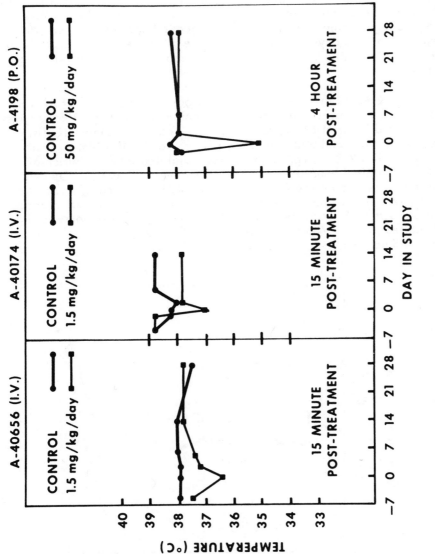

Figure 4 – Rectal Temperatures in Male Rats Treated with A–40174, A–40656, or A–41988

Drug- and dose-related behavioral signs of depression and hyper-reactivity to external stimuli were also observed in rats treated p.o. or i.v. with these three congeners. Rats treated orally with 20-50 mg/kg/day of Abbott-40174, Abbott-40656, or Abbott-41988 were inactive within 30 minutes after the first treatment, and vocalized persistently. Spontaneous, intermittent episodes of jerks and jumps occurred without stimulation in many treated rats. Intravenous treatments with Abbott-40174 or Abbott-40656 produced effects within one minute. Tolerance to behavioral effects was evident within 3-10 days. Generally, female rats were more susceptible to treatments as indicated by a faster onset and greater intensity of behavioral effects.

In a subacute toxicity study in dogs, oral administration of Abbott-41988 produced a dose-related sequence of ophthalmic changes that progressed from decreased lacrimation to corneal opacity, keratitis, conjunctivitis, corneal ulceration, and prolapse of the iris, especially in females. Female dogs treated with 2.8 mg/kg/day for 7 days exhibited total inhibition of lacrimation within 4 hours after the initial treatment (Figure 5). Decreased lacrimation persisted for the 7 days of treatment, but marked tolerance was evident in 2/3 treated dogs on day 5. Total recovery of lacrimation occurred within 24 hours after treatment termination. The pupillary response to light was inhibited in only 1/3 dogs treated with 2.8 mg/kg/day, and the affected dog also did not exhibit tolerance to lacrimal inhibition.

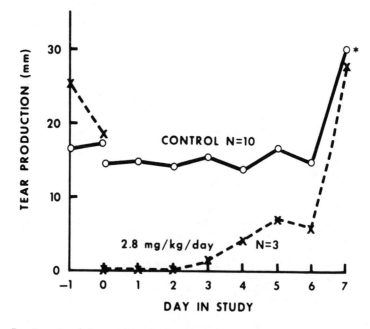

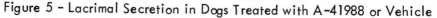

Figure 5 - Lacrimal Secretion in Dogs Treated with A-41988 or Vehicle

   Intraocular pressure was significantly decreased in a dose-related manner in dogs treated with Abbott-41988 (Figure 6). Decreased intraocular pressure first occurred one hour after the initial treatment and persisted for more than 6 hours. Affected dogs exhibited normal intraocular pressure within 24 hours after each treatment (Figure 7). The ophthalmic effects of Abbott-41988 were more pronounced in female dogs and did not occur in either of two subacute rhesus monkey studies or in one rat toxicity study with this compound. Therefore, ophthalmic effects in beagles treated with Abbott-41988 appeared to be species-specific and sex-related.

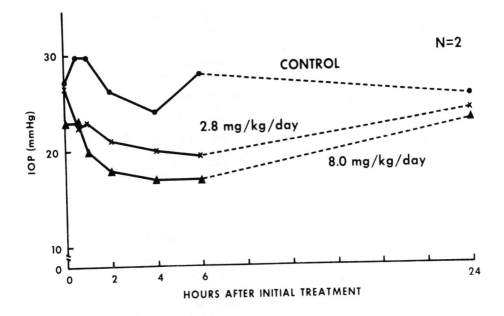

Figure 6 - Onset and Duration of Decreased Intraocular Pressure in Dogs Treated with A-41988 or Vehicle

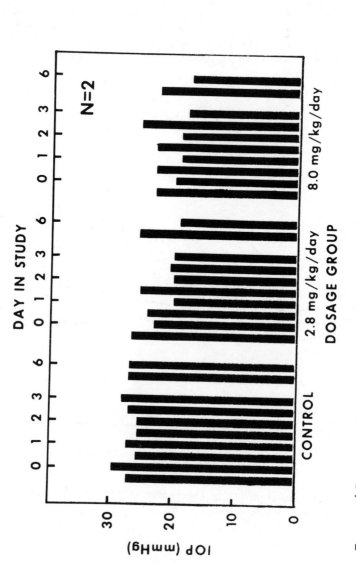

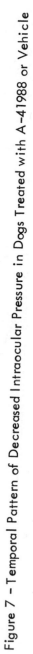

Figure 7 – Temporal Pattern of Decreased Intraocular Pressure in Dogs Treated with A-41988 or Vehicle

   Ophthalmic effects in dogs were further evaluated in 15 female dogs treated with equal molar dosages of all three congeners, and cannabinol, for 3 days (that is, days 0, 1, 2) (Table 3). The three congeners produced decreased intraocular pressure, lacrimal inhibition, and increased incidences of conjunctivitis. Cannabinol also decreased intraocular pressure and inhibited lacrimation, but conjunctivitis did <u>not</u> occur in dogs treated with this compound. Decreased intraocular pressure in female dogs treated with Abbott-40656 or Abbott-41988 occurred within one hour after each treatment for the 3 days of compound administration. Dogs treated with either Abbott-40174 or cannabinol did not exhibit decreased intraocular pressure until one hour after the second treatment. Most affected dogs exhibited normal intraocular pressure within 6 hours after each treatment.

   Increased incidences of conjunctivitis in dogs treated with Abbott-40656, Abbott-40174, or Abbott-41988 but not in dogs treated with cannabinol may have resulted from impaired lacrimation. All three congeners inhibited lacrimation within 4 hours after the initial treatment (Figure 8). Total lacrimal inhibition by Abbott-40656 persisted for the 3 days of treatment. However, partial tolerance to this effect was evident on day 1 in 3/3 and 2/3 dogs treated with Abbott-41988 and Abbott-40174, respectively. The persistence of lacrimal inhibition by Abbott-41988 in this 3-day study

Table 3

Ophthalmic Effects in Female Beagles Treated Per Os for Three Days
With A-40174, A-40656, A-41988 or Cannabinol

| Parameter | Test Compound | | | |
	A-40174	A-40656	A-41988	Cannabinol
Dosage (mg/kg/day)	7.3	10.8	8.0	5.7
Lacrimation[a]	-70% (1)[b]	-100% (3)	-96% (1)	-25% (1)
Intraocular Pressure[c]	-10% (1)	-39% (3)	-17% (3)	-17% (1)
Conjunctivitis	+33%	+33%	+66%	0

[a] Measured 4 hours after each treatment by the Schirmer Tear Test.

[b] Numbers in parenthesis indicate duration of the effect in days.

[c] Measured 1 hour after each treatment.

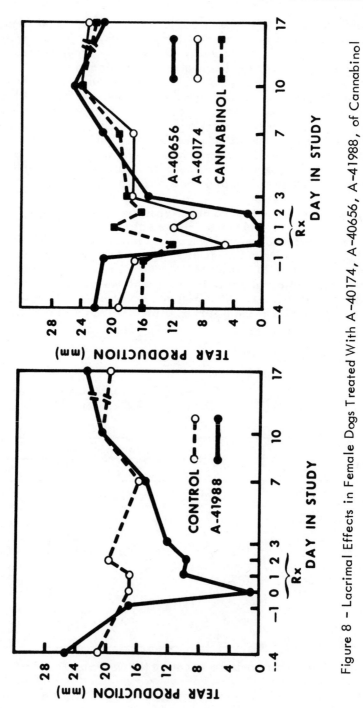

Figure 8 – Lacrimal Effects in Female Dogs Treated With A-40174, A-40656, A-41988, of Cannabinol

was much less than in a previous 6-day study (Figure 5). Total recovery of lacrimation in dogs treated with Abbott-40174 occurred within 24 hours after treatment termination. Total recovery in dogs treated with Abbott-40656 or Abbott-41988 did not occur until days 7-10 (that is, 5-8 days after treatment termination). Dogs treated with cannabinol were slightly affected on day 0 only.

The three congeners and cannabinol also produced behavioral and physical effects in the 3-day experiment. Ataxia and sedation occurred 4 hours after the initial treatment and lasted for approximately 24 hours. These effects were less pronounced in dogs treated with cannabinol. Tolerance was evident about two weeks after initiation of treatments. Decrements in body weights were evident in all dogs 24 hours after initial treatments. Body weight losses of 8-9% occurred after 3 days of treatment with Abbott-40656, Abbott-40174 or Abbott-41988. Cannabinol produced only about a 3% weight loss after three days of treatment. Effects on body weight persisted during the 2-week recovery period in all three dogs treated with Abbott-40656 and in 2/3 dogs treated with Abbott-40174 or Abbott-41988. Dogs treated with cannabinol exhibited normal body weights within the 2-week recovery period.

Patterns of behavioral and physiological effects produced by the three congeners were generally similar in monkeys. Behavioral changes in monkeys treated orally with Abbott-40656, Abbott-40174, or Abbott-41988 included ptosis, drowsiness, inactivity, and huddled posture. The times of onset for drowsiness and depression were dose-related, and occurred within 1-4 hours after treatment. These effects persisted for approximately 5 days, but tolerance was evident by days 6-8. Tolerance was manifested as a decreased daily duration of effects (in hours) or a complete cessation of the abnormal behavior.

Physiological effects produced by the congeners in monkeys included hypothermia, bradypnea, anorexia, and decreased growth rates (Table 4). The onset and severity of hypothermia and bradypnea in monkeys treated with these three congeners were dose-related. During the first 3 days of treatment, hypothermia and bradypnea usually occurred within 4 hours after treatment. Tolerance to these effects developed more rapidly in monkeys treated with lower dosages and was evident between days 7-21. Food consumption was slightly decreased in monkeys treated with 40 mg/kg/day of Abbott-41988. Normal food consumption was evident in affected animals by day 7. Only male monkeys treated with Abbott-40656 showed decreased food consumption during the first week of treatment, and tolerance was evident by day 14. Data for food consumption in monkeys treated with Abbott-40174 were not available. Male and female monkeys treated with Abbott-41988 and male monkeys treated with Abbott-40656 exhibited moderate body weight loss during the first week of treatment. All affected monkeys were generally normal by day 14. Effects on body weights did not occur in male or female monkeys treated with Abbott-40174.

Table 4

Physiological Effects in Rhesus Monkeys Treated Per Os
With A-40174, A-40656, or A-41988

	A-40174	A-40656	A-41988
Duration of Administration	30 days	30 days	35 days
Dosage (mg/kg/day)	30	50	40
Rectal Temperature[a]	no data	no data	F (−3%) M (−3%)
Respiration Rates[a]	no data	no data	F (−28%) M (−23%)
Food Consumption[b]	no data	F (−2%) M (−21%)	F (−16%) M (−17%)
Body Weight[b]	F (normal) M (normal)	F (normal) M (−9%)	F (−3%) M (−3%)
Hemorrhagic Diarrhea Incidence	0	F (0%) M (100%)	F (50%) M (100%)
Mortalities[c]	0	0	F (17%) M (50%)

[a]Measured 4 hours after the second treatment.
[b]Measured on day 7.
[c]Included animals sacrificed due to moribund condition.

Hemorrhagic diarrhea occurred in monkeys treated with Abbott-41988 or Abbott-40656, but resultant mortalities occurred only in monkeys treated with Abbott-41988 (Table 4). Neither hemorrhagic diarrhea nor mortalities occurred in monkeys treated with Abbott-40174. Rhesus monkeys treated with Abbott-41988 for one month exhibited dose-related morbidity, mortality, and onset time for severe colitis (Table 5). Monkeys treated with Abbott-41988 at 40 mg/kg/day exhibited hemorrhagic diarrhea as early as 4 days after the initial treatment. In the low-dose group (2.5 mg/kg/day) two animals had an onset of hemorrhagic diarrhea as late as 22 days after the initial treatment. Most of the animals with diarrhea had colitis at necropsy.

Drug- and dose-related incidences of mortalities also occurred in monkeys treated with Abbott-41988. Shigella were isolated from many of the animals in this study, and the intestinal lesions were characteristic of changes induced by this bacteria. Consequently, another 5-week oral

Table 5

Shigellosis Incidence, Morbidity, and Mortality in Rhesus Monkeys treated per Os with A-41988

Dosage (mg/kg/day)	No. of Animals Per Group	No. of Animals Exhibiting Isolated Shigella spp.	Incidence of Hemorrhagic Diarrhea	Incidence of Characteristic Lesions	Mortality[b]
0 (Vehicle Control)	6M & 6F	1	0	0	0
2.5	3M & 3F	4	3/6 (16)[a]	1/6	1
10.0	3M & 3F	5	5/6 (9)	4/6	2
40.0	6M & 6F	4	9/12 (4–14)	7/12	4

[a] Number in parenthesis indicates mean day of onset.

[b] Included animals that were sacrificed due to moribund condition.

toxicity study was performed with Abbott-41988 administered to rhesus monkeys that were free of fecal Shigella and Salmonella for three consecutive determinations. The absence of signs and lesions in the uninfected monkeys indicated that effects in the original study resulted from exacerbation of an infection with Shigella rather than from direct, primary intestinal toxicity produced by Abbott-41988. Since Abbott-41988 had no apparent direct effect on the Shigella organisms, or on immunological mechanisms, the mechanism for the chemical exacerbation of shigellosis was probably related to decreased gastro-intestinal motility. Similar hemorrhagic diarrhea occurred in rhesus monkeys treated with delta-9-THC (Thompson, Fleischman, Rosen-krantz and Braude, 1974).

No adverse clinical or anatomic pathology findings were observed in rats, dogs, or monkeys treated per os with Abbott-40174, Abbott-40656, or Abbott-41988 except for the ophthalmic effects in dogs and the exacerba-tion of shigellosis in monkeys treated with Abbott-41988. Behavioral and physiological changes predominated in all species, but tolerance generally developed to these effects during the first 3-21 days of treatment. The onset of tolerance was consistently inversely dose-related (that is, faster in animals treated with lower dosages). Chronic oral toxicity studies with these congeners have not been performed, and consequently the potential for cumulative behavioral and/or neurochemical changes similar to effects reported for cannabinoids (Ho, Taylor, Englert and McIsaac, 1971; Luthran and Rosenkrantz, 1974) remains to be evaluated.

Toxicity signs produced by the three congeners in rats, dogs, or monkeys were generally similar for all routes of administration. However, animals treated with Abbott-40656 by intramuscular administration exhibited muscle necrosis that was not observed for other treatment routes. Similar severe necrosis occurred in rabbits treated subcutaneously with delta-9-THC (Thompson, Rosenkrantz, Fleischman and Braude, 1975). Essentially all other behavioral and physiological effects occurred for both i.v. or p.o. treatment; only the temporal patterns and severities of effects were affected by changes in the route of administration.

Toxicity produced by Abbott-40174, Abbott-40656, or Abbott-41988 in rats, dogs, or monkeys was quite similar to that produced by cannabinoids. Behavioral and physiological effects produced by these three congeners were previously observed in animals similarly treated with cannabinoids. Only ophthalmic histopathological changes in dogs treated with Abbott-41988 have not previously been reported for the cannabinoids. The similarity of subacute toxicities for the tetrahydropyridobenzopyrans and cannabinoids suggests that neurochemical changes observed in rats and monkeys treated chronically with cannabinoids may also occur in animals treated chronically with these three congeners. This possibility will be evaluated in subsequent chronic toxicity studies.

Evaluation of the toxicity observed in experimental animals treated with the three congeners indicated that considerable safety margins could be anticipated for short-term clinical trials. Abbott-40174 produced essentially no persistent behavioral or physiological effects, and no histopathological changes occurred in rats, dogs, or monkeys treated with this compound. The only serious effect produced in three animal species by Abbott-41988 was hemorrhagic diarrhea in monkeys. Subsequent evaluations in monkeys treated with Abbott-41988 indicated that hemorrhagic diarrhea in this species resulted from exacerbation of shigellosis. Abbott-41988 also produced pathologic effects in the eyes of dogs which resulted from lacrimal inhibition. Exclusion of clinical subjects with Shigella and/or Salmonella would avoid the potential colitis, and cessation of clinical treatments in subjects exhibiting impaired lacrimation should prevent the development of ophthalmic effects. Consequently, preclinical toxicological evaluations with these three congeners permitted initiation of short-term clinical trials.

REFERENCES

Gaoni, V. & Mechoulam, R. Isolation, structure and partial synthesis of an active constituent of hashish. J. Amer. Chem. Soc. (1964), 86, 1646-1648.

Hively, R.L., Mosher, W.A., & Hoffman, F. Isolation of trans-delta-6-tetrahydrocannabinol from marihuana. J. Amer. Chem. Soc. (1966), 88, 1832-1833.

Ho, B.T., Taylor, D., Englert, L.F., & McIsaac, W.M. Neurochemical effects of L-delta-9-tetrahydrocannabinol in rats following repeated inhalation. Brain Res. (1971), 31, 233-236.

Litchfield, J.T. & Wilcoxon, F. A simplified method for evaluating dose-effect experiments. J. Pharmacol. Exp. Ther. (1949), 96, 99-113.

Luthra, Y.K. & Rosenkrantz, R. Cannabinoids: Neurochemical aspects after oral chronic administration to rats. Tox. Appl. Pharmacol. (1974), 27, 158-168.

Rossi, G.V. Pharmacological effects of drugs that are abused. Amer. J. Pharm. (1970), 142, 161-170.

Thompson, G.R., Fleischman, R.W., Rosenkrantz, R., & Braude, M.C. Oral and intravenous toxicity of delta-9-tetrahydrocannabinol in rhesus monkeys. Tox. Appl. Pharmacol. (1974), 27, 648-665.

Thompson, G.R., Mason, M.M., Rosenkrantz, R., & Braude, M.C. Chronic oral toxicity of cannabinoids in rats. Tox. Appl. Pharmacol. (1973), 25, 373-390.

Thompson, G.R., Rosenkrantz, R., Fleischman, R.W., & Braude, M.C. Effects of delta-9-tetrahydrocannabinol administered subcutaneously to rabbits for 28 days. Toxicology (1975), 4, 41-51.

Thompson, G.R., Rosenkrantz, R., Schaeppi, U.H., & Braude, M.C. Comparison of acute oral toxicity of cannabinoids in rats, dogs and monkeys. Tox. Appl. Pharmacol. (1973), 25, 363-372.

CHAPTER 28

NEW BENZOPYRANS: ANTICONVULSANT ACTIVITIES

Nicholas P. Plotnikoff

Pharmacology and Medicinal Chemistry Division
Abbott Laboratories

North Chicago, Illinois

NOTE: We would like to express our appreciation to
Dr. Harvey Kupferberg and the Anticonvulsant Advisory
Committee of the National Institute of Neurological
Diseases and Stroke for their encouragement of this
study (supported in part by contract N01-NS-3-2314.)

The authors are indebted to Dr. R. K. Razdan, B. Zitko
Terris, and H. G. Pars of the John C. Sheehan Institute
for Research and Sharps Associates (SISA), Cambridge,
Massachusetts, for the original chemical preparation of
the three derivatives of DMHP.

SUMMARY

Three new analogs of dimethylheptylpyran (DMHP) (SP-141, SP-143,
and SP-175) were found to exhibit significant anticonvulsant activity against
audiogenic, supramaximal electroshock, and maximal pentylentetrazol
induced seizures in mice. In rats, all three compounds were found to be
more active than diphenylhydantoin in the supramaximal electroshock test.
In particular, a different profile of anticonvulsant activity was demonstrated
for SP-175 compared to DMHP or delta-9-THC. It was discovered in 5-day
studies that dilantin, phenobarbital, DMHP, and SP-175 do not exhibit
tolerance development against audiogenic seizures in mice.

INTRODUCTION

Our interest in the benzopyrans as anticonvulsants stemmed from the pioneer animal studies of Loewe and Goodman (1947) and clinical studies of Davis and Ramsey (1949) on the isomers of dimethylheptylpyran analog (DMHP). Earlier O'Shaughnessy (1842) had introduced marihuana to Europe to treat various central nervous system disorders including epilepsy. Thus, it became of great interest to several investigators to study the anticonvulsant activity of the constituents of marihuana, for example, delta-9-THC, delta-8-THC, cannabidiol, cannabinol (4-16) (Garriott, Forney, Hughes and Richards, 1968; Sofia, Solomon and Barry, 1971; Man and Consroe, 1973; Boggan, Steele and Freedman, 1973; Corcoran, McCaughran and Wada, 1973; Wada, Sato and Corcoran, 1973; Karler, 1973; Karler, Cely and Turkanis, 1973; Carlini, Leite, Tannhauser and Berardi, 1973; Consroe and Man, 1973; Karler, Cely and Turkanis, 1974; Chesher and Jackson, 1974; Karler, Cely and Turkanis, 1974).

Our own interest has been to study new analogs of DMHP (Figure 1) in an attempt to find more specific anticonvulsant activity. A preliminary report on these compounds was presented recently (Plotnikoff, Zaugg, Petersen, Anderson and Ardensen, 1974).

METHODS

Experimental Animals, Drug Preparations, and Test Intervals

The test procedures were conducted with white male ARS/Sprague-Dawley strain mice, 18 to 24 grams, and male Long-Evans rats, 170 to 190 grams, unless otherwise stated. The test compounds were administered orally as a suspension in 10% olive oil and 90% Methocel (0.5%) to 10 animals per dose. All drugs were tested for activity at 1, 4, and 24 hours post drug administration in different groups of animals. Statistical analyses were carried out using simultaneous linear regression and probit techniques.

Audiogenic Seizures Test (Mouse)

Male O'Grady strain mice (14 to 16 grams) specially bred for susceptibility to audiogenic seizures were used as subjects. The audiogenic apparatus consisted of a wooden box enclosing a metal container with two doorbells attached to the upper section. After drug administration, the animals were placed in the audiogenic chamber and the bells activated for one minute and the animals were observed for convulsions (Plotnikoff and Green, 1957).

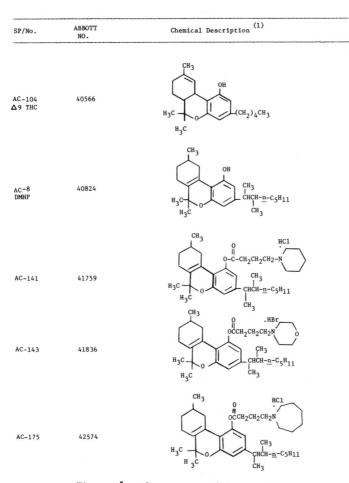

SP/No.	ABBOTT NO.	Chemical Description [1]
AC-104 Δ9 THC	40566	
AC-8 DMHP	40824	
AC-141	41759	
AC-143	41836	
AC-175	42574	

Figure 1. Structures of Benzopyrans

Chemistry

SP-141 (ABBOTT-41759)
3-(3-Methyl-2-octyl)-1-[4-(1-piperidine)butyryloxy]-6,6,9-trimethyl-7,8, 9,10-tetrahydro-6H-dibenzo[b,d] pyran hydrochloride

SP-143 (ABBOTT-41836)
3-(3-Methyl-2-octyl)-1-[4-(4-morpholine)butyryloxy]-6,6,9-trimethyl-7,8, 9,10-tetrahydro-6H-dibenzo[b,d]pyran hydrobromide

SP-175 (ABBOTT-42574)
3-(3-Methyl-2-octyl)-1-[4-(1-homopiperidine)butyryloxy]-6,6,9-trimethyl-7, 8,9,10-tetrahydro-6H-dibenzo[b,d]pyran hydrochloride
(Razdan, Terris, and Pars, 1975.)

Supramaximal Electroshock Test (Mouse and Rat)

After drug administration, each animal received an electroshock (mice received 100 cps., pulse duration 1.0 msec., at 140 volts for 0.3 sec.; rats received 150 ma at 0.2 sec.) through corneal electrodes to initiate a hindlimb tonic extension convulsion; anticonvulsant activity occurred when the above convulsion was blocked (Swinyard, Brown and Goodman, 1952; Toman and Everett, 1964).

Psychomotor Electroshock Test (Mouse)

After receiving drug, each animal was given an electroshock (6 cps., pulse duration 1.0 msec., at 70 volts for 3 sec.) through corneal electrode to initiate a psychomotor seizure. Protection from convulsions occurred when either the clonic forepaw activity or facial clonus was blocked (Toman and Everett, 1964).

Pentylenetetrazol Maximal Seizures Test -- Tonic Extension (Mouse)

After drug administration, each animal received pentylenetetrazol at 120 mg/kg subcutaneously to cause a tonic extension convulsion; anticonvulsant activity occurred when this convulsion was blocked (Toman and Everett, 1964).

Pentylenetetrazol Minimal Seizure Test (Mouse)

Following drug administration, each animal was given pentylenetetrazol at 85 mg/kg subcutaneously to elicit clonic convulsions; anticonvulsant action occurred when the convulsions were blocked (Swinyard, Brown and Goodman, 1952).

Supramaximal Electroshock Test (Rat)

Male Long-Evans rats (170-190 grams) are administered a single dose of test drug orally in a suspension in olive oil and 0.5% methocel for 4 consecutive days; on the fifth day various doses of the test drug (dose response) are orally administered to 10 rats per dose. At 4 hours post drug administration, the animals receive an electroshock (150 ma at 0.2 sec.) through corneal electrodes to initiate a hindlimb tonic extension and the animals are observed for protection from convulsion (Swinyard et al., 1952).

Rotarod Test (Mouse)

Mice were trained to remain on a rotating rod (16 revolutions per minute, Stoelting Company) for a maximum period of 100 seconds for two consecutive trials, modified after Kinnard and Carr (1957) procedure. After training, the animals were administered drug and again tested on the rotating rod. Motor deficit (TD50) was determined by a 50% reduction in the time the animals remained on the rod as compared to control time.

Inclined Screen Test (Rat)

After drug administration, each animal was placed in the center of a 14" x 16" wire mesh screen (1/2" hardware cloth) at an angle of 60 degrees for a period of 60 seconds. Motor deficit was determined by the length of time the animals remained on the inclined screen.

RESULTS

Audiogenic Seizures

Tonic extensor component. All compounds exhibited marked activity in preventing the hindlimb extensor component of the audiogenic seizure (Table 1). Thus, delta-9-THC was found to reduce the tonic extension component in 50% of the animals (ED50) at a dose of 5 mg/kg at the 1-hour test period. At later times (4 and 24 hours), delta-9-THC was considerably less active. In contrast, DMHP was found active over a prolonged period (24 hours) with ED50 values of 6.7, 2.9, and 15.1 mg/kg at 1, 4, and 24 hours, respectively. The new compounds exhibited potent activity at both the 1- and 4-hour periods but less at the 24-hour test time. Maximal effects were seen at the 4-hour test period with SP-141 with an ED50 of 2.8 mg/kg, SP-143 with an ED50 of 2.4 mg/kg, and SP-175 with an ED50 of 1.1 mg/kg. By way of comparison, diphenylhydantoin was quite effective at 1 and 4 hours and less so at 24 hours, the peak effect was seen at 1 hour with an ED50 of 1.7 mg/kg.

Five-day study. The oral administration of Abbott-42574 once daily to mice for 5 consecutive days showed marked activity in abolishing the hindlimb tonic extensor component of the audiogenic seizure; at 4 hours post drug administration on the fifth day, the ED50 was 0.7 mg/kg. In comparison with DMHP and diphenylhydantoin had estimated ED50's of 1.6 and <0.5 mg/kg, respectively, while phenobarbital was also very active with an ED50 of 0.1 mg/kg (Table 2).

Table 1

Effect of Various Benzopyran Compounds
And Diphenylhydantoin (DPH) on Audiogenic
Seizures in Mice

SP/No.	1 hr ED50* mg/kg (95% C.L.)	4 hr ED50* mg/kg (95% C.L.)	24 hr ED50* mg/kg (95% C.L.)
SP-104	5.0	38.8	
Delta-9-THC	2.4-77	29.1-49.3	100
SP-8	6.7	2.9	15.1
DMHP	2.1-11.0	1.8-4.9	8.2-26.3
SP-141	8.5	2.8	32.3
	5.1-13.8	1.4-6.8	20.0-48.8
SP-143	4.2	2.4	19.1
	2.1-8.0	1.2-5.5	12.5-27.0
SP-175	6.8	1.1	65.9
	4.1-11.3	0.5-2.4	27.0- --
DPH	1.7	3.3	11.0
	1.3-2.5	2.7-4.4	6.5-21.6

* Oral dose (mg/kg) at which 50% of the animals are protected
from hindlimb tonic extension.

Table 2

Comparison of Activity of ABBOTT-42574, DMHP,
Diphenylhydantoin (DPH) and Delta-9-THC in the
Audiogenic Seizure Tests at Various Times

SP/No. or Name	A/No.	4 Hr ED50* mg/kg (95% C.L.)	Five Day Chronic Audiogenic Seizure Test ED50 4 Hr*
SP-175	42574	1.1 (0.5-2.4)	0.7 (0.01-2.1)
SP-8 DMHP	40824	2.9 (1.8-4.9)	1.6 (0.01-4.9)
DPH	5538	3.3 (2.7-4.4)	ED50= 0.5
Phenobarbital		0.3 (0.1-0.9)	0.1 (0.01-0.2)

* Oral dose (mg/kg) at which 50% of the animals are protected
from hindlimb tonic extension.

Supramaximal Electroshock Studies

In mice the test compounds were found to be less potent than
diphenylhydantoin in antagonizing the tonic extensor component of supramaximal seizures (Table 3). Thus, delta-9-THC showed peak effects at 1 hour
with an ED50 of 31.9 mg/kg, while DMHP peaked at 4 hours with an ED50
of 57.2 mg/kg. The new compounds (SP-141 and SP-143) showed maximal
effects at 4 hours with ED50 values of 59.4 and 67.8 mg/kg, respectively.
SP-175, in contrast, was effective both at 1- and 4-hour test periods with
ED50 values of 68.3 and 75.9 mg/kg.

Table 3

Effect of Various Benzopyran Compounds and
Diphenylhydantoin (DPH) on Supramaximal
Electroshock Seizures in Mice and Rats

| | Mice | | | Rats |
SP/No.	1 hr ED50* mg/kg (95% C.L.)	4 hr ED50 mg/kg (95% C.L.)	24 hr ED50* mg/kg (95% C.L.)	4 hr ED50* mg/kg (95% C.L.)
SP-104	31.9	101.5	---	40.6
Delta-9-THC	29.1-34.5	96.4-106.6		24.1-142.7
SP-8	310.8	57.2		7.5
DMHP	230.7-587.5	35.1-80.1	>300	3.4-11.2
SP-141		59.4		4.6
	>300	41.6-81.4	>300	2.8-7.2
SP-143		67.8		25.2
	>300	41.0-150.3	>300	5.3-52.2
SP-175	68.3	75.9		7.4
	61.8-78.7	58.6-102	>300	4.2-13.4
DPH	8.1	7.6		62.2
	5.2-11	7.0-8.3	>20	57.0-67.3

* Oral dose (mg/kg) at which 50% of the animals are protected from
hindlimb tonic extension with 10 animals per dose.

In rats, DMHP and the new compounds appeared to be more potent than diphenylhydantoin in preventing hindlimb extension, whereas delta-9-THC was found to be approximately equal in potency to diphenylhydantoin (Table 3). At the peak time of 4 hours, the following ED50's were observed: DMHP, 7.5 mg/kg; SP-141, 4.6 mg/kg; SP-143, 25.2 mg/kg; and SP-175, 7.4 mg/kg. In contrast, diphenylhydantoin had a peak effect at 1 hour with an ED50 of 23 mg/kg and an ED50 of 62 mg/kg at 4 hours.

Supramaximal Electroshock Studies – Mice

Five-day study. The oral administration of Abbott-42574 and DMHP to mice for 5 consecutive days showed no activity in doses up to 300 mg/kg at 4 hours post drug administration in preventing hindlimb tonic extension component of the supramaximal seizure (Table 4).

Table 4

Comparison of Activity of ABBOTT-42574 and DMHP After Five Days Chronic Oral Dosing in the Supramaximal Electroshock Test in Mice (Daily Dose of 25 mg/kg for Four Days)

Compound	Fifth Day Oral Dose (mg/kg)	Percent Protection From Tonic Extension
Control	25	0
	50	0
	100	0
Abbott-42574	150	0
	200	0
	250	0
	300	0
Control	25	0
	50	0
	100	0
DMHP	150	0
	250	0
	300	0

Psychomotor Seizures

No significant activity was observed with the test agents in reducing facial forelimb clonus induced by low frequency electroshock except for slight activity with DMHP at high doses (Table 5).

Pentylenetetrazol Seizures

<u>Maximal seizures (tonic extension)</u>. All of the test agents effectively reduced the incidence of tonic extension with the exception of delta-9-THC (Table 6). DMHP was more effective than delta-9-THC or the new compounds with ED50 values of 9.5 and 10.2 at the 1 and 4 hour test periods. SP-141 and SP-143 were most effective at 1 hour with ED50 values of 20.2 and 31.1 mg/kg. SP-175 was effective at both the one and four hour tests with ED50 values of 41.8 and 38.2 mg/kg.

<u>Minimal seizures (clonus)</u>. No significant anticonvulsant activity with the test agents was observed against minimal (clonus) seizures, with the exception of DMHP and SP-141 (Table 6).

Table 5

Effects of Various Benzopyran Compounds and
Diphenylhydantoin (DPH) on Psychomotor
Electroshock Seizures in Mice

SP/No.	SP-104 Delta-9-THC	SP-8 DMHP	SP-141	SP-143	SP-175	DHP
4 hr ED50* mg/kg (95% C.L.)	> 300	186.3 (estimated)	> 300	> 300	> 300	> 240

* Oral dose (mg/kg) at which 50% of the animals are protected from facial and forelimb clonus.

Table 6

Effect of Various Benzopyran Compounds and
Diphenylhydantoin (DPH) on Pentylenetetrazol
Seizures in the Mouse
(Tonic Extension and Clonic Seizures)

SP/No.	Tonic Extension		Clonic Seizures	
	1 hr ED50* mg/kg (95% C.L.)	4 hr ED50* mg/kg (95% C.L.)	1 hr ED50* mg/kg (95% C.L.)	4 hr ED50* mg/kg (95% C.L.)
SP-104				
Delta-9-THC	300	>300	> 300	>300
SP-8	9.5	10.2		
DMHP	3.5-21.6	5.3-22.3	100=50%	>100
SP-141	20.2	54.9		
	10.0-41.0	29.4-113	100-70%	>300
SP-143	31.1	52.1		
	15.6-62.6	34.5-74.7	> 300	>300
SP-175	41.8	38.2		
	22.0-90.6	16.2-90.0	>100	>100
DPH	2.7	2.2		
	1.7-5.9	1.8-2.7	> 100	> 100

* Oral dose (mg/kg) at which 50% of the animals are protected from hindlimb tonic extension with 10 animals per dose.

RESULTS

Supramaximal Electroshock Seizures in Rats

<u>Single Doses</u>. The administration of Abbott-42574 in single oral doses demonstrated marked activity in preventing the hindlimb tonic extension feature of supramaximal electroshock. The ED50 for the peak time of drug activity (4 hours post administration) was 7.4 mg/kg, and the ED50 for DMHP was 7.5 mg/kg. In contrast, diphenylhydantoin was much less active with an ED50 of 62.2 mg/kg for the same time period (Table 7).

Table 7

Comparison of Activity of ABBOTT-42574, DMHP,
Delta-9-THC, and Diphenylhydantoin in the
Supramaximal Electroshock Test in Rats

SP/No. or Name	A/No.	1 hr ED50* mg/kg (95% C.L.)	4 hr ED50* mg/kg (95% C.L.)	24 hr ED50 mg/kg (95% C.L.)
SP-175	42574	60.6	7.4	
		(38.3-98.3)	(4.2-13.4)	$>$150
SP-8	DMHP	4.6	7.5	66.8
	40824	(3.0-6.9)	(3.4-11.2)	35---
DPH	5538	23.0	62.0	
		(32-51.4)	(57-67.3)	$>$200

* Oral dose (mg/kg) at which 50% of the animals are protected from hindlimb tonic extension.

Five-day study. The oral administration of 2.5 mg/kg of Abbott-42574 and DMHP to rats for 5 consecutive days showed moderate activity in abolishing the hindlimb tonic extensor component of the maximal electroshock seizure test; at 4 hours post drug administration on the fifth day the ED50 for Abbott-42574 and DMHP were 37.2 and 26.7 mg/kg, respectively (Table 8).

Table 8

Activity of ABBOTT-42574, DMHP, and Diphenylhydantoin After
Five Day Chronic Oral Administration of the
Supramaximal Electroshock Test in the Rat

SP/No.	A/No.	Oral Dose (mg/kg)	Percent Protection* or ED50**
SP-175	42574		
		ED50=	37.2*
Rats were dosed for 4 days at 2.5 mg/kg, on the fifth day a dose response was initiated.			(24.0-66.0)
DMHP			
		ED50=	26.7*
Rats were dosed for four days at 2.5 mg/kg, on the fifth day a dose response was initiated.			(5.4-118)
Diphenylhydantoin		10	40%
		25	20%
		50	40%
Rats were dosed for four days at 30 mg/kg, on the fifth day a dose response was initiated.		100	20%
		150	100%
		200	60%

*   Percent protection from tonic extension (N=10 animals/dose).

** Oral dose which protects 50% of the animals from tonic extension.

The activity of diphenylhydantoin was erratic and no ED50 could be calculated. When higher doses of Abbott-42574 (5.0 and 10.0 mg/kg) were administered daily, a certain degree of tolerance to anticonvulsant activity was observed (Table 9).

Table 9

Activity of ABBOTT-42574 After Chronic Oral Administration
on the Maximal Electroshock Test in the Rat.

SP/No.	Compound	Oral Dose (mg/kg)	Percent Protection*
SP-175	42574	20.0	60%
		40.0	30
Rats were dosed for four days at		80.0	60
5.0 mg/kg, on the fifth day a		100.0	40
dose response was initiated.		120.0	50
SP-175	42574	5.0	10%
		10.0	10
Rats were dosed for four days at		20.0	10
10.0 mg/kg, on the fifth day a		40.0	30
dose response was initiated.		80.0	15

* Percent protection from tonic extension.

Rotarod (Mice)

Therapeutic indices (TD50/ED50) were obtained when the anti-convulsant activity of the test agents against audiogenic seizures in mice was compared to the neurotoxicity of compounds tested on the rotarod (Table 10). At the 4 hour test period, delta-9-THC, DMHP, SP-141, SP-143, SP-175, and diphenylhydantoin showed ratios of 2, 7, 5, 8, 18, and 36, respectively.

Inclined Screen Test (Rat)

At peak time of anticonvulsant activity against supramaximal electro-shock (4 hours) no impairment of grip strength on the inclined screen was seen with either DMHP or SP-175 at doses up to 1280 mg/kg. (SP-141 and SP-143 at doses up to 640 mg/kg.)

DISCUSSION

The present study represents the first investigation of the profile of anticonvulsant activity of new benzopyran structures. In reviewing the anti-convulsant activity of delta-9-THC, it becomes apparent that it resembles diphenylhydantoin in profile (short duration) while DMHP appears to resemble trimethadione in profile (pentylenetetrazol antagonism). Thus, our new analog, SP-175, may represent a therapeutic advance in providing a longer duration of action than delta-9-THC and a diphenylhydantoin-like profile. In particular, SP-175 was found to be more active than diphenylhydantoin against supramaximal electroshock in the rat. DMHP and delta-9-THC in animal and human studies has been found to exhibit significant side effects,

Table 10

Effect of Various Benzopyran Compounds and
Diphenylhydantoin (DPH) on Rotarod
Performance in Mice

SP/No.	SP-104 delta-9-THC	SP-8 DMHP	SP-141	SP-143	SP-175	DPH
4 hr TD50* mg/kg	82.8	21.0	15.7	16.6	20.1	119.7
(95% C.L.)	46.6-321.7	3.4-39.0	0.3-31.8	7.1-42.8	11.5-29.5	82.3-164.7

* Oral dose (mg/kg) at which a 50% reduction occurs in the time the animals remain on the rotating rod.

not only in terms of neurotoxicity but also with respect to cardiovascular parameters (Hardman, Domino and Seevers, 1971; Domino, Hardman and Seevers, 1971; Domino, 1971). Most investigators have used the intravenous or intraperitoneal route of administration with delta-9-THC and DMHP. The new compounds, particularly SP-175, appear to exhibit a low degree of neurotoxicity by the oral route, particularly in the rat. It is our hope that this new compound will be evaluated in higher species, both alone and in combination with other known anticonvulsant agents.

Our studies in audiogenic seizures in mice showing no tolerance formation to the anticonvulsant activity to diphenylhydantoin or phenobarbital represent the first successful rodent model to correlate with clinical findings. Apparently little or no tolerance to the anticonvulsant activity of diphenyl-hydantoin or phenobarbital is seen clinically (Woodbury, Penry, and Schmidt, 1972). Thus, it has been difficult to predict tolerance formation from rodent studies up to now, in view of the marked tolerance observed with diphenyl-hydantoin and phenobarbital against maximal electroshock seizures (Frey and Kampmann, 1965; Fried and McIntyre, 1973; Karler, Cely and Turkanis, 1974). More recently, Karler, Cely, and Turkanis (1974) have reported tolerance to delta-9-tetrahydrocannabinol, cannabidiol, diphenylhydantoin, and phenobarbital against maximal electroshock seizures in mice, which they attribute to central adaptation.

In the case of our own compounds, Abbott-42574 exhibited no tolerance to the anticonvulsant activity against audiogenic seizures in mice, but did exhibit pronounced tolerance against supramaximal electroshock in mice. In rats, the rate of tolerance appeared to be somewhat less against supramaximal electroshock with both Abbott-42574 and DMHP. Thus, there may be species differences in the rates of tolerance formation to anticon-vulsants.

It would be extremely interesting to see whether higher species, such as the cat or monkey, would show less tolerance formation to anticonvulsants against supramaximal electroshock over a period of time.

REFERENCES

Boggan, W.O., Steele, R.A., & Freedman, D.X. Delta-9-tetrahydro-cannabinol effect on audiogenic seizure susceptibility. Psychopharmacologia, 1973, 29, 101-106.

Carlini, E.A., Leite, J.R., Tannhauser, M., & Berardi, A. C. Cannabidiol and Cannabis sativa extract protect mice and rats against convulsive agents. Psychopharmacologia, 1973, 25, 664-665.

Chesher, G.B., & Jackson, D.M. Anticonvulsant effects of cannabinoids in mice: Drug interactions within cannabinoids and cannabinoid interactions with phenytoin. Psychopharmacologia, 1974, 37, 255-264.

Consroe, P.F., & Man, D.P. Effects of delta-8- and delta-9-tetrahydro-cannabinol on experimentally induced seizures. Life Sci., 1973, 13, 429-439.

Corcoran, M.E., McCaughran, J.A., Jr., & Wada, J.A. Acute anti-epileptic effects of delta-9-tetrahydrocannabinol in rats with kindled seizures. Exp. Neurol., 1973, 40, 471-483.

Davis, J.P., & Ramsey, H.H. Antiepileptic action of marihuana-active substances. Fed. Proc., 1949, 8, 284-285.

Domino, E.F., Hardman, H.F., & Seevers, M.H. Central nervous system actions of some synthetic tetrahydrocannabinol derivatives. Pharmacol. Rev., 1971, 23, 317-336.

Domino, E.F. Neuropsychopharmacologic studies of marijuana: Some synthetic and natural THC derivatives in animals and man. Ann. N.Y. Acad. Sci., 1971, 191, 166-192.

Frey, H.H., & Kretschmer, B.H. Anticonvulsant effect of trimethadione during continued treatment in mice. Arch. Int. Pharmacodyn., 1971, 193, 181-190.

Frey, H.H., & Kampmann, E. Tolerance to anticonvulsant drugs. Acta Pharmacol. and Toxicol., 1965, 22, 159-171.

Fried, P.A., & McIntyre, D.C. Electrical and behavioral attenuation of the anticonvulsant properties of delta-9-THC following chronic administrations. Psychopharmacologia, 1973, 31, 215-227.

Garriott, J.D., Forney, R.B., Hughes, F.W., & Richards, A.B. Pharma-cological properties of some cannabis related compounds. Arch. Int. Pharmacodyn., 1968, 171, 425-434.

Hardman, H.F., Domino, E.F., & Seevers, M.H. General pharmacological actions of some synthetic tetrahydrocannabinol derivatives. Pharmacol. Rev., 1971, 23, 295-315.

Karler, R. Anticonvulsant activity of delta-9-tetrahydrocannabinol. Fed. Proc., 1973, 32, 756.

Karler, R., Cely, W., & Turkanis, S.A. The anticonvulsant activity of cannabidiol and cannabinol. Life Sci., 1973, 13, 1527-1531.

Karler, R., Cely, W., & Turkanis, S.A. A study of the relative anticonvulsant and toxic activities of delta-9-tetrahydrocannabinol and its congeners. Res. Commun. Chem. Pathol. Pharmac., 1974, 7, 353-358(a).

Karler, R., Cely, W., & Turkanis, S.A. Anticonvulsant properties of delta-9-tetrahydrocannabinol and other cannabinoids. Life Sci., 1974, 15, 931-947(b).

Karler, R., Cely, W., & Turkanis, S.A. A study of the development of tolerance to an anticonvulsant effect of delta-9-tetrahydrocannabinol and cannabidiol. Res. Commun. Chem. Path. Pharmac., 1974, 9, 23-39(c).

Killam, K.F., & Killam, E.K. The action of tetrahydrocannabinol on EEG and photomyoclonic seizures in the baboon. Fifth Int. Cong. Pharm., Basel, Switz., 1972, 124.

Kinnard, W.J., & Carr, C.J. A preliminary procedure for the evaluation of central nervous system depressants. J. Pharmacol. Exp. Therap., 1957, 121, 354-361.

Loewe, S., & Goodman, L.S. Anticonvulsant action of marijuana-active substances. Fed. Proc., 1947, 6, 352.

Man, D.P., & Consroe, P.F. Effects of delta-9-tetrahydrocannabinol on experimentally induced seizures. J. Int. Res. Commun., 1973, 1, 12.

O'Shaughnessy, W.B. On the preparation of the Indian hemp or gunjah (Cannabis indica): The effect on the animal system in health, and their utility in the treatment of tetanus and other convulsive diseases. Trans. Med. Phys. Soc., Bombay, 1842, 8, 421-461.

Plotnikoff, N.P., & Green, D.M. Bioassay of potential ataraxic agents against audiogenic seizures in mice. J. Pharmacol. Exp. Therapy, 1957, 119, 294-298.

Plotnikoff, N.P., Zaugg, H., Petersen, A.C., Anderson, R., & Arendsen, D. Anticonvulsant activity of new benzopyrans. Abstracts of 168th ACS National Meeting, Atlantic City, N.J., September 9-12, 1974.

Plotnikoff, N.P., Zaugg, H.E., Petersen, A.C., Arendsen, D.L., & Anderson, R.F. New benzopyrans: Anticonvulsant activities. The Pharmacologist, Fall, 1975, 17, 2, 177(a).

Plotnikoff, N.P., Zaugg, H.E., Petersen, A.C., Arendsen, D.L., & Anderson, R.F. New benzopyrans: Anticonvulsant activities. Life Sci., 1975, 17, 97-104(b).

Razdan, R.K., Terris, B.Z., & Pars, H.G. Manuscript in preparation (Compounds SP-175, SP-141, SP-143), 1975.

Sofia, R. D., Solomon, T.A., & Barry, H., III. The anticonvulsant activity of delta-9-tetrahydrocannabinol in mice. Pharmacologist, 1971, 13, 246.

Swinyard, E.A., Brown, W.C., & Goodman, L.S. Comparative assays of antiepileptic drugs in mice and rats, J. Pharmacol. Exp. Therapy, 1952, 106, 319-330.

Toman, E.P., & Everett, G.M. Anticonvulsants in evaluation of drug activities (Ch. 13), Pharmacometrics, vol. 1. New York: Academic Press, 1964.

Wada, J.A., Sato, M., & Corcoran, M.E. Antiepileptic properties of delta-9-tetrahydrocannabinol. Exp. Neurol., 1973, 39, 157-165.

Woodbury, D.M., Penry, J.K., & Schmidt, R.P. Antiepileptic drugs. New York: Raven Press, 1972.

DISCUSSION

Harshman: I would like to ask our chemists and pharmacologists -- particularly Dr. Mechoulam, who has on a number of occasions come up with a great enthusiasm and talked about the possibility of separating off and discarding the high effects from other effects of the cannabinoids -- whether or not you might also consider fiddling around with the molecules to begin to pull out some of the different components of the high itself.

Mechoulam: There are many, many compounds. If somebody's willing to do some serious work on that kind of psychological testing in animals, I am indeed anxious to send compounds and prepare some others; we may even have them. If you drop me a line, if you are interested, I will be glad to send you compounds.

Burstein: I just want to make one comment on structure activity relations. In the past couple of days we have seen an amazing array of substances, and I have been searching for one common structural feature. Obviously, it's the alkyl resorcinol moiety which just happens to coincide with our results on the prostaglandins.

*   *   *   *   *   *   *   *   *   *   *   *   *   *   *

EDITORS' NOTE: The following question by Dr. Ralph Karler and answer by Dr. Nicholas P. Plotnikoff were the result of discussion following the scheduled question and answer session and have been included in this volume for general reader interest and information.

Karler: On the basis of the data you have presented, I am forced to question all of your conclusions. For instance, you have focused attention on drug potencies throughout your paper until, finally, you imply in your discussion that because SP-175 is "more active than diphenylhydantoin against

495

supramaximal electroshock in the rat," it may represent a therapeutic advance. If you believe that potency is such an important pharmacological characteristic, why did you fail to compare the relative potencies of these two drugs in your other anticonvulsant tests? In Table 6, for example, DPH is clearly more potent than SP-175 against PTZ-induced tonic extension. Furthermore, in Table 3, DPH is again more potent than SP-175 in the maximal seizure test in mice. How did you decide, therefore, that the greater potency of SP-175 in the one test, but not in the others, represents a therapeutic advance?

I also question your assertion that SP-175 exhibits a low degree of neurotoxicity, because your own data do not support this conclusion. Your data do indicate that both DPH and SP-175 are relatively nontoxic if you calculate the therapeutic indices (T.I.'s) from your audiogenic seizure data (T.I. for DPH is 36 and for SP-175, 18); however, if you calculate the T.I.'s from your maximal electroshock data, DPH has a high T.I. of 16, whereas SP-175 has a value of only 0.3, indicating that it is a relatively toxic drug. How do you reconcile these data with your conclusion that SP-175, compared with DPH, is relatively nontoxic?

In your discussion, you also stress that tolerance did not develop to the anticonvulsant activity of DPH and phenobarbital in the audiogenic seizure test and, therefore, you propose that this particular test may have predictive value for the development of tolerance to anticonvulsants in humans. While your failure to observe the development of tolerance in one seizure test may fit the data that we reported last year and that I summarized in yesterday's session, your conclusion is not necessarily justified. For example, our studies of the influence of repeated drug treatment on activity in several anticonvulsant tests showed that tolerance did not develop in some tests; however, it still seems unsound to interpret such results as ours or yours as an indication that these tests may be used predictively for the development of tolerance in humans. In fact, tolerance is a function of several factors, including the nature of the test, the species, the length of exposure to the drug and, significantly, the daily dose which, incidentally, you neglected to specify in your audiogenic seizure test. Whether tolerance to an anticonvulsant dose of a cannabinoid administered for months or years will develop in humans will only be known when such a drug is clinically evaluated.

Finally, I have several questions regarding your methodology. The supramaximal electroshock parameters for mice suggest that your electroshock apparatus was not a constant voltage stimulator; as a consequence, the voltage would drop as a function of the electrode contact and animal resistance. Since these resistances vary from animal to animal, your voltage would likewise be variable; hence, the results of your maximal electroshock test in mice are probably meaningless.

Secondly, the data in Tables 8 and 9 strongly suggest that here, too, something is wrong with your methodology. It is well established in the literature that anticonvulsant activity is related to dose in the maximal electroshock test, but your data clearly demonstrate that you are unable to obtain a dose-response relationship with either DPH or SP-175. For example, you obtained 60 percent protection with a dose of 20 mg/kg SP-175 but only 30 percent protection with twice the dose.

Thirdly, your method of assessing neurotoxicity in mice is not comparable to that used in rats. The rotarod is generally employed to measure minimal neurotoxicity; the inclined screen test, on the other hand, is useless for this measurement. Animals can hang on the screen long after minimal toxicity develops; therefore, the significance of your data based on the inclined screen is doubtful.

In my view, all of the conclusions you have drawn from the data presented are highly questionable because of serious limitations in your methodology and in the design of your experiments. You have demonstrated only that the benzopyran derivatives, like the naturally occurring cannabinoids, have anticonvulsant activity in some laboratory tests. Your conclusion that SP-175 may represent a therapeutic advance is totally unwarranted.

Plotnikoff: The basic question raised appears to be a discussion of SP-175 as a therapeutic advance.

In our experience with the benzopyrans, we have found a close correlation in activity between rats as a species and man. In most tests, we have found less correlation in mice.

One of the conventional estimates of therapeutic advance is a measure of side effects compared to therapeutic activity. Our original study of neurotoxicity in rats was the use of the inclined screen (a test of maximal neurotoxicity). More recently, we have developed a functional rotarod test in rats with the following results for "minimal neurotoxicity."

SP-175 $\dfrac{\text{Rotarod ED50}}{\text{ECS ED50}} = \dfrac{47 \text{ mg/kg}}{7} = $ Approximately 7

DMHP $\dfrac{16}{8} = 2$

Phenobarbital $\dfrac{46.0}{4} = $ Approximately 12

	Rat Rotarod ED50	95% C.L.
SP-175	47	(35 – 65)
DMHP	16	(8 – 25)
Phenobarbital	46	(28 – 148)

	Rat ECS ED50	95% C.L.
SP-175	7 mg/kg	(4 - 13)
DMPH	8 mg/kg	(3 - 11)
Phenobarbital	4 mg/kg	(2 - 7)

In comparing the three compounds, it appears that SP-175 and phenobarbital are approximately equivalent in potency and minimal neurotoxicity
(sedation, atoxia as measured on the rotarod). However, it is extremely important to stress that SP-175 is not a barbiturate; SP-175 does not produce
hypnosis. Thus, SP-175 does not produce tolerance or withdrawal effects in
dogs as does phenobarbital on chronic medication. At the same time, SP-175
does not produce hypotension in dogs unlike DMPH which does.

In conclusion, we are proposing that SP-175 represents a therapeutic
advance because (1) it is a non-barbiturate structure, (2) SP-175 has an
adequate therapeutic margin as measured by minimal neurotoxicity test for
side effects, and (3) SP-175 has no cardiovascular side effects in dogs (unlike
DMPH).

CONCLUSIONS OF THE CONFERENCE

Sidney Cohen

University of California

Los Angeles, California

Twenty-eight papers dealing with the historical, preclinical, and clinical aspects of cannabinoid therapeutics were delivered at the Asilomar Conference. This figure, representative of the more advanced studies, is revealing. It means that despite the difficulties involved in research with cannabis, its therapeutic potential is actually being investigated. A number of additional studies are underway, and their results are not yet available. It would seem that no governmental policy exists, as some believe, to suppress investigations into the possible beneficial effects of cannabis. There is, however, a formidable bureaucracy in place with which one must contend.

Certain of the specific therapeutic indications reported upon appear to be more promising than others. It now is reasonable to believe that intra-ocular pressure is reduced in normal subjects and glaucoma patients with smoked marihuana or oral THC. THC is the most potent agent for this purpose, and when a safe, topically instilled ophthalmic preparation is developed, it may come to be a useful medication in the management of wide-angle glaucoma. Asthmatics seem to respond to oral, smoked, or aerosolized THC as well as to the conventional anti-asthmatic medications. The development of non-intoxicating bronchodilators and intraocular pressure reducers are a logical next step. Further studies will determine whether THC can play a role to ameliorate the nausea and vomiting of patients receiving cancer chemo-therapy. In such patients, the standard antiemetics are not very effective, and new agents are being sought. These patients could also be studied to evaluate the euphoriant and anxiolytic effects of THC.

No recent work has been done utilizing cannabis or some derivative for the treatment of epilepsy in humans. The animal data are encouraging, but the finding that THC is also a convulsant in certain animal strains requires clarification. Cannabidiol or one of the synthetic compounds may turn out to be the preferred agents in the convulsive disorders if the animal investigations can be extrapolated to the human convulsant syndromes.

In a number of conditions the evidence for clinical effectiveness is either ambiguous or still unproven. These include the utility of THC as an hypnotic, as a preanesthetic agent, for psychologic depression, and as a retarder of tumor growth. Likewise, its analgesic efficacy remains in doubt from the few available studies. An investigation into the use of cannabis as an adjunct in the treatment of alcoholism is in its preliminary stages.

The mechanism of action of the cannabinoids remains unsettled. A possible explanation of certain effects is by their inhibitory action on prostaglandin synthetase. Beta adrenergic stimulation has also been noted in certain end organs. The influence of the cannabinoids on neurotransmitters has been studied, but the findings are not definitive.

A large series of synthetic benzopyrans have been produced, and these or related structures may come to be the preferred chemicals to deliver certain of the therapeutic effects. They can be designed to provide a selective action with or without the psychic effects of cannabis. Further, some of them are soluble in water, permitting more reliable absorption from the gastrointestinal tract or making parenteral administration less difficult. In addition, they are stable, thereby avoiding the limited shelf life of cannabis and THC when they are kept under ordinary conditions.

Although some promising leads have been developed, a considerable amount of work will be necessary before any compound for any indication will find its way to the marketplace. Still, a promising start has been made. This conference, which assembled many of those working on the therapeutic aspects of the cannabinoids, will serve to focus attention on what has been done and what still needs to be accomplished.

Conference Chairman

Sidney Cohen, M. D.
Department of Psychiatry
UCLA

NIDA Project Officer and Conference
Co-chairman

Richard C. Stillman, M. D.
National Institute on Drug Abuse

SPEAKERS

Sumner Burstein, Ph.D.
Senior Scientist
The Worcester Foundation for
Experimental Biology

Joel R. Butler, Ph.D.
Professor and Chairman
Department of Psychology
North Texas State University

Paul F. Consroe, Ph.D.
Associate Professor
Department of Pharmacology
The University of Arizona

Paul Cooler, M. D.
McPherson Hospital
Durham, North Carolina

A. T. Dren, Ph.D.
Abbott Laboratories

Dennis M. Feeney, Ph.D.
Associate Professor
Department of Psychology
The University of New Mexico

Keith Green, Ph.D.
Associate Professor
School of Medicine
Department of Ophthalmology
Medical College of Georgia

John Hanley, M. D.
Brain Research Institute
UCLA

Louis S. Harris, Ph.D.
Chairman, Department of Pharmacology
Medical College of Virginia
Virginia Commonwealth University

Richard Harshman, Ph.D.
University of Western Ontario

Robert S. Hepler, M. D.
Jules Stein Eye Institute
UCLA

Shirley Y. Hill, Ph.D.
Assistant Professor of Neuropsychology
Washington University

Ralph Karler, Ph.D.
Associate Professor
College of Medicine
Department of Pharmacology
The University of Utah

Louis Lemberger, Ph.D., M. D.
Chief, Clinical Pharmacology
Lilly Research Laboratories

Raphael Mechoulam, Ph.D.
Department of Natural Products
The School of Pharmacy
Hebrew University of Jerusalem

Loren L. Miller, Ph.D.
Assistant Professor in Psychiatry
University of Kentucky

Carlos Neu, M. D.
Clinical Research Services Unit
I.R.R., Boston State Hospital

Harry G. Pars, Ph.D.
President
SISA Incorporated

N. P. Plotnikoff, Ph.D.
Head, Exploratory
  Neuropharmacology
Abbott Laboratories

Arthur Robins, M. D.
Boston University

Chaim M. Rosenberg, M. D., Ph.D.
Director, Division of Alcoholism
Boston City Hospital

Walton T. Roth, M. D.
Department of Psychiatry
Medical Center
Stanford University

Vera Rubin, Ph.D.
Director
Research Institute for the Study of Man

Stephen E. Sallan, M. D.
Sidney Farber Cancer Center
Harvard Medical School

Theodore C. Smith, M. D.
Department of Anesthesia
University of Pennsylvania

Donald P. Tashkin, M. D.
Assistant Professor of Medicine
Director, Pulmonary Function
  Laboratories
UCLA

Louis Vachon, M. D.
Department of Psychiatry
Boston University

Christine Yang, M. S.
Abbott Laboratories

SECTION CHAIRMEN

Sidney Cohen, M. D.
Department of Psychiatry
UCLA

Reese Jones, M. D.
Langley Porter Neuropsychiatric
  Institute
University of California at San
  Francisco

Robert C. Petersen, M. D.
National Institute on Drug Abuse

Richard C. Stillman, M. D.
National Institute on Drug Abuse

Stephen Szara, M. D.
National Institute on Drug Abuse

THOSE IN ATTENDANCE OTHER THAN SPEAKERS

Jack D. Blaine
National Institute on Drug Abuse

Monique C. Braude
National Institute on Drug Abuse

Reese T. Jones
Langley Porter Neuropsychiatric
  Institute
University of California
San Francisco

Phyllis Lessin
President's Biomedical Research Panel

Joseph Liftik
Boston University

Robert Nowlan
University of California
Los Angeles

James Olsen
University of North Carolina

Stephen Szara
National Institute on Drug Abuse

Edward C. Tocus
Food and Drug Administration

Stuart Turkanis
University of Utah

Eleanore Tyrell
University of California
Los Angeles

Gerald K. Weiss
University of New Mexico

Robert C. Peterson
National Institute on Drug Abuse

William Petrie
National Institute of Mental Health

Richard Phillipson
National Institute on Drug Abuse